The People's Health

Recent Titles in
Contributions in Medical Studies

Mother and Fetus: Changing Notions of Maternal Responsibility
Robert H. Blank

The Golden Wand of Medicine: A History of the Caduceus Symbol in Medicine
Walter J. Friedlander

Cancer Factories: America's Tragic Quest for Uranium Self-Sufficiency
Howard Ball

The AIDS Pandemic: Social Perspectives
Howard Ball

Childbed Fever: A Scientific Biography of Ignaz Semmelweis
K. Codell Carter and Barbara R. Carter

James Cook and the Conquest of Scurvy
Francis E. Cuppage

Romance, Poetry, and Surgical Sleep: Literature Influences Medicine
E. M. Papper

Sex, Disease, and Society
Milton Lewis, Scott Bamber, and M. Waugh, editors

Histories of Sexually Transmitted Diseases and HIV/AIDS in Sub-Saharan Africa
Philip W. Setel, Milton Lewis, and Maryinez Lyons, editors

The History of Modern Epilepsy: The Beginning, 1865–1914
Walter J. Friedlander

The Legend of Nietzsche's Syphilis
Richard Schain

Drama and Discovery: The Story of Histoplasmosis
Thomas M. Daniel and Gerald L. Baum

The People's Health

Public Health in Australia, 1788–1950

Milton J. Lewis

Contributions in Medical Studies, Number 49, Volume 1

PRAEGER

Westport, Connecticut
London

Library of Congress Cataloging-in-Publication Data

Lewis, Milton James.
The people's health : public health in Australia, 1788–1950 / Milton J. Lewis.
p. cm.—(Contributions in medical studies, ISSN 0886–8220 ; no. 49, volume 1)
Includes bibliographical references and index.
ISBN 0–313–31090–4 (alk. paper)
1. Public health—Australia—History. 2. Medical care—Australia—History.
3. Medicine—Australia—History. I. Title. II. Series.
RA553.L495 2003
362.1′0994—dc21 2001054099

British Library Cataloguing in Publication Data is available.

Library of Congress Catalog Card Number: 2001054099
ISBN: 0–313–31090–4 (Vol. 1)
0–313–32045–4 (Vol. 2)
0–313–32595–2 (Set)
ISSN: 0886–8220

First published in 2003

Praeger Publishers, 88 Post Road West, Westport, CT 06881
An imprint of Greenwood Publishing Group, Inc.
www.praeger.com

Printed in the United States of America

The paper used in this book complies with the Permanent Paper Standard issued by the National Information Standards Organization (Z39.48–1984).

10 9 8 7 6 5 4 3 2 1

Contents

Tables

Acknowledgments

I am grateful to the National Health and Medical Research Council for the research grant that made possible my inquiry into the history of public health in Australia. My thanks are also due to the many staff members of the Commonwealth Department of Health and Aged Care who assisted me during my researches. I wish to thank as well Charles Kerr, formerly professor of preventive and social medicine in the University of Sydney, for commenting on the first draft of the volume. The staff of the Burkitt-Ford, Medical, and Fisher Libraries at the University of Sydney, the Library of the Commonwealth Department of Health and Aged Care, the National Library of Australia, and the Noel Butlin Archives Center at the Australian National University have efficiently provided services essential to the whole enterprise. Finally, I want to thank the various people, too numerous to name here, whom I interviewed about the development of public health in Australia.

Introduction

What George Rosen saw as the biosocial nature of human beings requires that some area of social activity be devoted to the protection of the public's health. All societies have to arrange ways of dealing with such collective health matters as an adequate supply of quality water and food, cleaning of the physical environment, and control of communicable disease. What ways are pursued will depend, on the one hand, on how the causes of health and disease are understood, and on the other, on the social, economic, political, and cultural (including religious and ideological beliefs) context. In the most general terms, then, the history of public health is the record of the various ways in which the community has acted to deal with inescapable health problems that arise from the biosocial being of humans. These ways have changed with changing knowledge and changes in the social context in which that knowledge has been located.[1]

Modern public health evolved in Western Europe between about the sixteenth and the twentieth centuries, and it came to maturity in the last 150 to two hundred years. Unprecedented economic growth, industrialization and urbanization in a capitalist economic mode created the need for it, as well as the financial and material resources with which to construct it. The history of European settlement in Australia, from its inception in 1788, fits almost exactly into this period of maturation of modern public health in Europe; there was little or no time lag between the development of public health knowledge, practices and institutions in Australia and the development in the heartland of modern public health.

HEALTH IN THE PREMODERN ERA

Personal and environmental health were pursued in the classical world for both spiritual-cum-religious and material reasons. Conscious pursuit of personal health was the preserve of the well-to-do elite. Collective sanitary practises were pursued by the members of the governing classes for reasons of personal comfort and social prestige, and as part of the demonstration of their status as representatives of a civilized lifestyle. Salaried physicians had been employed by Greek communities to serve all citizens as early as the fourth century B.C., and Roman cities in the imperial era also employed public physicians. The Greek conception of philanthropy did not specifically focus on the poor; it embraced all members of the *polis,* all citizens. Early imperial Rome likewise did not make special collective provision for the sick poor. This classical "egalitarianism" contrasts with the tradition of obligatory good works for the poor arising from the religious beliefs of ancient Egypt and Israel. Developing out of this same religion-based concern for care of the disadvantaged came the Judeo-Christian focus on good works, and the Christian obligation to relieve the suffering of the indigent sick. True, the humanitarianism of Stoic philosophy helped engender a new sense of aristocratic obligation to the poor in the Roman imperial era. This translated sometimes into material gifts to support needy citizens. But Stoicism and other contemporary philosophical systems taught indifference to physical suffering, and special concern did not extend to the sick poor. Moreover, the fact of slavery's association with manual labor generally degraded the laboring free poor in the eyes of the leisured elite. Thus, the *valetudinaria,* the hostels or "hospitals" for treatment of sick slaves or sick soldiers, did not serve the needs of the free poor. The work of slaves and soldiers was vital to the economic and defence needs of the empire; both groups lacked the kinship networks that traditionally cared for sick and disabled Romans.[2]

By the 340s the Christian Church in Antioch was operating *xenodocheia,* or *xenones,* hostels to house the poor. Monasteries also cared for the poor and sick. One of the earliest figures to offer specifically medical care in these hospices was Aeteus, a Syrian physician. There was, however, no clear distinction between a *xenon,* a hostel, and a *nosokomeion,* a house for the sick. By the fifth and sixth centuries, towns in the Eastern Empire commonly had at least one hospital. The first *xenon* in the Latin West was founded in Rome by Fabiola in about 397. She had been inspired by Eastern examples. The first in Gaul was established after A.D. 500. The end of the empire in the West saw the infirmaries of monasteries carry on the care of the sick, and monastic medicine flourished from the fifth century to the tenth century. Larger hospitals in the 800s declined for lack of public revenue, consequent on the decline of Charlemagne's Holy Roman Empire. In the East some hospitals grew quite large. By A.D. 600, hospitals of six hundred beds existed in Antioch and Constantinople. From the ninth century, large specialized hospitals were established in the great cities of the Islamic world, like Baghdad and Cairo. With Christianity integral to the process of state formation in Western Europe after the fall of Rome, collective institutional provision for the sick poor became an established feature of Western society.[3]

Some ancient civilizations performed substantial public health engineering feats concerning drainage or conveyance of clean water to cities. But these works were undertaken for reasons of ritual cleanliness and for aesthetic rather than hygienic reasons. The ruins of Kohun (2100–1700 B.C.) and Tel-el-Amarna (1400 B.C.) in Egypt reveal that masonry gutters drained water from streets. The Cretan-Mycenean culture used conduits to supply water to cities. The palace at Knossos (2000 B.C.) had baths and flushing toilets. Half a world away, the Indus Valley cities of Harappa, Mohenjo-daro and Lothal (3000–1500 B.C.) possessed public water tanks, probably for communal bathing to purify ritually the inhabitants. Paved streets were drained by covered sewers. India's first great empire, the Mauryan State, was established in the fourth century B.C. Megasthenes, a Seleucid ambassador to the court of Chandragupta Maurya, noted public health practices carried out by committees of physicians, including concern with the statistics of births and deaths and with antenatal care.[4]

The bureaucratic feudalism of ancient China lent itself to preventive practices, and prevention was as highly valued in Chinese medicine as in statecraft and administration. *The Yellow Emperor's Treatise on Internal Medicine* (produced mainly in the early Han period, the second to first centuries B.C.) states, "The sage does not cure the sick only when they are such but he prevents the illness arising. In the same way he does not put right upheavals in the body politic, he prevents them from ever taking place."[5] The imperial court of the Chou dynasty (the middle of the first millennium B.C.) employed an "imperial dietitian" as well as an "imperial physician." The Confucian Analects (about 500 B.C.) forbade the consumption of damaged food. The practice of eating food cooked at high temperature (preventing the spread of food-borne infection) began about this time, and water to be consumed was always boiled. In the imperial capital, vermin exterminators were employed, rotting corpses of humans and animals were routinely removed from public areas, and streets were regularly swept. In the Chin and Han periods, some cities obtained water from a distance through bamboo, sometimes earthenware, conduits. The growth of Buddhist abbeys with bathing facilities from the second century reinforced existing bathing customs arising from Taoist purification ceremonies. In the Sung era, public bathhouses multiplied, and from the eleventh century commercial bathhouses became more common.

From ancient times, bamboo implements and water were employed to clean the body after defecation. Following the invention of paper about A.D. 100, improved lavatory hygiene spread more widely. Systematic removal of night soil each morning from cities dates from early times. As in Rome and other strongly hierarchical societies, those at the bottom of Chinese society were more exposed to environmental hazards. Helminth and other fecally transmitted infections were occupational dangers for peasants, who used human waste as crop fertilizer.[6]

Greek cities added water drawn from external sources—Athens obtained water from surrounding hills as early as the sixth century B.C.—to that obtained from wells and rainwater cisterns. But the Romans's public health engineering was unsurpassed in the ancient world. For Romans, clean water was part of everyday life and was not particularly connected with public or private health. Frontinus, water commissioner from A.D. 97, reported in *The Aquaducts of Rome* that the censor, Crassus, built the first aqueduct in 312 B.C. Nine aqueducts operated by Frontinus's time. Millions of gallons a day supplied public fountains and baths, but a private supply required imperial approval. Other cities throughout the empire were supplied by aqueducts. By the early imperial era, a board administered the water supply, and *aediles* supervised public baths, street cleaning and maintenance and the food markets, although how diligently is unclear.

The Roman sewerage system dated from republican times. In the time of Constantine, public latrines numbered as many as 150. But social inequality made for maldistribution of the benefits of public health engineering. The poor in the upper levels of Rome's slums still emptied chamber pots into the streets. Severe crowding and homelessness characterized slum life. Drainage in individual homes was often unconnected to public drains and sewers, as the ruins of Pompeii attest. Latrines did not have running water. Cesspits could contain dead bodies of the poor, carcasses of animals, sewage and garbage. It is worth remembering that for Romans, Greeks and other ethnic groups of the imperial world, average life expectancy was only twenty-five years.[7]

In Greco-Roman medicine, hygiene sought to preserve the health of the individual, by modification of lifestyle and of environmental factors. Classical hygiene did not seek to promote the health of the whole community. The ideal (male) citizen of the Greek *polis* was someone of cultivated mind possessing a physically fit and aesthetically pleasing body. Athletics brought fitness, and special instruction developed in bathing, massage, gymnastics, exercise and diet. The personal hygienic regimen recommended by Greco-Roman physicians was possible only for members of a leisured class, people whose lifestyles were supported by the labor of slaves.

The Hippocratic and Galenic texts on hygiene remained the source of ideas about individual health until at least the sixteenth century. They still influenced Western medicine in the nineteenth century, when the meaning of hygiene narrowed to equate with cleanliness but its focus widened from the individual to the group or population. The longevity of classical hygiene arose from various factors: because classical knowledge persisted due to the authority of the written text, the absorption of classical learning into medieval Christian culture, and the revival of interest in classical texts in the Renaissance; because the way of life of pre-industrial societies up to about the eighteenth century was not radically different from that of the ancient Greeks; and because before the development of scientific chemistry and bacteriology, the individual continued to have to rely on his or her own senses to assess the healthiness of air, food, and water.[8]

The Middle Ages and the Renaissance saw the promotion of the ideas of classical hygiene through the medium of new texts, the most famous of which was the thirteenth-century *Regimen Sanitatis Salernitanum,* attributed to the medical school of Salerno in Italy. The *Regimen,* like the illustrated handbooks on health, discussed Galen's "six non-naturals," or the categories of hygiene (air; food and drink; sleep and working; movement and rest; retention and evacuation; and the emotions) as well as therapeutics. Intended for the upper and "middle" classes, books on hygienic regimen were popular. In 1486–1604, they represented 115 of 392 editions published on medicine in English. Only when the state required the norms of hygiene to be observed by the whole population—a requirement expressed in nineteenth-century public health legislation (although it is foreshadowed in plague-control measures and intermittent use of quarantine from the fourteenth century)—was the transition to the focus on the group completed. The transition demanded not only the advent of new technologies (like cast-iron pipes) and state legislative and administrative action but a large-scale cultural transformation in hygienic habits. From the eighteenth century, the habit of personal cleanliness became more and more widely accepted. As a matter of routine, people washed their bodies and clothes, and in various other ways followed hygienic practices.[9]

FORERUNNERS OF MODERN PUBLIC HEALTH

In the aftermath of the fall of Rome, cities and trade gave way to a largely rural way of life. However, by the fourteenth century, cities of a hundred to 150,000 people were flourishing in Europe. Influenced by their reading of Roman legal texts, the governing elites of Italian cities reestablished the Greco-Roman office of public physician in the twelfth and thirteenth centuries. They also reestablished Roman public facilities like fountains, baths, and sewers, and the practice of regulating refuse disposal and food markets. Indeed, it was not until the creation of boards of public health in the fourteenth century that Italian cities moved beyond the classical world in public sanitation, although in medieval Europe both the church and the state organized care for lepers in residential hospitals.

Plague ravaged Europe in the fourteenth century. The republican city-states, Florence and Venice, introduced the innovation of lay health committees during epidemic crises. These oversaw the cleansing of the environment, kept public order, and implemented emergency legislation. A number of Italian city-states had established permanent health boards by the beginning of the sixteenth century; the boards now also attended to the regular sanitary supervision of their cities. Physicians acted usually only as advisers, and lay members of the governing classes continued to dominate the boards. The boards developed into significant arms of government in Italy and other parts of the Mediterranean region. They regularly gathered information about the health status of foreign states, in the light of which health magistracies could take strong action like imposing quarantine and destroying incoming goods (thought to convey contagion) in an effort to halt the ingress of epidemic disease. Quarantine was another city-state invention. In 1377 Ragusa, a Venetian colony, first imposed a suspension of trade and travel (then only thirty days, but later forty) to prevent incursion of plague. Originally, this was a passive procedure—"a cordon sanitaire"—but it subsequently came to involve action to isolate active cases of infection. Infected cases were collected in a *lazaretto,* or pesthouse. In the beginning a way of caring for the sick poor, from the mid-fifteenth century it was part of the system of isolating the infected from the healthy citizen.

The sanitary approach inherited from Rome reflected one explanation of disease—that polluted air (or exhalations) adversely changed the healthy "humoral" balance in humans and animals. Another explanation—that disease was spread by contact with diseased persons or with infected intermediate inanimate objects (contagion)—was, except in relation to lepers, not widely accepted among educated people in the classical or medieval periods. It became better established in the early modern period, as the growth of quarantine and isolation practices after the 1450s indicates. The human and material costs of plague in the late sixteenth and seventeenth century Mediterranean were huge. The damage wrought, together with the transfer of the center of trade and economic activity north of the Alps and the rise of strong monarchical states in northern Europe, meant that the future of public health development lay in France, Britain and Germany.[10] From Britain, modern public health spread later to British settlements, like the American and Australian colonies.

The northern European countries that pioneered modern public health did not simply reproduce the permanent public health magistracies of the Italian city-state type, although they did from time to time use such Italian epidemic-control measures as quarantine and temporary health boards. Seventeenth- and eighteenth-century ideological movements influenced in fundamental ways the evolving conception of public health. Mercantilism taught that to maximize national power and wealth the state had to "grow" a healthy and numerous population. The health of the people as a whole became a key objective of the state. Enlightenment rationalists would apply rational organization and collective responsibility to the prevention of disease, as they would apply them to other areas of human affairs. Good health for all became a matter of establishing rational social and political institutions and providing rational education for the individual.

Industrialization and urbanization under unregulated industrial-capitalist conditions in the early nineteenth century and the continuing threat of serious epidemic disease heightened the urgency of finding new mechanisms to protect the health of the laboring population, the living and working conditions of whom were degraded. Too many workers were falling, because of ill health, into unproductive penury and dependence on their parishes. Sanitation in Britain promised not only to advance the health of all the people but in doing so to relieve the financial burden on the propertied classes of supporting those in the lower classes reduced to poverty by sickness. Later in the nineteenth century, "neomercantilist" ideas of a numerous and healthy population as a vital resource in the growing economic and military "struggle for survival" among Western nation-states and empires came to influence public health strongly. At the same time, the rise to political power of the labor movement, and the more collectivist orientation of fin-de-siècle liberalism in a context of increasing democratization of the state, began to give rise to the conception of health as a right of citizenship rather than as a state resource, although the latter view remained alive at least up to the mid-twentieth century.

The severe international economic depression of the 1930s, the inhumanity of the totalitarian Fascist regimes, the destructiveness of World War II, and the postwar economic and political problems of many former colonies and Third World countries all promoted consciousness of human rights, including the right to health. The Universal Declaration of Human Rights (1948) included a right to a standard of living adequate for health. Notions of social justice and equity in postwar decades replaced, or at least overlaid, instrumentalist, healthy-population-as-productive-resource justifications for public health. Good health for all people (and peoples) as a matter of social justice was most fully recognized in formal terms at the international level in the 1970s, when the World Health Organization of the United Nations adopted its strategy of "Health for All by the Year 2000." In the 1980s, official acceptance of the WHO strategy by Australia reinforced, at least in principle, an emerging national commitment to better health for the whole population as an issue of social justice.

ORGANIZATION OF THIS VOLUME

A number of themes are addressed in this history of public health in Australia from the beginning of European settlement in 1788 to about 1950.

One important theme is the interaction between the internal history of ideas and practices in public health and medicine, and the changing social, political, economic and cultural context. A second theme concerns the institutional, professional and ideological relations between public health and clinical medicine—between disease prevention and health promotion addressed to the population as a whole, on the one hand, and treatment, rehabilitation and palliation directed to the individual, on the other.

Public health may refer to the professional knowledge and practices, social institutions, and public policy devoted to the advancement of the collective health. It may also refer to the actual state of health of the people—that is, the health status of the population as a whole. The health status of the Australian people has improved markedly over the last 150 years, the period in which modern public health was transplanted to, and matured in, that country. The reasons for this long-term improvement constitute the third theme.

A fourth theme involves the setting of the Australian history in international perspective. To this end much comparative material, especially from the British and American experiences, is presented. No other countries have had greater cultural influence on Australia than these two. Their influence has been substantial as well in the specific culture of public health and medicine. Britain, as the "mother country" and center of the empire and Commonwealth, was the key external reference point and examplar for Australia from 1788 to at least World War II. The United States increasingly assumed that position in the next fifty years. However, even in the early twentieth century, America had direct influence on the development of public health in Australia. A prime example is the critical role that the Rockefeller Foundation played in the establishment of the Federal Health Department in 1920. Moreover, because of the shared cultural, political, social and economic heritage of the three English-speaking countries, there are interesting, and perhaps instructive, similarities and differences between the history of public health here in Australia, in Britain and in the United States.

This volume ends chronologically at about 1950. A second volume will cover the period from 1950 to 2000. There is a certain unity to public health in the period from the nineteenth to the mid-twentieth century. First, the pattern of diseases with which public health dealt remained the same over most of this period. Infections bulked large as causes of mortality and morbidity. Only late in the period did chronic, "degenerative" disorders like cardiovascular disease and cancer begin to replace communicable illnesses as the main causes of death and disability. Even then, it took some years for public health experts and policy to "retool" in order to deal with the new epidemiological situation. Second, an instrumental approach to public health, as mentioned earlier, largely prevailed in those years. In the mid-nineteenth century spending on sanitary measures was thought worthwhile to reduce the cost of supporting the lower-class casualties of the diseases allegedly spread by filth in the environment. Later, it was considered worthwhile to spend on public health to produce a healthy and numerous population as a vital economic and military resource in a world of increasing international competition.

In the period after about 1950 as well, public health has a certain unity. The epidemiology fundamentally changed. The "diseases of affluence" have dominated the health agenda. By their nature they have called for different responses from public health. Health education and health promotion, persuading and working with people—not legislated mandatory action, the threat of legal sanction, or attempted control of behavior—are seen to be the way forward. The diseases themselves have required a more democratic, cooperative approach from professionals and the state alike, an approach that engaged, not forced, community compliance. At the same time, the extensive spread of democratic and "egalitarian" values fueled a quest for social justice and equity in health, a quest that had been initiated by the labor movement and social reformers in the earlier period. The difference in this post-1950 period is that the desire for social justice becomes a more central force of public health development.

Chapter 1 looks at the emergence of modern public health as a socially organized effort to protect the health of the whole population. This emergence took place in Western Europe between the sixteenth and the nineteenth centuries. As suggested earlier, its development depended on progress in understanding the nature and causes of disease, and on a conducive political, economic and social environment. Prominent in this environment were the rise of the strong, modern state; urbanization and industrialization in a capitalist mode; mercantilist ideas of population as a state resource; and Enlightenment-based faith in the educability of a rational humankind. These general forces were mediated by national cultures and political systems so that public health development followed particular national paths.

Chapter 2 discusses the transportation of European infections to Australia and their devastating impact on the Aboriginal tribes of Terra Australis. The Australian Aboriginal experience is compared with that of other indigenous peoples in the Americas and Oceania. The growth of public health measures in early colonial Australia is outlined against the backdrop of contemporary European public health, especially with respect to quarantine and smallpox vaccination.

Rapid urbanization and the growth of an industrial base in Australia in the second half of the nineteenth century resulted in serious deterioration in the quality of the urban environment and in public health problems similar to those of much older European cities. Chapter 3 discusses the transfer of the "sanitary idea" from Britain to the Australian colonies. The creation of classical public health administrations here, as in Britain and the United States, was spurred by the threat of epidemic. The role of public health measures in the decline of mortality in the United Kingdom, the United States and Australia is assessed. The advent of the first wave of public health professionals—the beginning of professionalization of public health—is recounted.

Chapter 4 focuses on an important turning point in public health development around the beginning of the twentieth century. In Australia, as in other parts of the Western world, public health began to expand into provision of personal services for social groups like mothers and babies. The organized medical profession ensured that the growth of such public services did not threaten the viability of private practice. “National efficiency” (as part of a “neomercantilist” climate) was a buzzword across the Western world at this time. This was a significant motive for the growth of state support for infant, maternal, and school health services. These new departures in public health in the United Kingdom and the United States, as well as in Australia, are outlined.

J.H.L. Cumpston, the first Commonwealth Director General of Health and the outstanding figure in Australian public health in the first half of the twentieth century, set out in the interwar years to construct a truly national public health system. This and other aspects of the interwar history of public health are discussed in chapter 5. Cumpston and his professional allies believed, reasonably enough, that more health gain was to be had at this time from prevention than from treatment. As in the United States, the federal division of powers between the center and states made it very difficult for the national health authorities to act effectively without the full cooperation of the states. In 1930, just before the economic depression severely restricted funds, the Commonwealth, at Cumpston’s urging, established a national school of public health at the University of Sydney to train public health professionals and to carry out research. In the following decade, the first mass immunization projects began with campaigns against diphtheria. Mass campaigns to control tuberculosis and poliomyelitis were to be pursued successfully two decades later.

The Labor Party began in the early twentieth century to feel its way toward the idea of equal access to health care as a right of citizenship. The period of 1941–49, which is covered in chapter 6, was marked by fierce debate about the merits of the federal Labor government’s plans for a tax-funded national health scheme. But it was Cumpston and other public health doctors who formulated the first detailed plan for a national health scheme integrating preventive and curative services. The plan called for a national salaried service, a concept opposed by the organized medical profession. After constitutional challenges and a bitter, protracted struggle between the Labor government and the medical community, the government finally enacted legislation establishing a national health service. This service supported fee-for-service practice. Still, the profession feared the government, even as part paymaster, and it rejected the scheme. Labor left office in late 1949.

By about 1950, in Australia, as in Britain and the United States, curative medicine’s star was rising. It took credit for the “defeat” of infectious diseases—when, in fact, well before it became effective, public health had been contributing significantly to the long-term decline in mortality from infection. Chapter 7, the last chapter, discusses this and other matters relating to the state of the health system in the middle years of the twentieth century.

Even in Britain, where the collective provision of health services was taken farther than in Australia or the United States, the new National Health Service was overwhelmingly focused on clinical services for the individual. However, changing disease and demographic patterns in the 1950s were bringing to the fore in affluent Western countries chronic "degenerative" conditions for which no cures existed. Government and health professionals became interested again in the behavioral and social causes of disease. The rocketing costs of technologically driven curative medicine reinforced interest in less costly preventive, public health measures. These and other issues relating to the period between 1950 and 2000 will be discussed at length in the second volume of this history of public health, *The People's Health: Public Health in Australia, 1950 to the Present.*

LIMITS TO THE SCOPE OF THIS HISTORY

The history of occupational health and safety in Australia, while closely connected with the history of public health, is not systematically discussed in this history of public health. So extensive and important a subject should be treated at length in a monograph of its own. Similarly, the history of psychiatric services, while touched upon, is by no means exhaustively discussed. Those interested in the latter might want to consult Milton Lewis, *Managing Madness: Psychiatry and Society in Australia, 1788–1980* (1988).

NOTES

1. G. Rosen, *From Medical Police to Social Medicine: Essays on the History of Health Care* (New York: Science History Publications, 1974), 176.

2. G.B. Risse, *Mending Bodies, Saving Souls: A History of Hospitals* (New York: Oxford University Press, 1999), 44–56; A.G. Carmichael, "History of Public Health and Sanitation in the West before 1700," in *The Cambridge World History of Human Disease*, ed. K.F. Kiple (Cambridge: Cambridge University Press, 1993), 195.

3. G.B. Risse, *Mending Bodies, Saving Souls: A History of Hospitals* (New York: Oxford University Press, 1999), 81–95; D. Porter, *Health, Civilization and the State: A History of Public Health from Ancient to Modern Times* (London: Routledge, 1999), 22–23.

4. G. Rosen, *A History of Public Health* (Baltimore: Johns Hopkins University Press, 1993), 1–3; S.C. Seal, "A Short History of Public Health in India," *Indian Journal of History of Medicine* 16 (1971), 26–28; R. Porter, *The Greatest Benefit to Mankind: A Medical History of Humanity from Antiquity to the Present* (London: HarperCollins, 1997), 84–85, 136–38.

5. Quoted in J. Needham and Lu Gwei-Djen, "Hygiene and Preventive Medicine in Ancient China," *Journal of History of Medicine and Allied Sciences* 17 (1962), 433.

6. J. Needham and Lu Gwei-Djen, "Hygiene and Preventive Medicine in Ancient China," *Journal of History of Medicine and Allied Sciences* 17 (1962), 435–38, 449–57, 463–67; I. Polunin, "Disease, Morbidity, and Mortality in China, India, and the Arab World," in *Asian Medical Systems: A Comparative Study*, ed. C. Leslie (Berkeley: University of California Press, 1976), 126–27.

7. Rosen, *A History of Public Health*, 14–25; A.G. Carmichael, "History of Public Health and Sanitation in the West before 1700," 193–94.

8. A. Wear, "The History of Personal Hygiene," in *Companion Encyclopedia of the History of Medicine*, Vol. 2, eds. W.F. Bynum and R. Porter (London: Routledge, 1993), 1283–90; Rosen, *A History of Public Health*, 6–13; Porter, *The Greatest Benefit to Mankind*, 84–85, 136–38.

9. Wear, "The History of Personal Hygiene," 1297, 1304–5.

10. A.G. Carmichael, "History of Public Health and Sanitation in the West before 1700," 196–99.

Chapter 1

The Emergence of Public Health in Europe and America

In his influential history of public health, originally published in 1958, Rosen sought to explain the rise of modern public health across Europe from the sixteenth century in terms of two basic factors: first, progress in understanding of the nature and causes of disease (especially infections), as the sine qua non of prevention; and second, the political, economic and social context that determined the application of such knowledge.[1] We might add a third factor, cultural change—a large-scale transformation in norms and behavior relating to cleanliness. In the eighteenth and nineteenth centuries, personal cleanliness became established as a social norm: "People washed their hands, their bodies, and their houses; learned not to spit in public, killed flies, kept food from going bad, and learned through education to do those things which today help to keep us well and alive and which we almost do automatically and without thinking."[2] More recent historical scholarship modifies Rosen's rather heroic interpretation of the development of public health, emphasising the "variation between national contexts of power in which political responsibility for health developed" and pointing to "its multiple and often contradictory dimensions."[3]

In the sixteenth and seventeenth centuries, epidemiological and clinical knowledge of diseases advanced. Old diseases like leprosy declined in prevalence, and new (or hitherto unobserved) diseases like typhus, malaria, the English sweat, scurvy, rickets, scarlet fever, chickenpox, smallpox and the ubiquitous syphilis appeared. To account for the waxing and waning of epidemics, two opposing explanations were offered. Each had roots in earlier epochs. The notion of epidemic constitution had roots in Hippocrates's emphasis on weather conditions and the seasons as the causes of disease outbreaks. Thomas Sydenham, an eminent English physician of the seventeenth century, divided acute fevers into epidemic distempers (plague, smallpox, dysentery) arising from the "epidemic constitution" (atmospheric changes) and intercurrent diseases (scarlet fever, pleurisy, rheumatism), which arose from bodily weaknesses. Miasmas (or exhalations) emanating from the earth were the alleged cause of atmospheric change. The rival explanation was contagion, which is associated with the work of Girolamo Fracastoro (1478–1533) on plague, typhus, syphilis and other epidemic diseases. He postulated the existence of seeds (infective agents), specific to particular diseases, which acted on the humors of the body in the fashion of chemical substances rather than of microorganisms. Contagion (infection) spread by person-to-person contact, by intermediate agents (fomites), and through the air. The conflict between the contagionist and atmospheric-miasmatic theories endured till bacteriology fundamentally changed understanding of the causes of infectious disease in the late nineteenth century.[4]

If growing understanding of epidemic disease was one force shaping the growth of modern public health, the emergence of the early modern state, resting on the centralization of national power and justified by the political philosophy of mercantilism, was another. Mercantilism aimed to subordinate society and the economy to the objectives of the centralized state, chief among which was maximization of national power and wealth. Considered necessary to this end was a substantial population, healthy and materially well supported, which would be a primary resource for the state in economic and military matters. "Political arithmetic," or national statistics, now became a vital tool in monitoring changes in the population and other resources of the state. William Petty (1623–87), English physician and economist, showed the importance of national statistical compilations and computations, but it was John Graunt (1620–74) who, examining the mortality returns for London, demonstrated that certain regularities in social and vital events could be identified. Others soon pursued the field, notably Christian Huygens, who in the 1660s concerned himself with determination of life expectancy at any age, and Edmund Halley, who constructed in the 1690s a life table that enabled life insurance to be more reliably based.[5]

The centralized nation-state, with its accompanying ideology of mercantilism, lent support to the emerging idea of public health. Enlightenment-based social and political reform, and its revolutionary expressions in America and France, created in the eighteenth and early nineteenth century another ideological and political context, one that encouraged the development of collective responsibility for prevention of disease and promotion of health. The enormous value placed upon reason in human affairs that had been the legacy of Locke and Newton and the late-seventeenth-century English Enlightenment had been taken up in France from the mid-eighteenth century by the "philosophes"—Diderot, d'Alembert, Voltaire and Rousseau—who looked to education, free institutions and improvement of social conditions to lift humankind toward perfection. Their aspirations to human improvement through applied knowledge were expressed in the *Encyclopédie des Arts, Sciences et Métiers* (1751–72), and the *Encyclopédie* addressed issues of public health such as life expectancy, population, political arithmetic, foundlings and hospitals. Revolutionary democracy in America and in France related health to the influence of free republican political and social institutions.

Thomas Jefferson and associates like the physician Benjamin Rush believed that the Creator intended that human health would flourish best under a free political order and good social institutions, although the Jeffersonians did not produce a systematic theory of the social relations of health. Rush said in 1799: "There is an indissoluble union between moral, political and physical happiness; and if it be true that elective and representative governments are most favourable to individual as well as national prosperity, it follows of course, that they are most favourable to animal life." The Jeffersonian position was the first approach to formulation of an American theory of social medicine, although it had no immediate impact and did not inform the development of public health in the soon-to-develop industrial and urban society.[6]

In France, the National Constituent Assembly and the National Convention, 1790–92, accepted that the people had a right to health. Revolutionaries argued that the right to health was part of democratic citizenship. Indeed, the health committee of the assembly devised an extensive plan for what amounted to a national public health system and universal access to medical care. But it was hardly pursued, and no Enlightenment state moved beyond rhetoric about, and plans to realize, the health rights of the citizen.[7]

Commonly, and in no small part because of the influence of Rosen, it has been argued that industrialization and urbanization and the high levels of disease associated with them almost inevitably elicited centralized state action in public health. Britain, as the first country to undergo in a capitalist mode industrialization and urbanization on a large scale, has been cited as the paradigmatic case. Certainly, the British response was an exemplar for Australia, other parts of the empire and the United States. But the development of public health in nineteenth-century Europe was not simply a response to socioeconomic modernization; the varying national cultures acted as mediating influences. The historical process was more problematic and contradictory than an abstracted, sociologically oriented explanation in terms of such broad social and economic forces would have it. The historical context was more complex and less straightforwardly determined.[8]

Thus, Sweden was not industrialized (indeed, it was to be more than a century before industrialization began) when a national preventive and curative health program was introduced there in the eighteenth century. In a country strongly influenced by mercantilist ideas, revelations in 1752 of the actual small size of the population (only two million), as indicated by the recently established national vital statistics system, caused considerable concern. Immigration, promotion of the birthrate, and health measures to reduce mortality were all explored as ways to boost population. Efforts quickly centered on health initiatives. Hospitals funded from local taxes and state subsidies began to be established throughout Sweden. A tax was levied to fund facilities for venereal disease patients. Medical care came under central control. District public medical officers and midwives were appointed. The poor were given free drugs and hospital care. A whole preventive program was introduced, with parish priests and other local notables involved in campaigns concerning personal hygiene, epidemics, venereal disease, infant care and breastfeeding. Vaccination against smallpox became compulsory in 1815. Health education was provided through cheap publications and through almanacs that resided in all homes.[9] While prevention of the type characteristic of the British sanitary revolution of the next century was absent, other significant preventive measures—publicly funded, state directed and national in range—were pursued. In a longer, broader perspective on public health, this was certainly a major national, public health initiative, almost a century before Chadwick and the British Public Health Act of 1848.

In France, from the seventeenth century, under the influence of mercantilism, the royal government accepted responsibility for the health of the whole population. Indeed, the last decades of the ancien régime saw the beginnings of a new public health system, directed by a medical bureaucracy (separate from the locally oriented medical police) and drawing on medical science. There was concern with control of epidemics and epizootics, and regulation of urban nuisances like waste disposal, although from the 1770s, with the foundation of the Royal Society of Medicine, public hygiene had come to mean anything to do with health. By the early 1800s, the Paris health council could list as its responsibilities control of epidemics; inspection of markets, rivers, cemeteries, slaughterhouses, horse butchering yards, dumps and public places; and also occupational hygiene, charlatans, lighting, secret remedies, adulteration of food and drinks, epizootics, prisons, and public assistance. As we have seen, the Revolution promised to protect the citizen's right to health and to provide assistance through a national health system, but in reality little was achieved, because the required state interventions conflicted with commitment to economic freedom and private property; also, and more fundamentally, the individualism expressed in the 1789 Declaration of the Rights of Man conflicted with the communitarianism of the radical revolutionaries. Moreover, the value placed on local autonomy in government early in the Revolution was incompatible with the centralized Jacobin state. Postrevolutionary society resolved these contradictions by allowing equality before the law but not allowing dangerous communitarianism, and by allowing a centralized state but not tolerating state intervention in social and economic life. The bitter conflicts of the Revolution limited public health development until well into the nineteenth century.[10]

Between 1820 and 1840, the French public health movement, national in scope and with its headquarters in Paris, led the way in Europe. Public hygiene was established as a professional, scientific activity. The Royal Academy of Medicine was established in 1820. Louis Villermé (1782–1863) produced his statistical studies. He found that none of the accepted environmental factors (climate, soil, altitude) explained mortality differences between Paris *arrondissements* but that economic status did. Indeed hygienists, like clinicians (notably Pierre Louis), now used statistics in their inquiries, seeking to turn hygiene into a medical science and to give it more credibility in an increasingly scientific culture. Alexandre Parent-Duchâtelet, the leading theorist of the movement, published a range of hygienic and sociological works on sewers and on prostitution in 1821–36. The *Annales d'hygiene publique et de médicine légale,* the first public health journal, was established in 1829. Cholera in 1832–35 brought reform of French quarantine, and the health council of Paris became the leading authority in the country. Hygienists believed health would advance *pari passu* with "civilization"—which for some meant greater wealth more justly distributed, and for others greater education or general enlightenment. Individuals would then attend to personal hygiene, and the state would take public health initiatives. Advancing "civilization" was expected to prevent epidemics too, and this was a reasonable position when the only specific disease preventive then available was vaccination against smallpox.

Another fundamental belief was that material improvement was interconnected with moral improvement. The teaching of middle-class values and habits would itself help raise working-class living standards. The "embourgeoisement" of the working class would advance its health. Public health in Britain and the United States shared this concern with moral improvement, as we shall see. The ultimate goal of the hygienists was a well-ordered society, necessary for national prosperity and security but also a desirable goal as such.

While the French movement continued to prosper in the 1840s and 1850s, this period saw the movement in Britain come to the fore. Under the leadership of men like Edwin Chadwick, William Farr and Thomas Southwood Smith, the British movement developed a different approach. In the 1830s France had been the source of ideas for Britain, but the roles were reversed by the 1850s.[11] Both theory and the political context worked in France against a greater role for the state (such as developed in Britain) in the middle decades of the nineteenth century. Local control was preferred to direction from the center. Further, disease continued to be explained more in social terms—in terms of poverty and individual behavior—than in Chadwickian, environmentalist terms. Also, degenerationism, associated with the work of A.B. Morel in particular, saw inheritance of morbid tendencies as the key to disease and looked to the family and local community rather than the state for answers. It was coming to enjoy an increasing influence in French medicine.[12]

The beginnings of the idea in Britain that the health of the people is a public responsibility are unclear, but according to Hamlin, after about 1750 a new humanitarianism, drawing on Enlightenment confidence in the capacity of ordinary people to improve, led many doctors and lay people to concern themselves with the health of the poor. The humanitarian movement expressed itself in practical terms through establishment of voluntary hospitals, dispensaries and charitable bodies. The prevention of fever and smallpox was the chief health concern; with inspiration from the teaching of John Pringle, William Cullen and William Pulteney Alison, the cause of fever was identified as debility arising from inadequate diet, clothing and housing, excess work, and dangerous fumes. In a climate of economic and political liberalism, the aim became to enable the individual to overcome the deleterious effects of the physical and social environment. While the nineteenth-century public health movement gave its primary attention to improvement of the physical environment, whether through water supply, sewerage or better housing, moral reformation of people remained an important objective.

In the first three decades of the nineteenth century, as British society was dislocated by the stresses of the long war with Napoleon, growing popular unrest, the massing of factory workers in the burgeoning towns, and the arrival of the first cholera epidemic in 1831, it was unclear what policy should be applied to the parlous condition of the working class. The response to yellow fever and cholera threats in 1805–1806 and 1831 was creation of temporary central boards of health under the Privy Council. Both boards ultimately failed, even though the 1831 board gave rise to 822 local boards in England and Wales, and about four hundred in Scotland, and so was national in scope. Local boards simply lacked the power to act effectively.[13] In 1818, local boards of health were created in Ireland in response to a typhus epidemic after a parliamentary select committee could not recommend a solution to the problem of poverty, which it identified as the basic cause of fever. The practical response was to institute street cleaning and the fumigation and disinfection of homes of infected people. As poverty and disease began to attract different solutions, the broad approach of the late-eighteenth-century humanitarian doctor to the health of the people narrowed to the sanitary idea of the mid-nineteenth-century public health movement.

The British sanitary movement, drawing on the earlier French public health movement's use of statistics and medical topography and the German idea of medical police, highlighted provision of an adequate water supply and sewerage. This solution to disease was taken up progressively in the rest of Europe, the United States and the British Empire—indeed, wherever industrialization and urbanization created similar health problems.[14] The French concern with vital statistics was carried forward in Britain by William Farr (1807–83), a former student of Pierre Louis and compiler of abstracts in the Registrar General's Department, which had been created after compulsory registration of births, deaths and marriages had been introduced in 1836. Mortality statistics, especially the infant mortality rate, were seen as indicators of the health of various districts. This tool became a basic component of the kit of the district medical officer of health when he emerged as a major figure in public health work in Britain and other parts of the English-speaking world. Farr believed knowledge of sanitation would reduce high death rates from "zymotic" (infectious) diseases. This belief was shared by other doctors who supported the Metropolitan Health of Towns Association (created by Southwood Smith in 1844) and other bodies that brought together social reformers, policy makers and politicians, such as the National Association for the Promotion of Social Science, the Royal Statistical Society and the London Epidemiological Society.[15]

It was Edwin Chadwick (1800–1890), barrister and sometime secretary to Jeremy Bentham (1748–1832), utilitarian philosopher and administrative reformer, who set the conceptual and institutional terms of public health in Britain for the rest of the nineteenth century. He essentially redefined the problem of the health of the people as one of engineering—a question of removing environmental filth by a system of glazed, small-diameter drains cleared by high-pressure water from an efficient and reliable water supply, and sewage farms to recycle the liquid sewage. Not only did this redefinition shift attention away from the health of individuals to physical infrastructure, but it made political, economic and moral issues seem insignificant. It deprecated a serious social question.

Chadwick had come to the sanitary idea via reform in 1834 of the long-established Poor Law, which, designed for a rural society in the sixteenth century and offering outdoor relief, promoted idle habits, according to Benthamites. Chadwick's new Poor Law established indoor workhouses, with conditions so unpleasant that they would deter applicants, thus cutting costs and forcing "idlers" onto the labor market. But when demand for relief was in fact not reduced, Chadwick was forced to accept that disease pushed many into poverty. In 1837 he arranged for Doctors Neill Arnott, James Phillip Kay-Shuttleworth and Southwood Smith to inquire into conditions in those parts of London having high mortality from typhus. Drawing on the reports of Poor Law medical officers, Chadwick himself produced in 1842 the *Report on the Sanitary Condition of the Labouring Population of Great Britain*. Environmental filth was held to be the cause of the ill health and premature death of laborers in London and other cities. Poverty resulting from preventable disease (disease caused by the miasmas or gases emanating from putrefaction) could be ended by sanitary measures that removed putrefying organic matter from the environment. Chadwick had little respect for the medical profession, though he worked closely with some sanitation-minded doctors. His skepticism was not unreasonable, given the medical disagreements of the time over the causes of disease and the caste wars that divided the profession. In the mid-nineteenth century, curative medicine had little to offer health advancement. The value of long-used, heroic treatments such as bleeding and blistering, and purging and emetics was being widely questioned, and there were very few specifics to hand—vaccination to prevent smallpox, quinine against malaria, and mercury compounds for syphilis.[16]

Chadwick's administrative solution involved establishment of a central health body to oversee local health boards as they instituted a clean water supply, drainage, environmental cleansing, and regulation of houses, public nuisances and noxious trades. After the Royal Commission on the Health of Towns, 1843–45, supported these proposed reforms, the sanitary idea began to be implemented. William Duncan became the first medical officer of health appointed by a local authority; he assumed that post in Liverpool in 1846. In 1846–47, a Nuisances Removal Act, a Common Lodging House Act and an Adulteration of Food Act were passed. But Chadwick's crowning achievement was the Public Health Act of 1848, the enactment of which was assisted by yet another cholera threat. This legislation created the General Board of Health, composed of Chadwick, the earl of Shaftesbury (an evangelical Christian as well as factory and lunacy reformer) and Southwood Smith.

With almost no coercive power, the board could only attempt to exercise influence over the local boards that were established by urban councils to carry out sanitary inspections, introduce drainage and water supplies, and raise local rates to finance this public health activity. The act was mainly permissive. Except where mortality was twenty-three or more per thousand of population, at which point the central board could force a town corporation to comply, establishment of a local board required 10 percent of rate payers to petition the central health authority. However, new houses had to be connected to the drainage system, and local medical officers of health were to be appointed (where boards existed) to regulate noxious trades, housing and cemeteries and to remove nuisances and other environmental risks. Five years after the passing of the act, 103 towns had local boards. London stood outside the new system, because it possessed a Metropolitan Commission of Sewers and a medical officer of health, John Simon (1816–1904). Chadwick's own assertiveness and perceived centralizing ambitions—Lord John Russell called him "Prussian"—and the enmity of vested interests made him and the Central Board vulnerable to attack. When in 1854 Chadwick lost office, the *Times* leader observed, "Aesculapius and Chiron, in the form of Mr Chadwick and Dr. Southwood Smith, have been deposed, and we prefer to take our chance of cholera and the rest than be bullied into health."[17] Chadwick's commitment to what proved to be an unreliable sewerage technology undermined his credibility with local authorities—which, after all, funded the sewers. His small-diameter sewer pipes too often blocked or broke, and his preferred soft-water supplies were sometimes not available in adequate volume.[18]

When the Central Board of Health was disestablished in 1858, its responsibilities were shared between the new Local Government Act Office (responsible for day-to-day local administration including oversight of public works loans) and the new medical department of the Privy Council, headed by John Simon (responsible for public health).

In Britain's seventeenth-century American colonies, public health was no more than quarantine, some sanitary controls (which had both aesthetic and health objectives) and regulation of the marketing of food. As early as 1611, the governor of Virginia, trying to deal with crowding in the Jamestown fort, forbade nuisances within twenty feet of the well or "necessities of nature" within a quarter of a mile of the palisade, and he required houses to be kept "sweete and cleane."[19] In the 1660s, Boston instituted scavenging for the removal of straying and dead animals from the streets; it quickly became a common practice in colonial towns. In the 1690s, the authorities in Charlestown, one of the three important towns of this era (about three thousand people in 1700), required slaughterhouses and cattle as well as sheep and pig pens to be located outside the town. In New York City (New Amsterdam) in the 1640s, bread content, size and price were regulated, because of concern about adulteration, and by the 1660s, when Britain took control of the colony from the Dutch, bread price and quality were government guaranteed. Since epidemics were believed to be sent as divine punishments, the response to the threat of imported disease was penitential, with resort to prayer and fasting. But quarantine was also employed from an early date. In the 1640s, with an epidemic from the West Indies in the offing, the Massachusetts General Court required ships from that area to delay docking until it was clear that they were free of infection.[20]

In the eighteenth century, the colonial population increased markedly—from about three hundred thousand in 1700 to 2.5 million in 1770, and trade with Europe and the West Indies also increased, so quarantine measures were made more stringent. In 1717, Massachusetts established a pesthouse on Spectacle Island in Boston Harbor and twenty years later built an improved one on Rainsford Island. Charleston, in what is now South Carolina, nearer to the West Indies, from whence yellow fever came, had from 1712 a port quarantine commissioner. In the 1740s the Carolina General Assembly appointed six physicians to be inspectors of ships arriving at Charleston. As labor-intensive cropping expanded in the southern colonies, demand for slaves grew; to prevent the ingress of smallpox, yellow fever and other communicable diseases with them, the African slaves were kept in quarantine for ten days in Charleston Harbor's Sullivan's Island pesthouse.

Pennsylvania experienced much Irish and German immigration in the 1730s and 1740s, and so a physician was appointed to check ships, while captains had the responsibility of providing for the sick outside city limits. New York instituted specific measures in the 1730s, requiring ships from infected ports to stay at a quarantine anchorage, and appointing a health officer. In 1760, a pesthouse was established. The much-feared smallpox, endemic by the eighteenth century, was partly restrained in Boston after inoculation was employed in 1721. But the practice did not become widespread until the 1770s. While Rev. Cotton Mather and Zabdiel Boyleston, a physician, introduced the practice in Boston, Benjamin Franklin and Philadelphia physicians helped popularize it in the 1750s. Inoculation and improved quarantine and isolation were important in lowering smallpox mortality in this period.[21] The Revolutionary War and the establishment of the republic brought little advance in public health. However, recurrent epidemics of yellow fever ravaged the eastern cities in 1793–1806 and heightened awareness of public health needs. Health commissions and health boards were created, quarantine measures strengthened and sanitation improved. The need for clean water and air, and pure food was widely recognized in health publications. But as the epidemic threat declined in the northern cities, the threat of higher taxes to pay for sanitary reform slowed its forward march.

Control of smallpox was one area where government remained active. Never a major health problem, it nonetheless provoked great anxiety. The practice of vaccination slowly increased with the support of medical societies and town councils—Milton, Massachusetts, set out to vaccinate in 1809 all its citizens—but by 1830 vaccination was very widely accepted, even if the more risky inoculation was also still practiced. Complacency in the face of a declining smallpox incidence soon led to neglect of vaccination, and incidence commenced to increase once more in the 1840s.[22]

Local government was becoming more involved in public health, as developments in New York illustrate. The first permanent post there in the sanitary area was that of city inspector (which was occupied by John Pintard in 1804). The inspector reported public nuisances and abuses; the problem was that he could not take rectifying action. Two other officials were involved in health administration: the health officer (quarantine) and the resident physician (identification of communicable disease cases). Authority in health was further fragmented, because from 1805 there existed an advisory Board of Health. Popular distrust of orthodox medicine and the medical profession's lack of credibility in light of its disputes about causes of disease in the first half of the century are reflected in the fact that most health boards were run by lay people. Almost all port cities had health officers concerned with quarantine, and almost all possessed a health board of some sort, although it was usually created only when major health crises loomed. However, large social and economic forces were changing the face of cities from the 1840s. Population growth and immigration made great demands on housing and water, sewage and drainage facilities. New York and Boston were first to experience the health problems of the city slum.

At the same time, western expansion saw the United States triple in size in 1800–1860. The sanitary state of the new towns and settlements was not much better than that of the eastern cities, as western migration transported smallpox, diphtheria, measles, scarlet fever and other diseases into new areas, while malaria and enteric and respiratory infections added to the disease burden.[23]

Rapid population growth—New York grew from about seventy-six thousand in 1805 to 515,000 in 1850—gave American cities slum health problems like those in older European cities. The work of sanitary reformers in Europe—Villermé's studies in France and Chadwick's reports in England—inspired reformers in the United States, although the period from the 1830s to the end of the Civil War in 1865 was one of preparation for achievements that were to be delayed until the later decades of the nineteenth century. Cholera epidemics in 1832–33 and 1849–54 also promoted community concern about public health.

The first significant health study of this era was Dr. Benjamin McCready's 1837 study of the impact of occupation on health. But the study that set out the principles that the sanitary reform movement was to pursue over the next decades was Dr. John Griscom's *The Sanitary Condition of the Laboring Population of New York* (1845). It originally was a supplement to his 1842 report as city inspector of New York City. Like other public health reformers of the time, Griscom saw sanitary improvement as linked to moral uplift of the poor. But while the sins of the poor predisposed them to disease, he argued, overcrowding and inadequate housing in turn promoted immorality. Griscom's report noted the immense amount of preventable illness and mortality among the poor and the cost-effectiveness for government of public health action. Indeed, the idea of preventable mortality was at the heart of sanitary reform. His work did not enjoy speedy results, but along with the voluntary health associations (similar to British bodies that proliferated after 1845), Griscom helped create a climate favorable to a sanitary revolution. In Providence, Rhode Island, Dr. Edwin Miller Snow enjoyed more immediate success. His report on cholera in 1854 condemned the city's lack of concern for sanitation and led to creation of a health department, headed by Snow. His energetic sanitary campaigns, including compulsory vaccination for schoolchildren, made Providence a leader in the quest for civic cleanliness.

The best known of the sanitary publications of this era is Lemuel Shattuck's *Report of the Sanitary Commission of Massachusetts* (1850). Shattuck and Dr. Edward Jarvis were pivotal in the establishment of the American Statistical Society in 1839 (in reality a local association, for some time), and together they secured legislation in 1842 creating statewide vital statistics registration. The Massachusetts law inspired similar systems in other States. Shattuck's *Census of Boston* (1845) established a reliable basis for the recording of statistics in the United States, but his wider report of his commission's sanitary survey of Massachusetts prefigured public health administration and practice in the country for the next century. It was in effect a health policy, which drew on the best of the sanitary movement, international and national.

Yet nothing concrete resulted in the short term. His proposed state health department (with local health boards) was not created for almost twenty years. He called for community sanitary surveys and detailed vital statistics machinery; communicable disease control, food and drug regulation, and environmental sanitation; monitoring of infant and school child health; and health education.

The growth of the urban sanitary movement is also indicated by the calling of four national quarantine and sanitary conventions in 1857–60. They prepared the way for establishment of the American Public Health Association in 1872. The conventions were initiated because of concern about effective quarantine against yellow fever and cholera. By the third convention, held in New York in 1859, there was much more interest in sanitary reform than in quarantine; President Griscom claimed that the danger from importation of disease (and therefore the need for quarantine) in relation to danger from local causes (and so the need for better sanitation) was about one to one hundred.

It was New York that pioneered reform. A Council of Hygiene, modeled on the French *conseil de salubrité* and made up of prominent doctors, was established in 1864 by the Citizens' Association, itself formed to eradicate corruption from city government. The council sponsored a sanitary survey, the results of which were published in a report of 1865. So disturbing were the findings that sanitary reform became prominent on the political agenda. Another arm of the Citizens' Association, the Council of Law, drew up a public health bill. Once enacted in 1866, it brought into being a Metropolitan Board of Health, which was inspired by English sanitary administration and was composed of a president, four doctors, the port health officer and four police commissioners. It could both draw up ordinances and enforce them. Four years later, the New York City Health Department was brought into being; four bureaus were established: sanitary, sanitary permits, street cleaning and vital statistics. The creation of the Metropolitan Board of Health and the City Health Department represented a major advance in public health in the United States, because an effective administrative base had thereby been established for the first time, and when in the late 1870s new bacteriological knowledge became available, it could be assimilated into public health practice more easily.[24]

European colonists took to the countries of the New World, in which they settled not only their ideas and practices concerning public health but their infections. These caused death and population decline on a large scale among indigenes. In the following chapter we will discuss the new disease environment created in Australia, America and other parts of Europe overseas.

NOTES

1. G. Rosen, *A History of Public Health* (Baltimore: Johns Hopkins University Press, 1993), chaps. 4–6.

2. A. Wear, "The History of Personal Hygiene," in *Companion Encyclopaedia of the History of Medicine,* vol. 2, ed. W.F. Bynum and R. Porter (London: Routledge, 1993), 1297, 1304–5.

3. D. Porter, "Introduction," in *The History of Public Health and the Modern State,* ed. D. Porter (Amsterdam, Atlanta: Editions Rodopi B.V., 1994), 5.

4. Rosen, *A History of Public Health,* 61–83.

5. Ibid., 85–90.

6. G. Rosen, "Political Order and Human Health in Jeffersonian Thought," *Bulletin of History of Medicine* 26 (1952), 32–44.

7. M. Ramsey, "Public Health in France," in *The History of Public Health and the Modern State,* ed. Porter, 48–49. D. Porter, "Introduction," 8.

8. Porter, "Introduction," 24.

9. K. Johannisson, "The People's Health: Public Health Policies in Sweden," in *The History of Public Health and the Modern State,* ed. Porter, 165–68.

10. A.F. La Berge, *Mission and Method: The Early Nineteenth-Century French Public Health Movement* (Cambridge: Cambridge University Press, 1992), 11, 44; Ramsey, "Public Health in France," 46–51.

11. La Berge, *Mission and Method,* 25–42.

12. Ramsey, "Public Health in France," 64–67.

13. F. Brockington, "Public Health at the Privy Council 1831–34," *Journal of History of Medicine and Allied Sciences* 16 (1961), 161–85; F. Brockington, "Public Health at the Privy Council 1805–6," *Medical History* 7 (1963), 13–24; C. Hamlin, "State Medicine in Great Britain," in *The History of Public Health and the Modern State,* ed. Porter, 134–39.

14. C. Hamlin, *Public Health and Social Justice in the Age of Chadwick: Britain, 1800–1854* (Cambridge: Cambridge University Press, 1998), 1–2.

15. R. Porter, *The Greatest Benefit to Mankind. A Medical History of Humanity from Antiquity to the Present* (London: HarperCollins, 1997), 407–8.

16. H.R. Woolcock, "'Our Salubrious Climate': Attitudes to Health in Colonial Queensland," in *Disease, Medicine and Empire: Perspectives on Western Medicine and the Experience of European Expansion,* ed. R. MacLeod and M. Lewis (London: Routledge, 1988), 183.

17. Quoted in W.W. Holland and S. Stewart, *Public Health: The Vision and the Challenge* (London: Nuffield Trust, 1998), 11.

18. Holland and Stewart, *Public Health: The Vision and the Challenge,* 9–11; C. Hamlin, "State Medicine in Great Britain," in *The History of Public Health and the Modern State,* ed. Porter, 147–48; Porter, *The Greatest Benefit to Mankind,* 411–12.

19. Quoted in J. Duffy, *The Sanitarians: A History of American Public Health* (Urbana: University of Illinois Press, 1990), 11.

20. Duffy, *The Sanitarians,* 11–15.

21. Ibid., 24–28; W.M. Reynolds, "Inoculation for the Smallpox in Colonial America," *Bulletin of History of Medicine* 22 (1948): 273.

22. Duffy, *The Sanitarians,* 38–56.

23. Rosen, *A History of Public Health,* 210–12; Duffy, *The Sanitarians,* 57–63; E. Fee, "Public Health and the State: The United States," in *The History of Public Health and the Modern State,* ed. Porter, 229.

24. Rosen, *A History of Public Health,* 213–22; Duffy, *The Sanitarians,* 95–105.

Chapter 2

Health and Disease in a New World

EUROPEAN DISEASES AND INDIGENES

Before discussing health and disease in early colonial Australia, we will look at the impact of Western expansion on the health of the indigenous peoples of the Americas, Australia, New Zealand and the Pacific islands. The major causes of death and disability in small-scale, isolated communities of hunter-gatherers, both Palaeolithic and historical, would appear to have been zoonoses ("accidentally" transmitted), chronic infections and infestations (which co-evolved with humans from the time of our primate forerunners), and violence, accidental and deliberate. Life expectancy at birth is estimated to have been twenty to thirty years. The viral infections present were those marked by latency and recurrent excretion, such as chickenpox and herpes zoster. The populations were too small to sustain smallpox, measles and rubella, which lack those characteristics. With the advent of sedentary agriculture about ten thousand years ago, and the rise of cities three to four thousand years ago, these and other crowd diseases could be sustained by the much larger, more concentrated populations. Agriculture supports population densities ten to a hundred times greater than does hunting and gathering. Moreover, the close proximity of domesticated animals meant that some of their pathogens appear to have evolved into specialized human pathogens: measles from rinderpest in cattle; smallpox from cowpox in cattle or related pox viruses in other livestock; influenza from pigs and ducks; pertussis from pigs and dogs; and tuberculosis from cattle. Farmers and city dwellers lived close to their wastes, unlike hunter-gatherers, and so were at greater risk of faecal-oral infections and worm infestations. They lived close to disease-bearing rodents attracted by stored foodstuffs. As the civilizations of the ancient world expanded, they began to share infections; by the Roman imperial era, Eurasia shared major pathogens with North Africa. In the plague of Antoninus, A.D. 165–80, smallpox killed vast numbers of Roman citizens. Bubonic plague reached Europe in the plague of Justinian, A.D. 542–43. But the indigenes of America, Australia and the Pacific islands remained isolated from this long-term exchange of deadly pathogens and so had no chance to build up resistance.[1]

The modern decline of mortality in Europe to today's historically unprecedented low levels may be broken up into four phases. The first covered the seventeenth century. It saw great peaks of mortality, in large part due to epidemics of plague and typhus (which were exacerbated by famine and which added to high mortality from endemic infections). The second, coterminous with the eighteenth century, saw these infections decline as a result of the capacity of the relatively centralized governments more effectively to quarantine plague, to unify grain markets so that the threat of famine was reduced, and to pursue less destructive forms of warfare. The crowd diseases, smallpox and measles, became less deadly. In the late eighteenth and nineteenth centuries—the third phase—growing urbanization of a poorly regulated type helped promote infant and child mortality from the diarrhea-pneumonia syndrome. The fourth phase began in the early to mid-twentieth century, when degenerative and other "lifestyle" diseases took the place of infections as the primary causes of death.

While epidemic diseases did not ravage pre-Columbian urban populations of America, endemic enteric and respiratory infections exacted heavy tolls, so life expectancy at birth was at about the same low level—the late teenage years to the early twenties—as in pre-industrial towns in Europe. Thus, neither sewerage nor water supply systems, whether in Rome or Teotihuacan, nor the evolution of more complex medical systems seem to have advanced the health of their populations over that of hunter-gatherers. But from the eighteenth century, health began to improve in Europe. Life expectancy improved as epidemic, then endemic, infections declined. Historians who believe industrialization initially lowered living standards for the working classes tend to identify public health measures as the explanation for rising life expectancy in the nineteenth century, whereas those convinced that living standards improved play down the significance of social interventions. Since the killing capacity of epidemic plague, typhus and smallpox is not enhanced by undernutrition, the issue of living standards (in income terms) is irrelevant. However, the severity of endemic infections like tuberculosis and infant diarrhea—major killers in nineteenth-century cities—is heightened by undernutrition, so their decline may have been related to better wages. Kunitz proposes that in England and in overseas offshoots like the United States, where individualism and liberalism prevailed, increasing living standards may have been significant in lowering mortality in the nineteenth century, but that in more authoritarian societies like Japan, public health imposed by bureaucrats may well have been more important.[2]

Smallpox and measles, which were introduced by European explorers, traders and colonizers, ravaged the immunologically virgin indigenous populations of the Americas and Oceania, as the West began its rise to world economic and political hegemony from the end of the fifteenth century. It was in truth a form of unintentional biological warfare. "Smallpox was the captain of the men of death in that war, typhus fever the first lieutenant and measles the second lieutenant. More terrible than the conquistadores on horseback, more deadly than sword and gunpowder, they made the conquest by the whites a walkover as compared with what it would have been without their aid. They were the forerunners of civilization, the companions of Christianity, the friends of the invader."[3]

The pre-Columbian population of the Americas has been variously estimated to have been from 8.4 million (Alfred Kroeber, 1939) to 112 million (Henry Dobyn, 1966). The huge decline in population after European colonization has been explained, especially by those opting for a larger precontact population estimate, in terms of high mortality and low reproductive rates, both due to infections. Smallpox undoubtedly assisted Hernán Cortes and his six hundred Spanish conquistadors to conquer the Aztec Empire after he invaded Mexico in 1519. A severe epidemic in 1520–21 killed the emperor Cuitlahuac and almost half the Aztec population. Smallpox (and perhaps measles) swept New Spain in 1531–32, and in 1545–48 another severe "plague" killed large numbers of natives. Further epidemics of smallpox, measles and mumps reduced population, and malaria that came from Africa with slaves barred settlement in the lowlands. Erysipelas, typhus, influenza and enteric diseases are all noted by the late sixteenth century. Venereal diseases (VD) became significant among both the Spanish and the Indians. At the end of the second decade of the seventeenth century, Mexico's population, estimated variously as five to twenty million, had declined to between one and 1.6 million.[4] In the 1530s, Pizarro with about 170 followers conquered the Incas of Peru, numbering in the millions. He was assisted by the fact that smallpox had swept through the empire not long before his arrival and killed a large proportion of the population.[5] In the colonies of the other European powers, smallpox had a similarly devastating effect. In New France, smallpox decimated the Indians in 1640, not long after missionary nuns settled in Quebec. In 1702–3, 1732–33 and 1755–57, significant epidemics ravaged the Canadian colony.[6] The last of these epidemics was so devastating for the Indians that they stopped their attacks on the English colonies in the French and Indian War, a factor that led to the loss of Quebec to the British in 1759. The war facilitated the diffusion of smallpox to the west as far as Niagara. French, British and colonial troops, and settlers, were infected as well as Indians.[7]

Early accounts of the New England Indians recognize their robust health. Capt. Bartholomew Gosnold recorded in 1602, "the people [are] of a perfect constitution of body, active, strong healthful, and very witty."[8] Locked in conflict for control of the land, the English saw the destruction of the Indians as God's answer to their prayers. In 1705, a missionary to New York wrote, "Ye Indians . . . they wast away and have done every since our first arrival . . . (as they themselves say.) like Snow agt. ye sun. . . . God's Providence . . . seems very wonderful, and no cause of their Decrease visible unless their drinking Rum, with some new Distempers we have brought amongst them."[9]

Smallpox or bubonic plague so reduced the New England tribes just before the Pilgrims settled in New England that they did not resist the invasion. Of the 1633 smallpox epidemic and Indian recalcitrance over land, Increase Mather said, "God ended the Controversy by sending the Smallpox amongst the Indians of Saugust who were before that time exceeding numerous."[10] The next year the infection destroyed the Narragansetts and the Connecticuts, but the settlers, immune from previous exposure, seemed under God's special protection. Epidemics then spread to the Great Lakes and the St. Lawrence area in 1634–41 (including Quebec as mentioned above). The destruction of the Huron, north of Lake Ontario, is captured in what follows: "Terror was universal. . . . Everywhere . . . the wail of the sick and dying children; and on or under the platforms at the sides of the house crouched squalid men and women, in all stages of the distemper."[11] In 1662–63, the Iroquois were ravaged: "The small-pox, which is America's pest, has wrought sad havoc . . . and as a result their villages are nearly deserted, and their fields are only half-tilled."[12] In what is now Hampton County, Virginia, in 1667, practically every tribe disappeared because of smallpox.[13] The devastation continued in the northern colonies in the late seventeenth century as well as in Virginia and the Carolinas, and it became worse in the following century.

In 1702–3, smallpox spread from New York to Quebec via the Indian tribes, and in 1716–17 the tribes of the Northwest were laid low. From Boston in 1730, it spread to nearby towns and to the Indians, and next spring was among the Indians of Eastern Canada. To the south, the governor of New York expressed regret to the Five Nations for the "great mortality among you by the smallpox."[14] When it struck Charleston in 1738, the Cherokee Indian population was reduced by half. The same year, a northern outbreak spread to the Indians of the Hudson Bay area. In the early 1750s it was among the Great Lakes Indians, and in the mid-1750s an outbreak spread to almost all Indians in Eastern Canada and the New England region. In 1759–60, the Indians of Georgia and South Carolina were badly affected by an epidemic. A 1760 colonial newspaper account said that seventy years earlier the Catawbas had been four thousand people but rum, war and smallpox had reduced them to fewer than a hundred "gunmen." Fighting between the English and French helped to disseminate the infection, apparently now endemic among the military. In 1764–65, Indian groups very distant from each other were reported infected. A New York newspaper said it was among the Creek, and a Pennsylvania publication reported it among the Choctaws and Chickasaws. It retreated until the movement of troops in the Revolutionary War spread it to Indians and colonists alike. Two great pandemics, 1801–2 and 1836–40, destroyed many tribes, and smallpox continued to reduce the North American Indian population through the nineteenth century, being brought under control only in the early twentieth century.[15]

The European colonization of the Americas linked the disease pools of that continent with those of Eurasia, but the indigenes of Australia, New Zealand and the Pacific islands remained until the late eighteenth century isolated from this process of microbiological unification. The same devastating effects of European-introduced infections as seen among the Amerindians can be seen at work among the Aborigines of Australia and the Polynesians and Melanesians of the Pacific islands. An epidemic era was inaugurated with the increasing intrusion of European ships into the Pacific Ocean from the eighteenth century, although island groups were differently affected, and the extent of depopulation and cultural dislocation was not uniform. One of the worst epidemics, in this case measles, was that which devastated the Melanesian population of the Fiji Islands in 1875. The paramount chief, King Cakobau and his two sons, returned from a visit to Sydney (at the invitation of the governor of New South Wales) infected with measles. On their return they were not quarantined, and at least forty thousand of approximately 150,000 Fijians died. A report to the Epidemiological Society of London said, "The attacks are so sudden and complete that every soul in a village will be down at once."[16] Hawaii's population declined from about five hundred thousand at the time of Capt. James Cook's visit in 1779 to eighty-four thousand in 1853. Syphilis, gonorrhoea, tuberculosis and influenza appear to have arrived with Cook. A serious epidemic of typhoid followed in 1804, and in 1853 about ten thousand people died from smallpox.[17] Dr. John Batty Tuke, writing of disease among the Maoris of New Zealand in 1863, said that the "grand cause" of population decline—"large villages are now either deserted or very thinly inhabited, which twenty-five or thirty years ago, teemed with inhabitants"—was tuberculosis. He claimed that 50 percent of Maoris showed evidence of the disease. Venereal disease had been introduced by Europeans. Influenza in 1844, whooping cough in 1847, mumps in 1851, and measles and scarlet fever in 1854 had "carried off multitudes."[18]

Even the remote Polynesian population of the Cook Islands was affected in the nineteenth century. In 1830, a violent cough (a *maki manuiri,* a "foreign disease") was prevalent after the visit of a ship; the Rarotongans had a phrase, *kua pai au,* "I am suffering from a disease brought by a ship." In 1824, a dysentery-like infection carried off one in twelve people on Mangaia. Three years later on Rarotonga, what may have been influenza killed "numbers" of those infected. Bacillary dysentery in 1830 raged for four months.

Mortality was variously estimated to be eight hundred to a thousand, and as high as 1,600, in an estimated population of six to eight thousand. From the 1830s, Cook Islanders traveled overseas, bringing back infections. Tuberculosis probably entered the population as early as 1835, and it was a significant cause of illness and death by the end of the century. Epidemics continued: dysentery in 1843 and 1846, the latter visitation combined with food shortages resulting from a hurricane's destruction of crops and food trees; scarlatina and whooping cough in 1848; and influenza and mumps in 1851–52. Measles struck in 1854, when food was short after hurricane damage. Evidence is very incomplete, but it is clear that on some islands population decline was marked. On Rarotonga, probably the worst-affected island, it fell from six to eight thousand when the first missions arrived, to three to four thousand by 1843. It bottomed out at 1,856 in 1867, and no population growth occurred before the 1900s.[19]

It was not, of course, just the high mortality from imported diseases that caused population decline in the Americas, New Zealand and the Pacific islands. Violence and deliberate killing by Europeans; famine from loss of crops or hunting grounds, social disorganization (lack of marriage partners and VD-induced infertility); and cultural demoralization in the face of proselytising Christianity and superior Western technology—all pushed indigenous societies toward collapse.[20] Australian Aborigines suffered similarly.

The natural obstacles to creating human societies in Australia were probably greater than in Eurasia, Africa and the Americas. Australia is drier, flatter, less fertile or biologically rich, and has a more unpredictable climate than these land masses (due to an irregular nonannual cycle, the El Niño Southern Oscillation, over most of the continent). The Aborigines, who have occupied Australia for at least forty thousand years, developed a lifestyle well adapted to the unpredictable availability of resources. Nomadic hunter-gatherers, they avoided the risk of dependence on a limited number of crops by using many wild foods. By nomadism and by limiting population, they could survive recurrent times of scarcity. Population was greatest in the areas where water was most abundant—the southeast, where the major river system, the Murray-Darling, is located; the southwest; and the eastern and northern coasts. Dryness and unpredictable climate limited Australia's indigenous population to hundreds of thousands, compared with the tens of millions on the American continent.[21]

Palaeolithic communities had high birthrates and high infant mortality rates, and precontact Aboriginal society very probably had similar demographic characteristics.[22] Estimates of the Aboriginal population in 1788, when European settlement began, have varied since that date. The first governor of New South Wales claimed the population was one million, but the very low figure of 150,000 appeared in official publications from 1881 to the end of the 1920s. The anthropologist A.R. Radcliffe-Brown attempted a careful analytical estimate and concluded in 1930 there had been 250,000 to 300,000. More recent estimates have hovered in that range: Davidson's (1938), of 253,000–303,000; Jones's (1970), of 227,000–231,000; and Smith's (1980), 314,500. But the prehistorians White and Mulvaney (1987) increased the figure to 750,000.[23]

The Aboriginal population declined drastically soon after European settlement and the downward trend continued for 150 years. Table 2.1 shows changes in the "revealed" Aboriginal population: those who were identified as Aborigines at censuses plus estimates of numbers in remote areas not enumerated. Because the figures exclude those of Aboriginal descent who were enumerated but not identified as Aborigines, both the decline and the later recovery are exaggerated.

The first demographic transition, from about 1800 to 1870, saw a sharp fall in population from a decline in the birthrate (drastic at first) and a steep rise in the death rate. Figures for the very early period are scanty, but William Thomas, Guardian of Aborigines, recorded them for two tribes near Melbourne (then Port Phillip) in 1839–49, when the European settlement was established. Population fell from 207 to seventy-six, and the average annual crude birthrate was only eight per thousand, while the death rate was seventy-one per thousand. Contemporary descriptions report a shortage of children in tribes dispossessed of their land, resulting possibly from infant or maternal illness or destruction of children; they note also a deficit of women, apparently a feature of precontact society but now a very great deal more pronounced. The second demographic transition was to a stationary state by about 1880, when birth and death rates balanced at about thirty-five per thousand. The third transition occurred in 1940–50, when the birthrate climbed to more than forty per thousand. By the 1960s the birthrate had fallen to thirty-five, and the death rate had declined farther to sixteen per thousand. Population growth increased in the 1970s to between 2 and 2.5 percent a year.

Population decline took place at different times and to different extents in the various colonies/states and territories. Of the first settled colonies (New South Wales [NSW], Victoria, Tasmania and South Australia), Victoria and Tasmania experienced more rapid decline, and their populations fell to lower levels. But they also experienced more rapid recoveries. The existence of comparatively fertile land and small geographical size resulted in close and complete European settlement. Policies toward Aborigines focused on collecting them in controlled institutions separate from the rest of the community. These factors produced a speedier decline of the tribes and growth of a part-Aboriginal population. Many part-Aboriginal people stopped identifying as Aborigines. The decline and recovery were similar in timing in NSW and South Australia; differences from Victoria and Tasmania were the product of less emphasis on assimilation and of the remote locations of populations of full Aboriginal descent. Queensland's experience is intermediate between that of the four "original" colonies and that of Western Australia and the

Table 2.1
Estimated Change in the "Revealed" Aboriginal Population of the States (Colonies), Territories and Australia, 1788–1971

Year	NSW	Vic	Qld	SA	WA	Tas	NT	ACT*	Aust
1788	48,000	15,000	120,000	15,000	62,000	4,500	50,000		314,500
1861	15,000	2,384	60,000	9,000	44,500	18	48,500		179,402
1871	12,000	1,700	50,000	7,500	40,000	85	44,000		155,285
1881	10,000	900	40,000	6,346	35,500	120	38,500		131,366
1891	8,280	731	32,000	5,500	31,000	139	33,500		111,150
1901	7,434	652	26,670	5,185	26,500	157	28,000		94,598
1911	6,524	643	22,508	4,692	22,498	230	23,500	18	80,613
1921	6,185	586	19,104	4,744	19,547	152	19,500	33	69,851
1933	9,546	865	17,967	4,800	17,290	270	16,500	68	67,314
1947	11,560	1,277	19,811	5,122	16,234	214	16,147	100	70,465
1954	12,215	1,395	22,813	5,500	16,215	93	17,163	173	75,567
1961	14,720	1,796	24,903	6,100	18,276	38	19,707	145	85,685
1966	20,618	2,715	28,262	6,584	21,238	80	22,312	169	101,978
1971	23,873	6,371	31,922	7,299	22,181	671	23,381	255	115,953

*The Australian Capital Territory (ACT) was established on territory ceded by NSW in 1911.

Source: *Population and Australia: A Demographic Analysis and Projection. First Report of the National Population Inquiry*, volume 2 (Canberra: Australian Government Publishing Service, 1975): 478.

Northern Territory. While Queensland was settled early, it is geographically extensive, with remotely located Aborigines of full descent, as in Western Australia and the Northern Territory. Moreover, policy was for a long time based on segregation into separate institutions under state control. Part-Aborigines were encouraged to marry into Aboriginal communities. Permission to assimilate was dependent on capacity to live a white lifestyle. By the 1950s, even so, many people of Aboriginal descent were not identifying with the Aboriginal community, as in the southeastern states.

European settlement of the north, northwest and center of the continent occurred only in the late nineteenth century, and the decline of Aboriginal populations in Western Australia and the Northern Territory took place later than in the other colonies/states.[24]

Attempts to explain the population decline have varied over time. When Social Darwinism was at a zenith in the late nineteenth and early twentieth centuries, the inherent inferiority of Aborigines explained all. What has not been established is what violence, disease, loss of lands, and social and cultural disorganization individually contributed, although it would seem there has been a tendency to play down the contribution of outright killing. In Queensland alone in 1850–1900, at least ten thousand Aborigines were killed by Europeans, but pacification, especially by the notorious Native Police, was widespread in remote areas, so the total was very probably a great deal higher. Early epidemics of, for example, smallpox were probably not so significant as endemic disease interacting with social and ecological dislocation; undernutrition, and sometimes starvation, because loss of land to pastoral development meant lack of access to native plants and animals; chest and bowel infections from an unhygienic and unfamiliar sedentary lifestyle; and sterility and proneness to abortion arising from widespread prevalence of sexually transmitted infections.[25]

Britain did not recognize Aboriginal tenure of the land. However, Capt. Arthur Phillip, first governor of the penal colony of NSW, had been officially instructed in 1787 to estimate numbers of Aborigines, to see how advantageous relations might be developed, and always to behave in a humanitarian way. Prior to and after landing in 1788, he ordered that they not be "molested on any account . . . and . . . be treated with every mark of friendship."[26] Unhappily, while he himself had good intentions, by his departure in 1792 European behavior already manifested the violence, indifference and contempt that was to mark relations with the indigenous people for the next 150 years. Within four years, Aborigines up to several days' march from Sydney had been alienated and degraded by contact.[27]

In the early years it was hoped that education, work and Christianity would allow assimilation. Governor Lachlan Macquarie opened in 1814 an institution for vocational training of Aboriginal children; the school did not succeed, and it closed in 1823. Land was granted for farming, but Aborigines, preferring a hunter-gatherer lifestyle, sold it. From the 1820s, church missions sought converts to Christianity and to a European way of life. When they attracted few adults, they focused on children. In what was to become Victoria, the Port Phillip Protectorate, 1839–49, was created to offer some degree of sanctuary amid the struggle for the land. The meager funds allocated were eaten up by staff salaries; there was little for food, clothing and medicine for Aborigines. Three church missions subsequently set up also lacked adequate funds and could not offer proper rations or medical care. Settlers condemned the protectorate on the self-interested grounds that Aboriginal independence would promote conflict and that native reserves locked up grazing land.

Policy in the Swan River settlement, Western Australia (1829), also began with good intentions. But having conceded the settler right to self-defense, Governor Sir James Stirling's superintendent of natives as early as 1833 was employing mounted police to punish Aborigines. Under Governor John Hindmarsh's proclamation of 1836, Aborigines in South Australia were to enjoy the same rights as other British subjects, and an 1842 act made possible establishment of reserves on crown land. The colonial administration here was more consistent in its pursuit of justice than those of the other Australian colonies, but settler land hunger was in conflict with protection of nomadic hunter-gatherers, and a colonization system that used funds from land sales to finance immigration of European labor was at odds with the provision of adequate reserves. From 1863, South Australia administered the Northern Territory. By now pessimistic about protecting Aborigines in more settled areas, the colonial government had almost no control over the vast lands to the north of South Australia. Indeed Protector Matthew Moorhouse argued that no more reserves should be created, because they would simply add to administrative problems when the Aboriginal race disappeared.[28]

A Select Committee of the Victorian Legislative Council, 1858–59, said that there had been a "great" and "almost unprecedented reduction" in the Aboriginal population. Numbers had almost halved in ten years. A Moravian Church missionary said that few babies were now being born in his district on the Murray River. Other witnesses blamed a combination of drink and disease for the decline in population. The Assistant Protector of Aboriginals, E.S. Parker, thought pulmonary disease was a primary cause of death. The select committee urged that reserves be created and that food and clothing be distributed regularly. A Board for the Protection of Aborigines was set up in 1860 to oversee occasional distribution of supplies to the aged, sick and orphaned. The able-bodied were expected to support their families as employees of settlers. Anglican and Presbyterian-Moravian stations, and later government stations, were established. In 1884, the board recommended that all fit "half-castes" be moved off the stations and merged into the general population; the 1886 Aborigines Act implemented this proposal. The economic depression of the 1890s and discrimination concerning housing and work undermined the policy of assimilation, but it continued to be applied, as children were placed in institutions and raised as whites, and marriage between "fullbloods" and "half-castes" was forbidden. Five of the six stations were shut down in 1904–24, and while from 1910 the board had discretion to provide residence, rations and clothing on a station to any person of "mixed blood," for thirty years from 1926 at Lake Tyers only indigent Aborigines of not less than "half-caste" could be residents. The state government would not participate in a major national Native Welfare conference in 1951, on the ground that there was "no native problem in Victoria."[29]

In the second half of the nineteenth century, in Victoria and NSW, frontier issues disappeared from policy, and in Tasmania there survived only a small community of people of mixed descent who had been removed from the main island to small Bass Strait islands. They were descendants of the remnants of the tribes that had been destroyed in the "Black Wars" or decimated by imported diseases. Only in South Australia, Western Australia and Queensland did confrontations on the frontier continue to be significant. NSW pursued a policy of segregating Aborigines on stations. From the 1880s, NSW looked to a board of protectors to channel public funds to private benevolent activities as well as government stations. The Aborigines Protection Board functioned without legislative backing until the 1909 Aborigines Protection Act was passed.[30]

By 1911, the mainland states had all passed legislation enshrining the principles of protection and restriction in Aboriginal policy. The "settled" states were primarily concerned with developing policy for people of part-Aboriginal descent. The "frontier" states wanted protective legislation, but not to the extent of removing from the European economy the cheap labor of the many "full-blood" people, who were essential to the success of the great primary industries of their outback regions.[31]

Epidemics of smallpox, measles and influenza were particularly dangerous for Aborigines, because everybody was at risk and likely to be sick at the same time, so that no one was able to care for the infected or provide food and water. This phenomenon on the colonial frontier was reproduced as the desert became the frontier in the twentieth century. Adults and children died in measles epidemics in the Western Desert in 1948 and in 1957. As well as smallpox, a number of diseases—influenza and measles, typhoid, chickenpox, whooping cough, mumps, scarlet fever, diphtheria, tuberculosis, gonorrhoea, granuloma venereum and syphilis—were introduced by Europeans, but tuberculosis and venereal disease were also introduced by Malaccans (Indonesians), Melanesians, Japanese and Chinese. Leprosy was introduced in the 1880s by Chinese immigrant laborers.[32] But Butlin claimed that much of the massive depopulation resulted from two diseases in particular—smallpox and venereal disease.[33] Two smallpox epidemics occurred among Aborigines in the early years—one in 1789–91 and the other in 1829–31. Col. David Collins, judge advocate of the colony of NSW, 1788–96, recorded: "In the year 1789, they were visited by a disorder which raged among them with all the appearance and virulence of the smallpox. The number that is swept off, by their own account, was incredible. . . . Notwithstanding the town of Sydney was at this time filled with children, many of whom visited the natives that were ill . . . , not one of them caught it, though a North-American Indian, a sailor belonging to Captain Ball's vessel, the *Supply*, sickened of it and died."[34] Butlin gave such weight to smallpox and venereal disease that he wrote, "Caught between smallpox and venereal disease, . . . the Australian aboriginals had little prospect except to do as the historians have proposed they did—to fade away."[35] Again, Collins noted very early cases of venereal disease in Aborigines: "The venereal disease also had got among them; but I fear our people have to answer for that; for though I believe none of our women had connection with them, yet there is no doubt but that several of the black women had not scrupled to connect themselves with the white men."[36]

While syphilis may produce abortions or stillborn and defective infants, chronic gonorrhoea of the fallopian tubes may significantly reduce fertility. Butlin, applying a model of gonorrhoea-induced infertility drawn from an African study, calculated that Aboriginal reproductive capacity between 1815 (after the Blue Mountains, the barrier to European expansion inland from Sydney, were crossed) and 1855 had been reduced by 40 percent.[37] Gray has argued that Butlin overestimated the extent of infertility in Aboriginal women. Perhaps 60 percent of gonorrhea-induced pelvic inflammatory disease cases, before antibiotics, became permanently sterile. However, only between 8 and 20 percent of untreated gonorrhea cases result in pelvic inflammatory disease. Chlamydia infections can also produce sterility, but again, only about 8 percent of infections result in pelvic inflammatory disease. Gray also challenged two other assumptions of Butlin. First, though very extensive, white sexual use of black women may have occurred on the frontier of settlement, it could not have taken place with Aborigines beyond the frontier. Second, the patterns of sexual behavior in the African model of gonorrhea-induced sterility upon which Butlin drew simply did not exist in Australia.[38]

There are some difficulties in assessing the impact on population decline of syphilis, the other major venereal disease of the time, because yaws, a closely related treponematosis, may well have been very prevalent in Aboriginal populations before European settlement. Certainly Hackett, an international expert on the treponematoses, thought that nineteenth-century European commentators mistook yaws for venereal syphilis and thereby overestimated the extent of syphilis in Aboriginal communities. Yaws would have blocked the progress of syphilis, because it offers some cross-immunity to syphilis. Indeed, Northern Territory Aborigines, among whom yaws was widespread until it was eradicated by antibiotics, seem to have been almost free of syphilis until the 1960s. Hackett suggested that the distribution of treponematoses in precontact Australia resembled that in Africa in the same southern latitudes. Osteological and serological evidence pointed to the presence of endemic (nonvenereal) syphilis in Aboriginal populations in central Australia and farther south, while yaws was prevalent in the tropical, coastal areas of northern Australia. He further suggested, "The aboriginal population . . . came into Australia in several waves from the north and northwest; thus yaws coming into northern Australia from Asia may have been the precursor of endemic syphilis in the semi-arid steppes of central Australia."[39]

Reports of explorers who observed the condition of the tribes beyond the frontier in the 1830s and 1840s raise the strong possibility that Aborigines in the temperate regions of the east and southeast were, despite Hackett's claims, free of the treponematoses altogether before European settlement. In 1830 Charles Stuart reached the Murray River and followed it to its mouth in South Australia. Of the tribes on the Murray beyond the junction with the Darling River, he wrote, "Leprosy of the most loathsome description, the most violent cutaneous eruptions, and glandular affections absolutely raged through the whole of them."[40] The "leprosy" that Stuart described is unlikely to have been true Hansen's disease, which is believed not have come to Australia till the 1880s, but it may have been, to follow Hackett's argument, yaws. A recent investigator, Dowling, has proposed that the disease was not yaws but rather epidemic venereal syphilis in a virgin population. He points out that yaws is found in humid, equatorial zones of the world, not in temperate areas; that the facts that it affected all age groups and that many victims experienced nasal erosions and blindness favored his hypothesis; and that after European settlement along the Murray River, venereal syphilis became rife.

Some support for Dowling's argument comes from Hackett's later work. Hackett's point that the geographical distribution of the treponematoses in Australia resembled that in southern Africa means that yaws was the treponematosis of the northern tropical areas of Australia, while endemic (nonvenereal) syphilis was dominant in the arid central and southern central areas. The temperate southeast (and southwest), the areas of earliest European settlement, may well have been quite free of any treponematoses. Hackett himself states that venereal syphilis was spread by European explorers and colonizers from the sixteenth century to areas of the world not "committed" to yaws, endemic syphilis and pinta. Venereal syphilis, introduced by Europeans, may have virulently infected the Aborigines of the southeast and southwest of the Australian continent because they had been previously unexposed to any of the treponematoses.[41] In the companion volume to this work, covering the second half of the twentieth century, the modern history of the health of Aboriginal people, including the impact of sexually transmitted infections, will be explored extensively.

PUBLIC HEALTH IN EARLY COLONIAL AUSTRALIA

The administration of William Pitt ("the Younger") did not decide to colonize New South Wales simply to empty Britain's prisons and prison hulks of convicts. Botany Bay was considered to be an advantageous location at which to use the labor of the convicts to build a settlement that could protect Britain's strategic and commercial interests in Asia. Among its advantages was its alleged healthiness. Capt. James Cook, who had "discovered" the east coast of Australia and claimed it for Britain in 1770, said that the Aborigines there lived "in a warm and fine climate and enjoy[ed] a very wholesome air." James Matra also extolled its healthiness, telling the House of Commons' Beauchamp committee, appointed to consider the question of resuming transportation of convicts overseas, that the experience of the Cook expedition had been that the climate was "perfectly agreeable to [the] European Constitution."[42] The 1,035 men, women and children (the majority male and female convicts, the remainder civil and military staff and dependants) of the First Fleet arrived in Botany Bay in January 1788 on six transports, three store ships and two naval ships of the line. Soon after, the fleet moved to Port Jackson (Sydney), just north of Botany Bay. The physical environment of Sydney was salubrious—a well drained site never having known permanent settlement, with a surface stream, called the Tank Stream, providing an adequate flow of clean water. Nonetheless, food shortages (in fact, dependence on food transported from Britain) marked the first years; scurvy was widespread. Once better land was settled inland from the coast, enough grain was produced and cattle raised to provide a more than adequate food supply.[43]

Although free immigrants began to arrive from 1802 to augment the continuing inflow of convicts, population growth was slow for some time. By 1809, the population of NSW had risen to 10,262, about ten times the number of first arrivals, and it had increased to 44,588 by 1830. Tasmania and Western Australia, settled as outposts in 1803 and 1829, respectively, had populations of 24,279 and 1,172 in 1830. By 1850, the population of NSW had grown to 267,000, and the nonconvict part of the population had become predominant. Tasmania had grown to just below sixty-nine thousand and Western Australia to almost six thousand. The last had grown slowly as a pastoral and agricultural, free settlement, but from 1850 to 1868 convicts were transported there to meet the labor and development needs of the colonists.

Tasmania received convicts from 1804. With transportation to NSW ended in 1840, Tasmania, a separate colony from 1835, received large numbers until transportation to Australia ceased altogether in 1868. Like Tasmania and Queensland, Victoria, where European settlement began in 1835, was originally part of NSW. Except for an aborted attempt to create a convict settlement in 1803, Victoria was a free colony, slowly developing as a pastoral economy until the finding of gold dramatically increased population and prosperity. It became a separate colony in the 1850s. South Australia from the outset in 1836 was a free colony, based on the pastoral industry. It steadily grew from 546 to almost sixty-four thousand in 1850. Queensland was a penal colony from 1824 until free settlers were welcomed at the close of the 1830s. Mainly pastoral, its population expanded from 2,258 in 1846 to 8,575 in 1851. Government-subsidised immigration from the 1830s—it continued to 1885—not only accelerated population growth in NSW but changed the nature of government and politics from deferential-authoritarian to democratic-populist. About 116,000 free immigrants had arrived by 1850. The new Poor Law—and indeed, the emergence of public health as state policy in the 1830s and '40s—were responses in part to the problem of poverty and social disorder in the United Kingdom, as we have seen. Subsidized migration was another response to the "politics of destitution."[44]

Typhus was extensive in London in 1787, when the First Fleet left, and cases of typhus (or typhoid—doctors confused them till well into the nineteenth century), dysentery, and "cholera morbus" occurred on the ships en route. The first five years of European settlement, 1788–92, were years of high mortality, the rates ranging from forty-seven per thousand to 152 per thousand population. This "crisis" mortality was characteristic of premodern Europe, when plague and other epidemic disease combined with famine and war to produce towering peaks of death. In Sydney, at times, extreme food shortages prevailed, but their contribution to mortality is unclear. The settlers were unwilling to experiment with the new flora and fauna, and they scorned the bush foods of the "primitive" (but well-nourished) Aborigines. Skills in gardening, farming and fishing were in short supply, and the seeds from Britain did not do well in the infertile coastal soil. Childhood mortality was high, deaths of infants and young children fluctuating between a low rate of 170 per thousand births in 1790 and a high of 490 per thousand in 1792.

Three waves of disease swept over the new colony in these "hungry years." The first, in 1788, which affected children and adults, involved dysentery and scurvy. In 1789, as we have noted, smallpox decimated Aborigines but left the European community untouched. The second disease wave broke with the arrival of the Second Fleet in 1790, and only adults were involved. Dysentery, typhus and scurvy had ravaged three of the four ships on the way, with 26 percent of convicts dying in the course of the journey from Britain. The third wave, lasting from August 1791 to July 1792, was consequent on the arrival of the Third Fleet, which had lost 11 percent of members en route. The chief disease was dysentery, and both children and adults perished.[45]

For the remainder of the 1790s, such epidemic waves were absent. Although causes of death were not regularly recorded, it is clear that enteric infections and typhus continued to be important sources of illness and death; this reflected the lack of adequate sanitary measures at the community level. The case books of Sydney Hospital, 1808–19, show that dysentery (probably many cases were typhoid) and VD were the most prevalent diseases.[46] In the period 1819–36, dysentery was the most prevalent disease, but rheumatism, venereal disease, and "dropsy" were almost as common. In the summer, ophthalmia and erysipelas were prevalent; in the winter and early spring, simple continued fever. An epidemic of influenza hit the colony in 1820 and again in 1825; a mumps epidemic struck in 1824. Intermittent fever manifested itself for the first time in 1825, and whooping cough, which was introduced by the *Morely* (about which more below), was epidemic for the first time in 1828.[47]

Two other sources of information are available for the 1820s. Peter Miller Cunningham was a surgeon-superintendent on convict ships from 1819 to 1828 and then lived until 1830 in NSW. His 1827 account of the colony included an assessment of its health. Reflecting the significance placed at this time on climate as a determinant of health, he wrote: "The extraordinary healthiness of the climate of New South Wales must be of no trifling importance in the eyes of a European, considering how unhealthy most other countries are. . . . Dysentery is the most prevalent and fatal disease[,] . . . yet deaths . . . are exceeding rare among the sober-living portion of the community . . . and on reaching the age of puberty, phthisis is liable to supervene from the rapid sprouting out in stature. . . . [B]ut the European phthisis is . . . at least relieved, by a removal hither, if early resorted to. . . . True syphilis among the whites . . . appears to be unknown; but gonorrhea is exceedingly common."[48] In 1830, in response to an inquiry by the Royal College of Physicians, James Bowman, Inspector of Hospitals, and Donald McLeod, Deputy Inspector of Military Hospitals, listed the diseases prevalent in the colony. McLeod identified "dysenteric affections," "erysipelatous affections" and "inflammation of the eyes" as the most common, recurrent diseases. Dysentery was the "most prevalent and fatal disease[;] . . . it carries off above one-half of the convicts." It was especially severe in 1788, '90, '91 and '99, and again in 1823. "Consumption of the lungs . . . is much more frequent than from the mildness of the climate might be expected."[49] Bowman identified a similar range of diseases and thought that the high prevalence of dropsy "may be accounted for by the dissipated lives most of the prison population have led previous to their conviction."[50]

In 1830–50, the rising tide of free immigrants had profound effects on the colony's health. The incidence of infectious disease increased as shipping arrivals increased. The pool of susceptible infants and children increased as the number of young families arriving increased and from the high local birthrate. Overcrowding, lack of ventilation, dampness, and inadequate food and water supplies on immigrant ships reproduced the disease-producing conditions earlier found on convict transports. Normalization of the population-age structure, more than the incidence of epidemics, determined the mortality trends. An ever-growing mortality among infants and children was a key feature; by the 1840s infants accounted for about 29 percent of all deaths. The ubiquitous gastrointestinal infections and skin diseases dominated the everyday morbidity and mortality pattern.[51]

From the mid-1830s, the major childhood infections established themselves in Sydney and other colonial concentrations of population as contact with the outside world and immigration numbers increased. Whooping cough was present first in Sydney in 1828, prevalent in Tasmania five years later, then was taken to Western Australia by a military detachment. Henceforth it became established, being very prevalent in Sydney in 1838–39, in Tasmania in 1838 and 1842, and in Western Australia and South Australia in 1848. Victoria was touched by it soon after. The first known case of scarlet fever was in Tasmania in 1833, and the first cases in NSW and Victoria occurred in 1841. It seems to have become established in the other colonies later: South Australia by 1859; Queensland, 1858; and Western Australia, 1865. Epidemics scourged Tasmania in 1843 and 1853, with deaths occurring again in four of the five years, 1857–61. The ship *America* was quarantined in Sydney in 1829 because of measles, and the first epidemic occurred there in 1834. It was established in all the Australian colonies by the 1850s. Whether the 1789 "smallpox" epidemic (which killed so many Aborigines near Sydney) was in fact chickenpox, as Curson claims, has not been settled, but cases of chickenpox in the European-child population of Sydney were certainly recorded by 1844. Croup was first identified in Australia sometime between the late 1820s and 1840s. Diphtheria was prevalent in England in 1858, and, as Cumpston pointed out, the first appearance in Australia—in Victoria in October 1858—was consistent with introduction by English immigrants who departed England in June, when the infection was raging. At this time immigrants were pouring into gold-rich Victoria.

Thus, the common infections of childhood became established from the mid-1830s in irregular cycles of occurrence. The accumulation of susceptible persons and their aggregation in sufficient numbers produced this tendency toward cyclical epidemics. Measles, for example, introduced to Victoria in 1850, became epidemic only in 1853, by which time the population had risen from 97,000 (1851) to about 222,000 (1853). Influenza epidemics in 1836–53 in the Australian colonies were linked to pandemics and regional epidemics overseas. For the first time Australia became caught up in international epidemics. Urban growth from the 1850s produced explosive outbreaks of enteric infections. These and the irregular cycles of childhood disease helped produce the short-term fluctuations in mortality characteristic of the nineteenth-century mortality trend until the 1880s, when the modern decline in mortality began.[52]

In the early colonial period the main kinds of state intervention to control infectious diseases, as was the case in Britain and Europe more generally, were vaccination against smallpox and quarantine of ships carrying disease. Some protosanitation measures were adopted, but these were more in the nature of protection of amenities and eradication of "annoyances" or "nuisances" than real sanitary legislation aimed at improving health. Also, there was an early attempt to control food standards, in legislation to regulate bread. Capt. Watkin Tench, who published in 1793 an account of the first years of the settlement at Port Jackson (Sydney), mentions in connection with the causes of the 1789 "smallpox" epidemic that the surgeons of the First Fleet had bought with them variolous matter in bottles. But no mention of such material is made in the list of medicines for use in the new colony. Variolation involved the inoculation of smallpox matter from an infected person, whereas vaccination employed matter from the related but harmless cowpox to produce immunity against smallpox. Variolation was introduced to England in the 1720s, but its use was restricted to the children of the upper classes, of whom fewer than a thousand were inoculated in 1721–29. It was probably not employed widely until the 1740s. The safer technique of vaccination did not became available until a decade after the first settlement of NSW. In 1796, Edward Jenner successfully performed his first vaccination, and in 1798, following further experiments, he published his results. The new technique spread very quickly in Britain and on the Continent. By 1801, more than a hundred thousand children had been vaccinated in the United Kingdom.[53]

It is possible that the First Fleet surgeons used the variolous matter on Europeans or Aborigines or both, but no record exists of this happening. In 1803, Governor Philip Gidley King requested the Secretary of State for the Colonies to have vaccine matter forwarded; in May 1804 a supply arrived from the recently established Royal Jennerian Society. Children were immediately vaccinated. By January 1806, more than a thousand persons in a population of seven thousand had been vaccinated. Vaccine supplies were sent for vaccination of children on Norfolk Island, a secondary penal station, and in Tasmania.[54]

The rapid spread of vaccination in Britain and the rest of Europe resulted from governments' eager embrace of the first, population-based, effective measure for control of a major infectious threat. On the Continent, still-surviving mercantilist ideas about promotion of population growth as a military and fiscal resource were an additional impetus. Vaccination in England and Wales passed through a number of phases in the nineteenth century: 1808–40, partial state provision; 1840–53, universal state provision but without compulsion; 1853–71, compulsion; 1871–83, consummation; and 1883–1907, gradual breakdown of the system as smallpox disappeared.[55] According to Cumpston, in New South Wales in the period to 1850 the colonial surgeons were markedly successful in persuading people to allow themselves and their children to be vaccinated, but as long as the person-to-person method was used, there were occasions when the virus became inactive and fresh vaccine matter had to be imported. At the Moreton Bay (Queensland) penal colony, efforts were made to ensure vaccinations were carried out. In 1841, David Ballow, a colonial surgeon, was instructed by his superiors in Sydney to maintain a supply of vaccine matter and to work at persuading parents to allow their children to receive free vaccination at the colonial hospital.[56] In South Australia, promotion of free vaccination began soon after the colony was established. In 1839, Governor George Gawler instructed the colonial surgeon to "perform vaccination gratuitously for the Emigrants every Tuesday . . . with pure vaccine lymph obtained in the Colony," and every Wednesday to do the same for "the Native Inhabitants at the Native huts on the Torrens."[57] In Western Australia, the colonial surgeon mentioned in a letter of early 1840 to the Secretary of State for the Colonies that despite earlier failures, vaccination was now effectively being carried out in the colony.[58] Because of distance from endemic foci of smallpox, Australia in the nineteenth century came to rely more on quarantine than on vaccination for protection from infection.

The use of quarantine to prevent infectious disease from entering the country had been long practiced in Britain. It was very early employed in the colony of NSW, although at first on an ad hoc basis using temporary locations in Sydney's large harbor. Governor King, responding to illness on convict transports in 1800 and 1802, instituted in the latter year a system of medical inspection of recently arrived ships. In May 1804, the first quarantine regulation was proclaimed after information about "an infectious Distemper [yellow fever] then raging in the State of New York" reached the colony. In 1805 the whaler *Richard and Mary*, with crew members "infected with a dangerous fever," became the first ship to be quarantined officially. The next quarantine was not till March 1828, when the convict vessel *Morely* brought whooping cough into the colony after failing to notify authorities of illness on board. Among those who died was Governor Darling's son. In July, the *Bussorah Merchant* arrived with smallpox, and again there was contact with shore before the fact was made known. In August, Governor Darling ordered that arriving vessels (except coastal boats and those from Tasmania) were to anchor well away from shore until the harbormaster permitted communication with the town. Hitherto, the legality of quarantine had flowed from the extensive legislative and executive powers vested in the governor—*quod gubernatori placet, legis habet vigorem* (the governor's pleasure has the force of law). But by the early 1830s, the influx of free immigrants was increasing notably—thirty-four ships from Britain and Ireland in 1831, and eighty-three in 1832. A profitable export trade in wool, tallow and whale oil was developing; more and more challenges to quarantine (because of the prospect of lost time) might be expected. Moreover, there was much concern about Asiatic cholera. In 1831, a cholera epidemic had reach Britain from India and from there North America on overcrowded immigrant vessels. In 1832, Governor Sir Richard Bourke, aware of these facts and the fact that cholera had broken out on a convict vessel en route to Sydney, had enacted, after consultation with his Legislative Council, the first Quarantine Act. Based on the British Act of 1825, it required any ship coming from a port where cholera or any disease "highly dangerous to the health of His Majesty's subjects in the Colony of New South Wales" had been proclaimed prevalent to perform quarantine. A dispatch from the Secretary of State for Colonies arrived soon after, enclosing the London-based Central Board of Health's arguments against quarantine. The Secretary of State himself, however, while recognizing the failure of quarantine to stop the entry of cholera to Britain, appreciated the commercial reasons for applying quarantine and accepted the colony's decision to use quarantine, except that British ships were not to be unnecessarily restricted. He preferred "to err on the side of caution from deference to popular feelings, than on that of temerity from respect to any Scientific authorities, however eminent."

The harbor's North Head, which had been occupied by dispossessed Aborigines, was chosen as the site for a quarantine station, and by 1838 work on a permanent station was complete. In 1828–1984, about 580 ships (and in excess of thirteen thousand people) were quarantined in the station's Spring Cove.[59] The 1832 act was amended in 1841 to provide for health officers at Port Jackson (Sydney) and Port Phillip (Melbourne), and further amended in 1849 to allow police magistrates at other ports to act as health officers. The health officer had power to order quarantine of any ship that had been infected or had called at an infected port and represented a reasonable "danger." Governor Sir John Franklin of Tasmania had passed a Quarantine Act in 1838, when it was realized no legal power existed to keep passengers isolated, because there was no quarantine law—the master of a quarantined ship extracted large compensation in demurrage. But the British Superintendent General of Quarantine argued that since plague was no threat to Tasmania and quarantine of vessels did not prohibit entry of cholera and smallpox, he would recommend only medical inspection of all vessels by a health officer and, where disease existed, removal of people, clothing and bedding to a hulk or shore station. The 1838 act was refused royal assent, but a further act two years later was allowed.

The first ship to be quarantined in Victoria was the *Glen Huntly,* in 1840. Lieutenant Governor Charles La Trobe notified the colonists of Port Phillip that "the 'Glen Huntly,' Government Emigrant Ship from Greenock, is declared under quarantine and that infringement of the quarantine Laws and regulations will subject the offending parties to the pains and penalties of the same." The independent colony of Victoria passed its own Quarantine Act in 1865. With free immigration to Moreton Bay (Queensland) increasing in the 1840s, a quarantine station was proclaimed at Dunwich in 1849, the northern section of Stradbroke Island having been gazetted as a site for quarantine. Quarantine work was normally not demanding, but one of the first health officers, David Ballow, died from typhus contracted in the course of his duties. Queensland, independent of its mother colony, NSW, from 1859, passed its own act in 1863. South Australia passed a Quarantine Act in 1850, but it was over two decades before the traditional method of isolating an infected vessel there was replaced by a special quarantine station. In 1876 the *Fitzjames,* which first came to Australia in 1854 as an immigrant ship, was brought from Melbourne as a hulk and, after refitting, anchored in Largs Bay; no longer would the colonial government face the risk of costly compensation for ships delayed by quarantine. In the early 1880s, the Torrens Island quarantine station was established. In Western Australia, the first Quarantine Act was passed very early—in 1833—only a year after the Legislative Council (the governor and four unelected senior officials) came into being. Further acts were passed in the 1840s, '50s, '60s and '80s. Reliance there on quarantine to protect the public health is clear from the response of the colonial surgeon, James Crichton, to a report of epidemic typhus in Hobart and its likely introduction to the Swan River colony by troops from Hobart. Crichton proposed strict application of quarantine so that absolutely no ship-to-shore contact would take place until precautions were in place.[60]

In the first years of settlement in Australia, there were scattered instances of official concern with what, from a modern viewpoint, would be seen as public health matters. Governor Arthur Phillip, reviewing the plans of Sydney and concerned to avoid overcrowding, insisted that no more than one house be built on an allotment. He also wished to promote ventilation; "Streets [were to be] laid out in such a manner as to afford a free [circulation of] air."[61] In the 1790s, orders were promulgated to protect the Tank Stream from being fouled by hogs or by human access at unauthorized points. In 1803, anyone found to have polluted the stream was made liable to a year in prison at hard labor. By the mid-1820s, the need for a clean and adequate water supply had become pressing. An official report pointed out that Sydney relied on tanks, private wells, and swamps and lagoons but that "the water is so contaminated by impurities from the streets and other sources, as to be unfit for almost every other purpose."[62] John Busby, specially brought out from England, completed in 1837 a tunnel from the Lachlan Swamp (now Centennial Park) to Hyde Park in the town. Mains were laid down to the harbor at Circular Quay, and public fountains were installed. Not only, however, did the supply prove inadequate, but the mains were built of lead, which presented a health threat to those using the service.[63]

The beginnings of a system of vital statistics registration can be seen in the requirements of an 1825 act that obliged all clergy to register every baptism, burial and marriage and forward a copy of each registration to the registrar of the Archdeacon's Court. In 1828, an act required each householder to state the name, age and "condition" of each person resident in his house at a designated time, and so was initiated the practice of census taking. An act "for abating the Nuisance occasioned by the great number of dogs which are loose in the streets of Sydney" of 1830 represented the first time the term "nuisance" was employed in legislation, although it had here the meaning of "obstruction" or "annoyance" rather than the later public health sense of a threat to the health of the community. In the 1830s and early '40s, other acts were passed that had varying implications for community health: in 1830, cattle slaughtering was regulated (though the act was mainly concerned with identifying stolen cattle); in 1833, it was made an offence to deposit filth in the tunnel that carried Sydney's water supply; in 1834, a range of measures was enacted concerning disposal of rubbish, offal, and cleansing of slaughterhouses and private hog styes; in the same year, it was required that slaughterhouses be located near natural water supplies, like creeks, for cleansing purposes; in 1837, buildings "so irregularly built as to become a common nuisance" could be demolished; in 1838, requirements were established concerning the ingredients, quality and weight of bread put up for sale; in 1839, an inspector was appointed to confiscate unwholesome provisions in market situations; in 1842, a Sydney city council was created with powers to build sewers, force owners of manufacturing and slaughtering establishments, and of privies, to cleanse them, and to regulate butchers' shops, all "with a view to promote the health and comfort of the inhabitants of the city." An act of 1850 on the sewerage and drainage of Sydney contained three new public health conceptions: of a "public nuisance" as something threatening or likely to injure community health; of the doctor as an agent or guardian of community health (two doctors might certify that the condition of a house was such that the health of any person was at risk—a provision taken from the 1848 English Public Health Act); and of factories (for the first time) as establishments with responsibilities for the health of their employees—they were to provide adequate numbers of water closets.[64]

In the following chapter we will trace the development of public health beyond these early attempts to protect the health of the Australian colonists, to the creation of classical public health administrations in the second half of the nineteenth century.

NOTES

1. F. Fenner, "Infectious Disease and Social Change," *Medical Journal of Australia* 1 (1971), 1099–1102; S.J. Kunitz, "Medicine, Mortality and Morbidity," in *Companion Encyclopedia of the History of Medicine,* Vol. 2, eds. W.F. Bynum and R. Porter (London: Routledge, 1993), 1694–95; J. Diamond, *Guns, Germs and Steel: A Short History of Everybody for the Last 13,000 Years* (London: Jonathan Cape, 1997), 205–207.

2. S.J. Kunitz, "Medicine, Mortality and Morbidity," 1695–97.

3. D. Joralemon, "New World Depopulation and the Case of Disease," *Journal of Anthropological Research* 37 (1981), 112.

4. Diamond, *Guns, Germs and Steel,* 210; G.B. Risse, "Medicine in New Spain," in *Medicine in the New World: New Spain, New France, and New England,* ed. R.L. Numbers (Knoxville: University of Tennessee Press, 1987), 27–28.

5. Diamond, *Guns, Germs and Steel,* 210–11.

6. T. Gelfand, "Medicine in New France," in *Medicine in the New World,* ed. Numbers, 77.

7. D.R. Hopkins, *Princes and Peasants: Smallpox in History* (Chicago: University of Chicago Press, 1983), 245.

8. Quoted in J. Duffy, "Smallpox and the Indians in the American Colonies," *Bulletin of History of Medicine* (1951), 326.

9. Quoted in ibid., 326.

10. Quoted in ibid., 327.

11. Quoted in ibid., 328.

12. Quoted in ibid., 329.

13. Ibid., 330.

14. Quoted in ibid., 335.

15. Ibid., 332–41; Hopkins, *Princes and Peasants,* 270–71.

16. Quoted in A.G. Carmichael, "Measles: The Red Menace," in *Plague, Pox and Pestilence,* ed. K.F. Kiple (London: Weidenfeld and Nicolson, 1997), 83.

17. Diamond, *Guns, Germs and Steel,* 214.

18. J.B. Tuke, "Medical Notes on New Zealand," *Edinburgh Medical Journal* 9 (1863–64), 221, 227.

19. R. Lange, "Plagues and Pestilence in Polynesia: The Nineteenth-Century Cook Islands Experience," *Bulletin of History of Medicine* 58 (1984), 326–46.

20. S.J. Kunitz, *Disease and Social Diversity: The European Impact on the Health of Non-Europeans* (New York: Oxford University Press, 1994), 12.

21. Diamond, *Guns, Germs and Steel,* 308–11.

22. E.J. Beck, *The Enigma of Aboriginal Health. Interaction between Biological, Social and Economic Factors in Alice Spring Town-Camps* (Canberra: Australian Institute of Aboriginal Studies, 1985), 6.

23. L.R. Smith, *The Aboriginal Population of Australia* (Canberra: Australian National University [hereafter ANU] Press, 1980), 68–69; J.P. White and D.J. Mulvaney, "How Many People?" in *Australians to 1788* (Broadway, Australia: Fairfax, Syme and Weldon Associates, 1987), 117.

24. *Population and Australia: A Demographic Analysis and Projection. First Report of the National Population Inquiry* (Canberra: Australian Government Publishing Service [hereafter AGPS], 1975), vol. 2, 479–81; Smith, *The Aboriginal Population of Australia,* 226–29.

25. Ibid., 227–28.

26. Quoted in W.E.H. Stanner, "The History of Indifference Thus Begins," *Aboriginal History* 1(1) (1977), 3.

27. Ibid., 3–25.

28. See M. Lewis, *A Rum State: Alcohol and State Policy in Australia* (Canberra: AGPS, 1992), 153–54; D.E. Barwick, "Changes in the Aboriginal Population of Victoria, 1863–1966," in *Aboriginal Man and Environment in Australia,* eds. D.J. Mulvaney and J. Golson (Canberra: ANU Press, 1971), 288.

29. Barwick, "Changes in the Aboriginal Population of Victoria, 1863–1966," 289–91; and see Lewis, *A Rum State,* 154.

30. Lewis, *A Rum State,* 154–55.

31. C.D. Rowley, *The Destruction of Aboriginal Society: Aboriginal Policy and Practice* (Canberra: ANU Press, 1970), 227.

32. See M. Lewis, *Thorns on the Rose: The History of Sexually Transmitted Diseases in Australia in International Perspective* (Canberra: AGPS, 1998), 354, 379–81.

33. N.B. Butlin, *Our Original Aggression: Aboriginal Populations of Southeastern Australia, 1788–1850* (Sydney: George Allen and Unwin, 1983), 175–76.

34. D. Collins, *An Account of the English Colony in New South Wales,* ed. B.H. Fletcher (originally published 1798; repr. Sydney: A.H. and A.W. Reed, 1975), vol. 1, 496.

35. Butlin, *Our Original Aggression,* 41.

36. Collins, *An Account of the English Colony in New South Wales,* vol. 1, 495–96.

37. Butlin, *Our Original Aggression,* 40, 78–79.

38. A. Gray, "Some Myths in the Demography of Aboriginal Australians," *Journal of Australian Population Association* 2 (1985), 138–39.

39. C.J. Hackett, "On the Origin of the Human Treponematoses," *Bulletin WHO* 29 (1963), 16–17.

40. Quoted in J.B. Cleland, "Disease amongst the Australian Aborigines," *Journal of Tropical Medicine and Hygiene* 31(12) (1928), 141.

41. See Lewis, *Thorns on the Rose,* 357–59.

42. Quoted in A. Frost, "Towards Australia: the Coming of the Europeans 1400 to 1788," in *Australians to 1788,* ed. White and Mulvaney, 395.

43. J.H.L. Cumpston, *Health and Disease in Australia: A History,* ed. M.J. Lewis (Canberra: AGPS, 1989), 37.

44. Cumpston, *Health and Disease in Australia,* 37–39, 52; D. Coward, *Out of Sight: Sydney's Environmental History 1851–1981* (Canberra: Department of Economic History, Research School of Social Sciences, Australian National University, 1988), 9.

45. B. Gandevia and J. Cobley, "Mortality at Sydney Cove, 1788–1792," *Australian and New Zealand Journal of Medicine* 4 (1974), 111–25; B. Gandevia and S. Gandevia, "Childhood Mortality and Its Social Background in the First Settlement at Sydney Cove, 1788–1792," *Australian Paediatric Journal* 11 (1975), 13; R. Taylor, M. Lewis and J. Powles, "The Australian Mortality Decline: All-Cause Mortality 1788–1990," *Australian and New Zealand Journal of Public Health* 22(1) (1998), 31; B. Wood, "Food and Alcohol in Australia. An Historical Overview: 1788–1938," in *Food Habits in Australia,* ed. A.S. Truswell and M.L. Wahlquist (North Balwyn, Australia: R. Gordon, 1988), 163; Cumpston, *Health and Disease in Australia,* 39–40.

46. Cumpston, *Health and Disease in Australia,* 41–42.

47. J.F. Watson, *The History of the Sydney Hospital from 1811 to 1911* (Sydney: Government Printer, 1911), 65.

48. Quoted in Cumpston, *Health and Disease in Australia,* 43.

49. *Historical Records of Australia,* series 1, vol. 15, 371–78; Cumpston, *Health and Disease in Australia,* 42.

50. Quoted in M. O'Connor, "A Socio-Historical Study of Health and Medical Care in New South Wales from 1788 to 1850" (Ph.D. dissertation, University of Queensland, Brisbane, 1991), 82.

51. Ibid., 83–84.

52. Taylor, Lewis and Powles, "The Australian Mortality Decline," 31; Cumpston, *Health and Disease in Australia,* 56–57, 306–307, 292–93, 300–301; P.H. Curson,

Times of Crisis: Epidemics in Sydney 1788–1900 (Sydney: Sydney University Press, 1985), 52–53.

53. A.J. Mercer, "Smallpox and Epidemiological-Demographic Change in Europe: The Role of Vaccination," *Population Studies* 39 (1985), 287; C. Huerkamp, "The History of Smallpox Vaccination in Germany: A First Step in the Medicalization of the General Public," *Journal of Contemporary History* 20(4) (1985), 619–20; O'Connor, "A Socio-Historical Study of Health and Medical Care in New South Wales from 1788 to 1850," 134–38.

54. O'Connor, "A Socio-Historical Study of Health and Medical Care in New South Wales from 1788 to 1850," 138; Cumpston, *Health and Disease in Australia,* 43.

55. R.J. Lambert, "A Victorian National Health Service: State Vaccination 1855–71," *The Historical Journal* 5(1) (1962), 1.

56. Cumpston, *Health and Disease in Australia,* 34.

57. Quoted in P. Woodruff, *Two Million South Australians* (Kent Town, Australia: Peacock Publications, 1984), 15–16.

58. D. Snow, *The Progress of Public Health in Western Australia 1829–1977* (Perth: University of Western Australia Press, 1981), 12.

59. J.D. Foley, *In Quarantine: A History of Sydney's Quarantine Station 1828–1984* (Kenthurst, Australia: Kangaroo Press, 1995), 10–11, 17–37; Cumpston, *Health and Disease in Australia,* 44.

60. Cumpston, *Health and Disease in Australia,* 408–409; C.R. Wiburd, "Notes on the History of Maritime Quarantine in Queensland, 19th Century," *Journal of Historical Society of Queensland* 3(5) (1945), 373; R. Patrick, *A History of Health and Medicine in Queensland* (St. Lucia, Australia: University of Queensland Press, 1987), 35; Woodruff, *Two Million South Australians,* 17; Snow, *The Progress of Public Health in Western Australia 1829–1977,* 12.

61. O'Connor, "A Socio-Historical Study of Health and Medical Care in New South Wales from 1788 to 1850," 52.

62. Quoted in Cumpston, *Health and Disease in Australia,* 43–44.

63. D. Clark, "'Worse than Physic': Sydney's Water Supply 1788–1888," in *Nineteenth-Century Sydney: Essays in Urban History* (Sydney: Sydney University Press, 1978), 55.

64. Cumpston, *Health and Disease in Australia,* 382–83.

Chapter 3

The Sanitary Revolution: Public Health, 1850–1900

THE MODERN DECLINE OF MORTALITY IN EUROPE, THE UNITED STATES AND AUSTRALASIA

By the eighteenth century, peaks of crisis mortality resulting from periodic epidemics of plague, smallpox and typhus were disappearing from Europe. Endemic infections, now comparatively more significant, slowed the mortality decline, and the decline did not became marked again until the later nineteenth century, when falls in mortality from, especially, diarrheal disease and tuberculosis produced gains in life expectancy, particularly for younger age groups.

The most influential recent work on the modern decline of mortality in Europe has been that of Thomas McKeown and colleagues. Concerned to show that mortality decline rather than fertility promoted the significant population growth that occurred in England and Wales from the eighteenth century, he was also eager to explain the causes of the mortality decline in the nineteenth century, which led to our contemporary low levels of mortality. Relying on the returns for death after the introduction of civil registration in 1837, he found that the average annual crude death rate per thousand population was 22.2 in the 1850s; 22.4 in the 1860s; 21.3 in the 1870s; 19.1 in the 1880s; and 18.2 in the 1890s. Standardized to the age and sex distribution of the 1901 population, the average death rate declined from 21.2 per thousand in the 1850s to 18.1 per thousand in the 1890s. Apart from the period of World War II, both male and female mortality continued to fall in 1901–71.The standardized death rate fell for males and females in 1901 from 18.1 and 15.8 per thousand, respectively, to 6.4 and 4.4 in 1971. About 75 percent of the reduction related to infectious disease, and the rest was from "conditions not attributable to micro-organisms." Diseases due to airborne pathogens (particularly tuberculosis) accounted for a considerable part of the decline in the nineteenth and twentieth centuries; diseases associated with water and food-borne pathogens were the next most significant contributors to the decline. Using argument by exclusion, McKeown pointed out that medicine would not have offered much; except for smallpox and diphtheria, most significant diseases were declining prior to the advent of effective therapy. Similarly, public health, although a more important contributor to the decline than clinical medicine, was not in his view effective until the late nineteenth century. Because airborne infections were the source of the bulk of mortality decline, he argued that attenuation of the virulence of pathogens and a reduction in exposure to infection accounted for little of the decline in infections. It followed that it was better host resistance, arising from improved nutrition, that was the major mechanism in reducing mortality.[1]

In 1962, McKeown and R.G. Record summarized their position on the mortality decline in nineteenth century England and Wales: "In order of their relative importance the influences responsible for the decline . . . in the second half of the nineteenth century were (a) a rising standard of living, of which the most significant feature was improved diet (responsible mainly for the decline in tuberculosis and less certainly, and to a lesser extent, of typhus); (b) the hygienic changes introduced by the sanitary reformers (responsible for the decline of the typhus-typhoid and cholera groups); and (c) a favourable trend in the relationship between infectious agent and the human host (which accounted for the decline . . . from scarlet fever and may have contributed to that from tuberculosis, typhus and cholera). . . . [T]herapy . . . had only a trivial effect on the total reduction of the death-rate."[2]

The powerful McKeown thesis generated much controversy about the causes of the decline and, more recently, much Europe-wide research to see if his England (and Wales) pattern is true for other Western European countries. Moreover, many have questioned whether a secular mortality decline occurred in England and Wales itself from the eighteenth century. In 1740–1820, life expectancy increased markedly (life expectancy at birth increased from 31.7 to 39.2 years), but it remained static in the middle part of the nineteenth century; a secular decline took place only from around 1870. England shared this experience of increased life expectancy from the eighteenth century with Sweden, Denmark, Norway and France, but national mortality trends began to differ between 1820 and 1830. In Scandinavia, mortality continued to decline, although in central and other parts of northern Europe it remained more or less static until 1870, when the modern health transition got under way. But the transition was delayed in Mediterranean countries. In Italy, mortality did not begin to decline notably until the 1880s; life expectancy at birth rose from thirty-three to thirty-eight years in 1881–91.[3]

If McKeown's picture of a continuous decline in mortality from the eighteenth century no longer holds up, even for England, his emphasis on nutritional improvement as the prime cause of the decline still has weight, although it is subject to much criticism. From a European perspective, the emergence in the eighteenth and early nineteenth centuries of national grain markets smoothed the fluctuations in supply and differences in distribution, but McKeown supposed nutrition and living standards were improving before 1850—when living standards may have in fact been worsening, or at best stagnating. For England, stagnation in living standards prevailed to the 1820s, after which real wages increased. But since it seems very unlikely that public health measures were significant in Europe until at least the second half of the nineteenth century, we are left with no explanation of the first part of the modern decline, other than to see it as the last phase of the period of premodern fluctuations in mortality.

The question of primacy of cause aside, both nutrition and public health are clearly involved in any explanation. But then, a range of other factors are directly or indirectly connected with them: living and working conditions, urbanization, education, aetiology of diseases, doctors and medical knowledge, mothers' attitudes, knowledge and behavior, infant rearing, politics and reformers, and climate. For infants and children, poor nutritional status may result from the fact that the disease environment is so closely connected with sanitation and personal hygiene habits. Low body weight makes a child more likely to succumb to recurrent diarrheal disease, and the latter in turn reduces growth and capacity to resist infection. For the population generally, the diseases that retreated in the nineteenth century—diphtheria, whooping cough, scarlet fever, tuberculosis and cholera—are to a greater or lesser extent related to nutrition, because resistance is poorer in the poorly fed. Equally, exposure is affected by public health and sanitary action—most obviously in the case of water-borne infections, but even tuberculosis and other airborne diseases are influenced by housing, hygienic standards and isolation of patients. The problem is assigning weights to different causal factors.[4]

The most telling criticism of McKeown's relative weighting of nutrition and public health has come from Simon Szreter. First, Szreter shows that McKeown's epidemiological history is unreliable, and he argues, contrary to McKeown, that respiratory tuberculosis improvement was not "the chronologically prior or the quantitatively predominant feature" of the nineteenth-century decline in mortality. Tuberculosis deaths were the end product of a disease burden resulting from the primary impact of other infectious and sanitary diseases. The first threats to life were, as William Farr noted, "convulsions" and "teething" (both frequently related to diarrheal disease), diarrheal disease, "typhus" (prior to 1860s typhus was not differentiated from typhoid), smallpox, measles and bronchitis. The last was often the result of the frequent urban outbreaks of measles and influenza. Second, in the growing cities, "the relative insalubrity" had greater influence on the national death rate than did increasing real wages or the more abundant food supply, and these cities, lacking social overhead capital for health preservation, needed a new social and political response to their health problems. The 1830s to 1875 are seen as the years when that response was made—years of activism in public health legislation and other activities, ending when the central government allowed its Local Government Board's subordination of public health interventionism to the conservatism of an administration heavily drawn from the Poor Law Board. The years from 1875 to 1900 are seen as years of budgetary constraint and limited activism. There appears, then, to be no fit between the period of activism in public health to 1875 and the period from the 1870s, when infectious disease mortality declined; the impact of public health on the decline is thus minimized.

But, as Szreter emphasises, this is to ignore the extent of municipal sanitation and local activism in the last three decades of the century. Public health then becomes a major influence reducing mortality. A pure water supply was put in place as urban local authorities came to run local waterworks—415 urban local authorities in 1879, but more than 66 percent of 1,138 urban authorities in 1905. The urban food supply was increasingly regulated as local authorities monitored adulterated and defective foods (especially meat and milk). Sanitary facilities and services were increasingly provided by local authorities. A good barometer is the increase in central government loans for such purposes—from eleven million pounds in 1858–70 to eighty-four million in 1871–97. The decline in mortality from the 1870s can thus be attributed to these achievements of "the politically and ideologically negotiated movement for public health" more than to any other factor.[5]

While the general death rate declined from the 1870s, the infant mortality rate remained substantial. But around 1900 it fell notably, dropping to 110 per thousand births by 1910–12 and eighty per thousand ten years later. The problem before 1900 was diarrheal diseases, spread mainly by contamination of food. They were a major contributor to infant mortality but fell much less rapidly than the enteric diseases, which were spread mainly by water at this time. The municipal sanitary movement could bring down the latter, but pure water, paved streets, garbage disposal and mains sewerage did not compensate for poor hygiene in food preparation in overcrowded working-class houses. Changes began to occur in the first decade of this century. Housing quantity and quality increased as stricter standards of design and hygiene were enforced, and philanthropic and municipal housing and town-planning activities expanded. Local infant and maternity services increased. There were few clinics until after World War I, but health visiting spread widely in England, and midwives and health visitors became an integral part of local health services. The 1907 Notification of Births Acts (compulsory for local authorities from 1913) enabled speedy contact with mothers after births. Greater regulation of urban milk supplies was important, but its effect was limited by unhygienic domestic conditions in preparation of milk for infant feeding, with the result that better housing and hygiene education were more fundamental factors in the decline of infant mortality. McKeown's greater nutritional intake does not promote infant health if it is both inappropriate in type and covered in pathogens. As Szreter points out, once the public health movement had occupied the territory of the urban environment outside the home, the working-class domestic environment became the "last frontier" for traditional public health. Better "living standards cease to have the leading role as historical guarantor of the nation's mortality decline[, and] . . . purposive human agency is returned to centre stage in this account of the mortality decline."[6]

Incomplete death registration bedevils attempts to talk about national mortality trends in the United States in the nineteenth century. Indeed, mortality statistics for the country as a whole are not easily computed before 1933. By 1900, the death registration area comprised only ten states, the District of Columbia and a number of cities in nonregistration states. It included 40.5 percent of the population of continental United States; the population covered was predominantly urban and white. But from the eighteenth to the middle years of the nineteenth century, it seems, urban death rates were greater than rural ones. Commonly cited causes of death in some rural areas were "consumption" (tuberculosis) and "dysentery" (diarrheal disease or typhoid). In contrast, in Boston in this period, epidemics of smallpox, measles and diphtheria occurred.[7] While historians have been in agreement that mortality declined in the late nineteenth century, they do not agree about the timing. Some claim there was a steady decline from midcentury. Others see little decline until 1880, after which it was rapid. Some explain the decline in mortality as due to better nutrition; others, to better living standards; yet others, to the sanitary movement, or to genetically based changes in people or pathogens. Robert Higgs, drawing on earlier work by Frederick L. Hoffman, examined the mortality experience of eighteen large American cities in 1871–1900. These cities had 10 percent of the total (and 42 percent of the urban) population in 1870, and in 1900 14 percent and 34 percent, respectively. The prevailing pattern of mortality for most of the cities was fluctuation around a declining trend, with a high peak in the early 1870s, another high peak in the early 1880s, a moderate peak in the early 1890s, a steady fall to the late 1890s and a slight rebound to 1900. The greatest declines in percentage terms were in Minneapolis, Milwaukee, Pittsburgh and Chicago. The average decline was about 25 percent (see table 3.1).

Higgs examines and rejects a changing age-gender-race structure of the population as the generally applicable cause of the decline. Public health measures as (collectively) an alternate explanation of the decline do not fit the timing of changes in the death rate or the shape of the trend line. Only from the 1880s were public health measures being implemented in the large cities, and these steadily increased to the 1920s, by which time all enjoyed proper sewerage and water supply systems, effective quarantine, well-enforced

Table 3.1
Crude Death Rate, U.S. Cities, 1870–1900

City	1870	1900	Percentage Reduction
New York	30.3	22.1	27.1
Brooklyn	25.6	20.9	18.2
Chicago	24.2	15.1	37.7
Philadelphia	23.7	19.8	16.6
St. Louis	22.0	17.6	19.9
Boston	25.3	21.6	14.6
Baltimore (whites)	25.3	17.5	30.9
Baltimore (blacks)	36.8	29.8	19.0
San Francisco	21.8	19.6	10.1
Cincinnati	24.2	18.1	25.2
Pittsburgh	28.0	16.5	40.9
New Orleans (whites)	29.4	22.1	24.9
New Orleans (black)	43.3	36.6	15.4
Milwaukee	24.5	14.0	42.7
Newark	29.2	19.7	32.5
Minneapolis	23.3	11.0	52.7
Providence	19.5	20.0	–2.6
Toledo	17.5	13.8	20.9
Worcester	23.4	15.9	32.0
Fall River	26.4	21.3	19.2

Source: R. Higgs, "Cycles and Trends of Mortality in 18 Large American Cities, 1871–1900," *Explorations in Economic History* 16 (1979): 394.

building codes and adequate vaccination programs. Even so, public health as a causal factor cannot be dismissed; if not predominant, it was influential. Another significant influence was a rising living standard, in which better housing and nutrition were particularly important. Consumption of goods per capita increased more than twice as quickly in the 1870s as in the 1880s and 1890s. Improving living standards, then, were pulling down the death rate in cities before the implementation of effective public health measures. Improved living standards, in conjunction with public health programs, were the key factors behind the downward tend in urban mortality in 1870–1900.[8]

In their study of age and cause-specific mortality in Philadelphia for the period 1870–1930, G.A. Condran and R.A. Cheney conclude that no single factor can explain the mortality decline in that city or, a fortiori, in the country as a whole. Rising per capita incomes, public health developments, more effective medical care and changes in disease virulence were coexisting and interconnected causes of the decline. Thus, higher incomes may well have improved health not only by increasing personal purchases of goods, like better food, but by increasing tax revenue available for public spending on health. Further, some developments—like changes in food inspection, quarantine procedures and other public health measures, which increased the quantum of community health per tax dollar spent—would have influenced mortality rates.[9]

Urban death rates remained higher than rural rates for some time after the mortality decline began in the United States (and in the United Kingdom and Australia). In the fifty years from 1870, the rural population of America—the large majority of the American people—also enjoyed mortality decline. There was a fall of about one-third in the crude death rate. This was historically unprecedented, and it is very probable that rural mortality in the mid-nineteenth century was significantly lower than a century before. Changes in the age and gender structure of the population were not factors in the decline. Also, before 1920, medical therapy contributed almost nothing; neither the diphtheria nor the typhoid antitoxin, developed in the 1890s, was very effective. In any case, rural areas were chronically short of doctors. Public health developments like cleaner water, pasteurized milk and safe sewage disposal occurred almost wholly in urban areas. Further, as late as 1920 only forty-three counties had full-time county health units; public health progress can have contributed little to the rural mortality transition. Changes in the virulence of diphtheria and scarlet fever, which according to McKeown occurred in Britain in this era, probably contributed only in a small way to the decline. They accounted for about 6 percent of deaths in Massachusetts in 1876–95 and for fewer than 2 percent in the rural population of the registration states in 1900; only 5 percent in the overall decline of 30 percent in the general death rate for 1870–1920 can be explained by this factor.

It seems very likely that to a large extent rising incomes produced the mortality decline. Net farm output per person rose by more than 50 percent in 1869–1919. The connection between higher incomes and better health would have been better housing and nutrition. With the ending of frontier conditions, better housing would have protected people more effectively against winter cold and so helped reduce influenza and pneumonia mortality. More spacious houses would have reduced the chances of domestic spread of diphtheria and tuberculosis. Better and more varied diet was made possible by the railroad and its refrigerator cars. Fresh meat, fruit, vegetables and dairy products were available nationwide by 1900. G.K. Holmes told the Industrial Commission in 1899, "The farmer's table is better[;] . . . his food is more varied and more of it is bought by him and less of it raised on his farm."[10]

New Zealand's death rates in the last three decades of the nineteenth century compare well with those in Britain. The mortality experience of the European population of New Zealand resembles in many ways that of European Australia, except that New Zealand, being located in more southern latitudes, was free of tropical diseases. With no excessive poverty and no very large cities, New Zealand had a mortality experience in the nineteenth century less harsh than that of Europe. The history of infectious diseases was shaped, like that of Australia, very much by the fact of isolation from Europe and Asia and by small overall population size. The comparative healthiness of New Zealand is reflected in its infant mortality rate, perhaps the best in the nineteenth-century world. From 110 per thousand births in 1871–75, it declined (except for a slight increase in 1891–95) to eighty in 1896–1900. It continued to decline in the first four decades of this century. The Australian rate was 118 in 1871–75, rose to 125 in 1881–85 and then (except for a small increase in 1896–1900) entered on a steady decline. In contrast, the infant death rate in England and Wales stayed reasonably steady around 153 per thousand births during the second half of the nineteenth century. But cities like London, Manchester, Liverpool and Birmingham suffered rates as high as two hundred in the 1890s.

New Zealand cities, like cities elsewhere in the Western world, in this period were more unhealthy than the countryside. The unhealthiest of the four main cities in the 1870s was Christchurch, with an infant mortality rate of 184 per thousand births. Over the next three decades or so, the mortality picture in Christchurch improved markedly. By 1911, the crude death rate of Christchurch city and adjacent boroughs had fallen by almost two-thirds, to 10.4 per thousand. By 1910, "zymotic" (infectious) disease mortality had declined to 4.4 percent of all mortality (30.3 percent in 1875) and respiratory mortality was steady at about 10 percent, while heart disease and cancer mortality accounted for 25 percent. From 1873 Canterbury (the province in which Christchurch is situated) had a central board of health. Unable to get the City Council to cooperate, however, the board limited its activities to quarantine. From 1876 to 1887, Christchurch itself had a health board and full-time medical officer of health, but from 1887 to the turn of the century council parsimony meant the city was without a board or medical officer. The notable mortality decline in the years 1875–80 (30.4 to 17.8 per thousand) took place before the sewers were completed (their construction began in 1878).

The continued decline from 1885, then, took place in the absence of a board or medical officer of health. McKeown's rising standard of living rather than sanitary measures seems the better explanation of the decline. But to accept it would be to ignore the sharp fall in zymotic-disease mortality related to the medical officer of health's and the local authorities' campaigns to banish cesspits from the city (and in so doing eliminate contamination of drinking-water wells) in the late 1870s and early 1880s. These measures were reinforced by the completion of the first sewer network, which improved drainage and lowered the water table. These public health interventions of the 1870s and '80s must have made a large contribution to the decline in death rates from the excessive levels of the mid-1870s, but high diarrheal mortality for those under five years in 1899 and 1907 indicates that these classic public health measures needed to be supplemented by improvements in domestic hygiene and infant-feeding practices.[11]

As we have noted earlier, an epidemic periodicity marked infectious disease morbidity and mortality in Australia for much of the nineteenth century. This was related to the rise and fall of immigration from Britain, the number of susceptibles and population densities. These primary cycles were followed by secondary ones as infections spread from the major port cities to regional centers and other colonies. Pandemics like the influenza pandemics of 1836–38, 1847 and 1850 could sometimes affect Australia despite its geographical isolation and comparatively small population. From the late 1830s, extensive free immigration, commonly involving young families, made epidemics of childhood infections common. Measles epidemics occurred in one or more colonies in 1834–35, 1854, 1860, 1867, 1875, 1880, 1888, 1893–94, 1898, 1902 and 1912. Scarlet fever epidemics occurred in 1840–41, 1849–50, 1858–59, 1863–64, 1875–76, 1893 and 1898. Whooping cough epidemics took place in 1838–39, 1845, 1859–60, 1867, 1878, 1889, 1901–1902 and 1907; and chickenpox, mumps and diphtheria also became common. Later in the nineteenth century other major epidemic diseases were present: influenza, typhoid, smallpox and bubonic plague. Typhoid epidemics became frequent occurrences. In 1900–25, 1,371 cases of plague, with 535 deaths, were recorded. Major smallpox epidemics occurred in Victoria, in 1857 and 1868–69; in NSW, Victoria and South Australia in 1881–85; in Tasmania, 1887–88 and 1903; and in Western Australia in 1893, while a large epidemic of "varioloid" occurred in NSW in 1913–18, extending itself to Queensland in 1913. Epidemics of mosquito-borne disease occurred in Queensland and the Northern Territory: Townsville in 1879, and Charters Towers and Rockhampton in 1885 (even penetrating to temperate Victoria in 1886). Dengue became established in southern Queensland from the 1890s and flared up below the border, in northern NSW, in 1898, 1904 and 1916. In 1925–26, a large epidemic, involving more than half a million cases, occurred, and it reached down to the central coast of NSW.[12]

In the years of crisis of the First Settlement at Sydney Cove, 1788–92, crude death rates climbed as high as 47 to 152 per thousand population, while fluctuations reaching up to twenty continued until the 1870s, after which a steady decline occurred, except for a marked rise in 1919 as a result of the influenza pandemic. Age-standardized death rates for both sexes fall from 1860, but the rate of fall diminishes from 1930. Male mortality at all ages is higher than female after 1900, and this differential expands in 1945–70. Male age-standardized mortality plateaus in the 1930s and in 1945–70. That for females levels off in 1960–70. After 1970 both sexes experience a progressive decline in mortality, but since the fall is steeper for males, the sex differential becomes narrower. Life expectancy at birth in NSW for males in 1856–66 was forty-four years and for females forty-seven years; in 1860–75 the figures were forty-seven and fifty, respectively. For Australia as a whole, life expectancy at birth increased from forty-seven years for males and fifty years for females in 1875 to seventy-four and seventy-nine, respectively, in

1990. By the latter date, Australia ranked for life expectancy in the highest third of Organization for Economic Cooperation and Development (OECD) countries, equal to Canada and above the United States and the United Kingdom.

The infant death rate fell from substantially above a hundred per thousand live births in the nineteenth century to below ten in 1990. About 40 percent of the decline took place by 1910, 70 percent by the mid-1940s. The maternal death rate showed no such downward trend, remaining at 450 to six hundred per hundred thousand births until 1937, when it fell dramatically, after which it continued to do so. It had fallen to 109 by 1950, and to ten by 1975. As observed earlier, the pattern of irregular fluctuations in general mortality very probably reflected epidemics and the waxing and waning of endemic infections like typhoid. Measles epidemics, sometimes accompanied by scarlet fever, contributed to mortality peaks. The speedy growth of cities from the 1850s produced recurrent typhoid outbreaks. The decline of tuberculosis mortality from the late nineteenth century paralleled the decline of general mortality.

The extent of the fall in infant mortality in Australia in the 1900s is remarkable, although similar falls occurred in England and Wales, other European countries and New Zealand. It fell from 116 in 1899 to seventy-two in 1909, and there is in all states of Australia a particularly marked decline in 1904 that cannot be explained by changes in statistical nomenclature or medical diagnosis, or by organized infant welfare work, as almost all of it was done after this time.[13] W.F. Litchfield, a well-known Sydney pediatrician of this era, could offer no clear solution to the puzzle: "There has been some agency in operation that has reduced very considerably infant mortalities. . . . [I]t has operated by diminishing the number of deaths from infective processes, especially those affecting the bowels and lungs. . . . It has been independent of public health and welfare schemes and there has been no great change in the habits of the people during the period of occurrence. The only thing I can attribute it to is a widespread but obscure climate effect."[14]

Modern commentators have suggested that decline in the virulence of the microorganism(s) causing diarrheal disease was responsible for the remarkable fall or that the breaking, in 1903, of Australia's worst drought reduced opportunities for the spread of microorganisms. The longer-term contributions of public health measures like cleaner water, better sewage disposal, and milk and other food regulation, as well as declining fertility and smaller families, the infant welfare movement and informal health education (especially about the importance of breast-feeding), will be discussed later. Better education of women was an "exogenous" factor of considerable significance. Mothers of this period were the first cohort of Australian women to have enjoyed universal primary education. In NSW in 1861, 24.6 percent of all who married signed with a cross, but by 1911 this group was only 0.55 percent.

A strong connection between infant mortality and female literacy has been shown to exist by research over the last two decades relating to modern developing nations. An education system communicating the value of science and fostering the idea that parents can influence the health of their children was producing graduates more ready to listen to medical and nursing experts who were spearheading the medicalization of infant and child care in Australia, as in Western Europe and the United States. In America, the federal government went beyond promoting propaganda supporting medicalization to collect, through the Children's Bureau from 1909, systematic data that permitted study of differences between ethnic and social groups as well as the effect of medicalization on behavior. State health authorities in Australia collected similar data in this period.[15]

URBANIZATION AND HEALTH PROBLEMS

Although it was clear from the early decades of the nineteenth century that the natural environment and the small population made Australia ideal for pastoral development and the export of wool to English mills, colonial governors—and later, after the coming of responsible government, colonial parliaments—put much effort, particularly in Victoria, New South Wales and South Australia, into encouraging creation of small-scale farming enterprises. Drawing on the ancient and rich concept of the British yeoman farmer, the rhetoric evoked the picture of small self-supporting, family-operated freehold farms. The *Argus* of Melbourne proclaimed in 1853: "If we . . . boldly throw open our lands to the occupation of the energetic, willing and intelligent minds now flocking in upon us, we may create a little England in Australia."[16] The Arcadian myth was resilient, but the reality turned out to be largely different. In the course of the nineteenth century, Australia became one of the most urbanized countries in the world. The American urban sociologist Adna Weber noted in 1899 that "the most remarkable concentration, or rather centralization, of population occurs in the newest product of civilization, Australia."[17] The NSW statistician, T.A. Coghlan, observed in 1901 that there was an "abnormal aggregation of the population into their capital cities."[18]

Australian economic development from 1860 is not simply an Antipodean appendage to the Industrial Revolution in Europe. It has a peculiarly modern face, not only in its exceptional rate of urbanization but in its very early focus on commercial-industrial specialization and the tertiary services of urban society:

> By 1891, two-thirds of the Australian population lived in cities and towns, a fraction matched by the United States only by 1920 and by Canada not until 1950. Most Australian capital equipment went into growing towns, most of the expanding workforce was employed in urban occupations and the greater part of gross product

came from urban activity. . . . The process of urbanisation is the central feature of Australian history, overshadowing rural economic development and creating a fundamental contrast with economic development of other "new" countries.[19]

In the last four decades of the nineteenth century, Australia's larger cities expanded considerably. The two largest, Sydney and Melbourne, were by the turn of the century noteworthy even by international standards. At this time, there were perhaps twenty cities of about half a million or more people in the world: four were in Britain, three were in the United States, and two—Sydney and Melbourne—were in Australia. Sydney had grown from ninety-six thousand in 1861 to 496,000 in 1901, and Melbourne from 125,000 to 478,000. Even the smaller colonial capitals experienced considerable growth. Brisbane, for example, expanded from a mere six thousand inhabitants in 1861 to 119,000 in 1901. The capitals dominated the hinterland. Twenty-seven percent of the population of NSW was located in Sydney in 1861, 37 percent at the turn of the century. Where 23 percent of Victoria's population dwelled in Melbourne in 1861, forty years later 40 percent lived there. Brisbane's share of Queensland's population in the same period grew from 20 to 24 percent.[20]

The three decades from 1860 were the period of the "long boom" in the Australian economy before the country entered six years of serious economic depression in the 1890s. Per capita income and consumption were at least as high as in Britain and the United States; Australians, at the aggregate level, were among the wealthiest peoples in the world. Modern economic historians talk of "a seller's market for labor" and "extraordinarily high" wages; expansion of construction and extractive industries created high demand.[21] Spokesmen for the colonial bourgeoisie, eager to attract investment and immigrants, talked of a "workingman's paradise." The editor of the *Victorian Review* observed in 1881 that "to the operative classes, Australia is a veritable land of promise."[22] Coghlan claimed in 1887 that "the contrast between rich and poor, which seems so peculiar a phase of modern civilization, finds no parallel in these southern lands."[23] In 1902 he pointed out that in Australia it required 111 days of labor a year for a working man to earn the cost of his food, whereas in Britain it took 127, in Germany 148, and in France 142.[24] However, the bright picture based on the economic historians' per capita income and consumption figures relates to averages and tells us nothing about distribution. Almost all of their evidence is from wage rates, which say nothing about regularity of employment. Detailed inquiry into social conditions, such as that carried out by urban historians concerning working-class life in the main cities, suggests that a good proportion of the working class did not enjoy the benefits of the long boom and that poverty of an order similar to that of their English cousins was their lot.[25]

One urban historian has written of late nineteenth-century Sydney, "The much vaunted high level of living standard was an illusion for a large proportion of working class families. . . . This claim presumes that the quality of housing is one of the most immediate, as well as one of the most potent, determinants of 'quality of life.'"[26] Shirley Fisher, a social historian, has argued that colonial society displayed marked inequalities and that many workers in local economies, especially in the construction and pastoral industries, were long-term victims of high levels of fluctuation in economic activity. Indeed, the prevalence of casual labor in these industries may be identified as the basic cause of much working-class poverty. The seasonal nature of employment in key industries like pastoralism helps explain this economic insecurity, but other factors operated as well: the small size and undercapitalization of manufacturing firms, the large number employed in dockside labor, and the importance of the construction industry.[27] The untrammeled growth of the major cities, often fuelled by property speculation, and the extent of working-class poverty, despite the high level of economic growth, pushed Australian cities toward death rates not so different from those of the much older cities of Europe and the United States. In table 3.2, the comparative mortality for two infectious diseases significant in this era is, although unstandardized, at the least suggestive. Australian and English urban death rates are not so different.

Pooley and Pooley point out that one of the most distinctive features of Victorian English cities was their unhealthiness, especially the extent to which high morbidity and mortality rates were concentrated in poorer districts. They point out that influential public health reformers failed to understand the social structural causes underlying the spatial concentration: poverty from fluctuations in employment and low wages brought malnutrition, while poor accommodation lowered resistance, as it increased exposure, to infection.[28] We have suggested that urban poverty was worse in later nineteenth-century Australia than might be inferred from the optimistic pronouncements of the colonial boosters or from the aggregative statistics of income and consumption of contemporary economic historians.

The larger Australian cities had much substandard working-class housing. In Sydney it did not become substandard through neglect over time; it was substandard when built, in the 1850s, 1860s or 1870s. W.S. Jevons, an English economist working in Sydney as an assayer at the mint in the late 1850s, considered the housing of laborers in the inner city odious even in comparison with the worst parts of London, Paris and Liverpool: "Nowhere have I seen such a retreat for filth and vice as the Rocks of Sydney. . . . [N]owhere are the country and the beauty of nature so painfully contrasted with the misery and deformity that lie to the charge of man."[29] It is worth remembering that Sydney was then seventy years old. The root cause was speculative building in a time of high economic growth. Houses were not only inadequate but often grossly overcrowded. Brougham Place, representative of working-class areas (according to the *Sydney Morning Herald*) and located between two of the main city streets, had small, mean houses, each of four rooms, with an average of sixteen persons in each house.[30]

Table 3.2
Deaths from Significant Infectious Diseases per 1,000 Population in Australian and English Cities, 1860–1900

	1860	1865	1870	1875	1880	1885	1890	1895	1900
SYDNEY									
Phthisis	1.1	1.0	0.9	1.9	1.9	2.1	1.5	1.1	1.0
Gastro-Intestinal Infections*	3.2	2.2	1.7	3.8	3.0	2.9	1.2	1.0	0.5
MELBOURNE									
Phthisis	2.3	2.2	2.2	2.1	2.4	2.4	2.0	1.8	1.4
Gastro-Intestinal Infections	3.2	3.6	2.1	2.8	1.6	2.0	1.6	0.7	0.4
BRISBANE									
Phthisis	NA	NA	1.0	2.7	1.2	2.2	1.1	0.8	0.6
Gastro-Intestinal Infections	NA	NA	1.3	12.2	1.5	4.1	1.2	0.8	0.6
LONDON									
Phthisis	2.7	3.1	2.7	2.8	2.2	2.2	2.1	1.8	1.7
Gastro-Intestinal Infections	1.0	2.5	1.7	1.3	1.2	0.9	9.8	1.0	1.0
BIRMINGHAM									
Phthisis	2.3	3.1	2.6	2.7	2.1	2.4	2.5	2.0	2.1
Gastro-Intestinal Infections	1.2	3.3	2.5	3.2	2.1	1.0	1.3	1.5	1.8
LEEDS									
Phthisis	2.9	3.0	2.5	2.8	1.9	2.2	1.9	1.9	1.7
Gastro-Intestinal Infections	2.4	5.5	3.8	2.7	2.2	1.0	1.1	1.8	1.3

*Include typhoid fever, diarrhea, dysentery and cholera, and, for 1860–80, typhus. NA = not available.

Source: M. Lewis and R. MacLeod, "A Workingman's Paradise? Reflections on Urban Mortality in Colonial Australia, 1860–1900," *Medical History* 31(1987): 391.

The chairman of a select committee on the condition of the working classes of the metropolis (1859–60), Henry Parkes (later Sir Henry, five times premier of NSW), said that generally, working-class housing was deplorable. The health officer of the city of Sydney, the English-born Henry Graham, told the inquiry that housing was worse than any he had seen elsewhere in the world—worse even than in parts of London. Overcrowding combined with poor sanitary facilities to promote the spread of infections. Other witnesses appearing before the committee attributed the poor personal hygiene of the working classes to the lack of water in the home. The administrators of the water supply had gradually withdrawn street fountains, in order to force house connections—but many landlords refused to connect to the mains. The committee was also told that sewerage facilities were poor. Of 1,446 house inspected, only 356 had water closets. Three houses in George Street had closets draining into cellars that also received drainage from higher houses at the rear.[31] The Sewage and Health Board, a board of inquiry set up in 1875, said in its first report that 4,700 of Sydney's water closets were connected with the water mains in such a way that pollution of drinking water was inevitable.[32] The three laws that followed from the inquiry—the Water Pollution Prevention Act, the Nuisances Prevention Act, and the City of Sydney Improvement Act (1879)—had almost no impact on the problem of substandard housing. By 1881, only about 350 "unwholesome tenements" had been demolished.

When bubonic plague arrived in Sydney for the first time in 1900 and 103 people, mostly from working-class areas, died, the chief medical officer, John Ashburton Thompson, criticized the health authorities for failure to do anything about the state of houses: "The house to house inspection showed that the Board [of Health] had fallen into a deplorable state from long continued omission of the local authority to execute the ample powers to preserve the public health . . . under its own Act of Incorporation, 1879 and under the Public Health Act, 1896."[33] In 1901, first medical officer of health for Sydney, W.G. Armstrong, said that in a year's work in the poorest part of London, Whitechapel, he had not seen dwellings in as parlous a structural condition as some in Sydney. But for Australia's better climate, the "damp, ill-ventilated and overcrowded hovels" occupied by so many-working class people would have raised the death rate from pneumonia and tuberculosis.[34] R.F. Irvine, who chaired an NSW inquiry into provision of workers' housing in Europe and the United States in 1912, observed that in parts of inner-city districts, like Redfern and Surry Hills, the quality of houses was as poor as anywhere in Europe: "But for our good climate there would be little to choose between life under these conditions and life in the worst existing slums of London." The streets and lanes were not clean but were preferable to small, dark, unventilated rooms.[35]

In the 1850s, Melbourne grew dramatically as immigrants from all over the world flooded into the southern colony in search of gold. When gold was discovered in 1851, the total population of Melbourne was only twenty-nine thousand; in 1852, almost a hundred thousand immigrants arrived. Considerable sanitary problems quickly developed. Night soil deposited in the immediate environs of the city became a "fearful nuisance." The manure depot, the answer of the authorities to the problem of human-waste disposal, was said in 1858 to be "the most offensive object in the vicinity of the city."[36] Certain conditions common to many of the rapidly growing nineteenth-century cities in the Western world soon developed. There was increased density of population, and the poor were pushed into the most congested districts, sometimes low-lying and badly drained. Domestic fires, factories and railways created great smoke pollution. Carts, coaches and cabs created a dust nuisance in summer and a mud problem in winter. The many horses, which provided locomotion, were stabled in the city, and manure accumulations were a health as well as aesthetic hazard. Compared with larger European and American cities, Melbourne may have had small-scale, "clean" industries and low population densities, but the hectic growth of inner Melbourne created a stock of jerry-built, ill-ventilated dwellings. Without an underground sewerage system for many years, industrial and domestic waste presented threats to health (and a stench assailing the nostrils) at least as great as in overseas cities.[37] Marvellous "Smelbourne" offered striking contrasts. By the 1880s, when the city was celebrating its mounting of an international exhibition, the inner area was "wallowing in its own filth."[38]

Typhoid had become endemic by the 1870s and was a more lethal threat to life and limb than the automobile was to be in the mid-twentieth century.[39] A Melbourne doctor, J.E. Neild, said of working-class conditions: "I know from experience something of the chronic domestic dirt that prevails among the lower classes in the manufacturing towns of England but nothing that I ever witnessed in the West Riding of Yorkshire and in South Lancashire equaled in repulsiveness what I found in Melbourne."[40] In the land boom of the 1880s, many poorly constructed dwellings were built on or near deposits of refuse, even of night soil. D.A. Gresswell, medical inspector to the Board of Public Health, inquired into the sanitary condition of Melbourne in 1890 and concluded that little had changed in the poorer districts since the 1860s.[41]

Not much more than a small town in the 1860s, Brisbane had grown quickly by the 1880s. Wishing to maximize profits, speculators subdivided land to create the largest possible number of building blocks. Consequently, many houses, particularly in working-class districts, were built on very small blocks in narrow streets. The prosperous households were generally located on the summits of Brisbane's many hills, because such locations were considered healthful in a semitropical climate. The working class lived in the valleys and on the river flats. Since there was no proper drainage or sewerage system, sewerage from houses higher up the slopes washed down to those at the bottom. The drainage was so inadequate that when it rained heavily, one part of the town would become cut off from another by impassable pools. In the 1850s one observer wrote, "In Adelaide-street, Elizabeth-street, Charlotte-street and Mary-street, the passenger in rainy weather may take his choice of wading through the muddy water, or balancing himself with the ingenuity of a tight-rope dancer, on some narrow pole placed across by some benevolent inhabitant."[42] In the 1860s, cesspits were everywhere; often, not having been emptied for years, they filled with rainwater or seepage (the latter the result of location on a floodplain with high water tables). One correspondent said in the *Courier* in 1866, "The pits [were] more or less full, and landlords and tenants in a chronic state of warfare as to emptying them; vile smells everywhere; with nothing but the inherent goodness of the climate and the mercy of God to ward off fever and similar dangers."[43] In the early 1890s, a sanitary engineer noted that from his own house he could see thirteen tenements, with their closets thirty feet from their kitchens and only a narrow passage between each house. Slop water had to be scattered on yard surfaces.[44]

In 1849, the resident commissioner in South Australia, J.H. Fisher, sought the views of doctors on the sanitary condition of Adelaide. Dr. Woodforde said that the city was filthy, that in particular there were problems with cesspits overflowing, pigsties, tanneries and failure to dispose of offal from animals slaughtered for meat. The colonial surgeon, Dr. Thomas Cotter, agreed that the city was filthy, declaring that what was immediately needed was a program of cleaning, paving, draining and pumping away of stagnant water, and the appointment of a health officer to pursue those responsible for nuisances. The City corporation through the 1850s and 1860s expressed concern about disposal of liquid wastes, but the sanitary state continued to be awful. The town clerk of Adelaide, displaying a miasmatic conception of disease causation, in 1872 recorded: "The fluid filth permeates the porous soil, and (I doubt not) in many instances the very foundations of the houses suffer from such fluid of the vilest description draining under them that the occupiers of the premises are inhaling deadly gases resulting in certain death."[45] Crude death rates in Adelaide were five to ten per thousand population, higher in the last three decades or so of the nineteenth century than in the colony as a whole.[46] The cause of this excess mortality was the deterioration of living conditions in Adelaide. Infant mortality rates (table 3.3) reveal this urban excess very clearly.

Western Australia, before the 1880s, was a slow-growing Crown colony with a paternalistic form of government. Then came the gold discoveries and the building of railways—by the end of the first decade of the twentieth century, the population had increased tenfold. But sanitary improvement in Perth was slow to come. Alfred Waylen, the colonial surgeon, expressed concern in 1875 about the high death rate from "zymotic" diseases in Perth: "Most of the cases . . . were from the low-lying portions of the City[,]

Table 3.3
Infant Deaths per 1,000 Live Births, Adelaide and South Australia

Year	1861		1881		1901	
	Male	Female	Male	Female	Male	Female
South Australia	161	132	146	131	105	90
Adelaide	NA	NA	174	169	173	121

NA = not available.
Source: T. Stevenson, "Miasmas, Morbidity and Milieu: Mortality in Victorian South Australia," *Proceedings of Royal Geographical Society* (South Australian Branch) 81 (1980): 43, 46.

. . . inhabited chiefly by artizans and laborers, who live in cottages built with little regard for sanitation. There is often a total absence of ventilation, as well as of drainage, and it is to these defects that, when towards the middle of winter the ground becomes saturated with water, the presence of fever may be ascribed."[47] At the end of the 1870s, H.C. Barnett, medical officer at Fremantle, Perth's port, called for regular collection of night soil, because wells, the universal sources of water, were often polluted by overflow or seepage from cesspits: "Wells are sunk in close proximity to one or more cesspools; the well pierces the porous and filth-soaked soil to a greater depth than its foul neighbour, and becomes poisoned and abominable beyond description."[48] A commission of inquiry, chaired by Waylen and set up in 1884, found that urban sanitation had not improved and called for a clean, reliable water supply to deal with the problem of polluted wells. But the scheme initiated to that end in 1890 was the responsibility of a private water company, which found it difficult to provide an adequate supply to a quickly growing Perth. A tolerable service was provided to affluent new districts, but new, working-class suburbs did less well. In the canvas towns on the goldfields, water was obtained from wells and swamps. Typhoid fever cases proliferated. In 1893, twenty-nine deaths occurred in the whole colony, but in Perth alone, in 1895–1900, deaths fluctuated between a low of nineteen in 1899 and a high of 134 in 1897. In 1896, Premier Sir John Forrest purchased the metropolitan supply for 220,000 pounds. Indeed, the government had little choice, having just agreed to spend 2.5 million pounds on a water supply for the distant Coolgardie goldfields.[49]

Hobart, Australia's second-oldest capital city, did not experience the considerable growth that the larger, mainland cities did in the later nineteenth century. While growing steadily, it remained comparatively small, although it suffered similar problems of poor housing and insanitation. From six thousand in 1830 it expanded to almost fifteen thousand in 1841, but its population was only just over nineteen thousand by 1870. It was almost thirty-five thousand in 1891 and remained at this level in 1901. In an authoritative report, rare for the 1840s, Robert Officer, medical officer of Hobart, decried the sanitary condition of the city: "Dunghills, pigsties, neglected privies, stagnant water and other accumulations of offensive matters are everywhere to be seen and exert a most unfavourable influence on the public health."[50] E.S. Hall, a vocal advocate of public health improvement from the mid-1850s and well-known Hobart medical practitioner, compiled from 1856 monthly reports on the city's health. In 1872 he stated that Tasmanian mortality had in recent years fallen notably and suggested that a better water supply had been a significant factor, because of its impact on intestinal diseases. Yet the city environment remained polluted. The City Council from 1888 removed household refuse from the business district, the landlords of which could afford the service (refuse removal remained limited to this area in 1900). In the mid-1890s, stagnant pools of water still existed in parts of the city, and polluted and foul-smelling rivulets ran through various areas. From the 1880s, water closets discharged into the largest of them, the Hobart Rivulet. The *Tasmanian News* observed in 1895 that "health and drainage matters are only half-attended to where the poor live."[51]

In 1886, 3,500 of the city's 4,500 houses still used cesspits. The following year a duplicate-pan system was instituted. But various problems plagued the pan system even after the City Council took it over from private contractors. The royal commission of 1901 on the municipal government of Hobart concluded that while the system represented an advance on the use of cesspits, it should be abandoned when the metropolitan drainage scheme was completed, because it was impossible to render the pan system safe. The drainage scheme was completed in 1912. Deaths from typhoid had reached as high as 224 per 100,000 population in Hobart in 1887 and 168 in 1891. There was a trend downward from 37 per 100,000 in 1903 to eight in 1914.

The 1881 Police Amendment Act gave the Hobart Council power to require repair or demolition of defective buildings. The act resulted in little improvement in housing, however, because even with new houses, the council did not apply the law vigorously, as it did not want to alienate builders or landlords. The *Tasmanian News* said in 1886 that there were "far too many hovels yet remaining in the City, which are altogether unfit for human habitation."[52] The 1901 royal commission took evidence from the city surveyor, R.S. Milles, who said there was "a great number" of buildings fit for demolition but that he had never reported them to the City corporation, because such a report had never been requested. A more socially progressive corporation from 1903 moved to have defective working-class houses identified and either repair or demolition initiated. The health officer, Gerard Smith, who had had long experience of workers' housing in East London, warned that "immorality and vice go along with ill-health and poor physique, which is caused by insanitary dwellings"; he predicted that the "businessmen of Tasmania" would find "money is to be made in Hobart, as in England, by erecting workmen's dwellings."[53]

INFANT MORTALITY

Infant mortality rates, particularly the post-neonatal rates, have long been recognised sensitive indicators of the quality of life of a historical population. The statistics of infant mortality in later nineteenth-century Australia support the documentary evidence of the impact of poor living and working conditions on the health and well-being of the urban working classes. Infant death rates in large colonial cities were often of much the same order as those reported by English cities. It is not unreasonable to suggest that in the light of the nature of colonial cause-specific mortality, much of it due to diarrheal and associated illness, poor living conditions were important influences on Australian infant mortality.

At the turn of the century, in Australia as in Britain, public health experts regularly argued that high infant death rates were a function more of "maternal ignorance" than of poverty. Historian Jane Lewis has pointed out that in Britain, government and philanthropy chose to deploy this argument rather than confront the larger problems of urban poverty and gross economic inequality.[54] Before 1900, those involved in infant welfare work subscribed to an implicit framework of values in which state provision of a "social minimum" had no place. So widespread was the doctrine that Arthur (later Sir Arthur) Newsholme, medical officer to the Local Government Board in Britain, felt called upon to point out that ignorance of proper infant care, while not limited to working-class mothers, was much more dangerous for them and their children, given an environment of inadequate housing and sanitary facilities, and minimal medical assistance.[55]

Colonial observers reported with satisfaction that infant mortality was comparatively low. In 1867, NSW had a rate of 106 per thousand births, when that of England was 150.[56] However, the urban rate was high; it was the low rural rate that kept down the figure for NSW as a whole. Sydney's rate in 1871–75 was 157, the rural rate only 83, and the NSW rate 103. As Sydney grew, its infant death rate rose: 160 in 1876–80, when the rate in rural areas was 98; in 1886–90, 154 and 92; and in 1896–1900, 130 and 105. Indeed, the urban rate was greater than the rural rate until the early 1930s.[57] The same pattern is to be seen in Melbourne. In 1870–90, the infant death rate was mostly above 150 per thousand births. In the 1890s, it fell markedly, although it rose well above 150 in two years. The small capitals had the same experience. The city of Adelaide in 1881–1901 had higher rates—as much as fifty per thousand higher—than the rest of South Australia.[58] Brisbane had an infant death rate of 180 per thousand births in 1876–85, when Darling Downs (rural) had a rate of 106. In 1886–95, the figures were 143 and 76 respectively, and in 1896–1905, 128 and 84.[59]

Sydney, Melbourne and London had the same order of infant death rates until the early 1890s, after which those of Sydney and Melbourne fell below those of London. The gap, however, was not great (see table 3.4).

High infant mortality from diarrheal disease was as common in Australia as in England, other parts of Europe and the United States. As early as 1854–57, when the infant death rate in Melbourne was two hundred per thousand births as compared with 130 in the rest of Victoria, W.H. Archer showed that diarrhea and dysentery were significant causes of infant deaths.[60] In Sydney, 1875–1900, mortality from diarrhea stood at thirty-two or more per thousand births for most years. The Victorian Board of Health draws attention to the fact in 1885 that five-sixths of diarrheal deaths in the colony were of children under five years. In New York in the same year, infant diarrheal mortality was a huge eighty-four per thousand. By 1901 it had fallen to forty-five. The average mortality of forty-two German cities as late as 1906 was 198 per thousand, and diarrheal conditions accounted for more than 80

Table 3.4
Infant Death Rates, Sydney, Melbourne and London, 1876–80 to 1901–5

Sydney		Melbourne		London	
Year	Number per 1,000 Births	Year	Number per 1,000 Births	Year	Number per 1,000 Births
1876–1880	160	1880–1884	170	1871–1880	158
1886–1890	154	1885–1889	179	1881–1890	152
1891–1895	138	1890–1894	140	1891–1900	160
1896–1900	130	1895–1899	132	1901–1905	141
1901–1905	106	1900–1904	117		

Sources: W. G. Armstrong, "The Infant Welfare Movement in Australia," *Medical Journal of Australia* 2 (1939): 647; *Report of Commission of Public Health, Victoria, 1939–40* (Melbourne: Government Printer, 1940), 6; G. Newman, *Infant Mortality, A Social Problem* (London: Methuen, 1906), 3.

percent of infant deaths. During the 1880s and 1890s, London's infant diarrheal rate averaged over twenty-three per thousand. In the Midlands, Leicester had an average of forty-eight for the same period, while Preston in the north of England returned 60 per thousand.[61] G.F. McCleary, historian of the infant welfare movement in Britain, said in 1935 that the "annual visitation [of epidemic diarrhea] was an impressive event, the tragic significance of which it is difficult at this time to realize."[62] G.J. Cuthbert, sometime Director of Maternal and Infant Welfare in the NSW Health Department, wrote in 1950: "The greatest over-all improvement in rates . . . is in the decline of diarrhoea and enteritis, which together, during the first quarter of the century . . . represented a dreaded community scourge with the return of every summer."[63] Indeed, falling diarrheal and associated mortality was the most notable contributor to the great decline in infant mortality in Sydney, and in Australia as a whole, in the early 1900s. From thirty-seven per thousand in 1901, diarrheal mortality fell to thirty-one in 1904, the great turning point in the downward trend of infant deaths. The rate was down to just twenty in 1911, fell to just over two in 1933, and was under one by 1947.[64]

But mortality reported as due to diarrhea was only the most obvious aspect of this health threat. In contemporary third world countries, diarrhea and malnutrition interact to decimate infant life. Weanling diarrhea involves a synergism between nutrition and infection when contaminated, weaning and post-weaning foods introduce infection; and malnutrition from a poor weaning diet reduces resistance. At the same time, diarrhea reduces appetite and gives rise to further restriction of the diet.[65] The problem of weanling diarrhea existed in Sydney and other cities of the Western world where diarrheal mortality was high in the later nineteenth and early twentieth centuries, although it was perhaps not as severe as in some poor countries today. Weanling diarrhea implies that mortality returned under the heading of "failure to thrive" or a synonym is as significant as that directly returned under diarrhea. In 1905, W.F. Litchfield, a distinguished Sydney pediatrician, argued that deaths from "dentition" (teething) and "atrophy," together with most deaths from "convulsions," should from his experience have been included in diarrheal mortality. A Brisbane doctor, W.S. Byrne, claimed that many deaths arising from gastroenteritis were returned under "dentition" and "convulsions."

W.G. Armstrong, first medical officer of health for Sydney and pioneer of organized infant welfare work in Australasia, pointed out that mortality in Sydney from convulsions, teething and atrophy had considerably declined from the mid-1870s. The decline is only comprehensible if more accurate diagnosis and certification meant that most such deaths had been transferred to other categories. Given mortality trends, the only categories to which they could have shifted were diarrhea and enteritis. Moreover, close seasonal correlations existed between the high points in the death rates ascribed to diarrhea, atrophy, convulsions and teething. Others agreed. R.R. Stawell, a Melbourne paediatrician, criticized the "pernicious belief" that diarrhea resulted from teething, as well as the practices of describing a baby's condition as "marasmus" (wasting) and of reporting the cause of death as "congestion of the brain." Reviewing the causes of infant deaths in eight American cities in 1911–16, R.M. Woodbury noted that many deaths of infants older than one month from "debility," "malnutrition" and "marasmus" were classified in vital statistics under "congenital debility" and thereby wrongly exaggerated mortality from causes peculiar to earlier infancy (developmental conditions).[66]

The seasonality of infant diarrheal mortality was noted in other Australian cities. In the 1870s Dr. C.D. Hunter, on behalf of the Australian Health Society, warned Melbourne mothers against weaning in the summer.[67] S.J. Magarey, a leading Adelaide doctor, noted in 1879 that as many babies died in the warmer months of December to March as in the whole of the rest of the year.[68] The same seasonality is clear in Perth in 1870–1914. The trends there are not so marked until the mid-1880s, because the small number of vital events allowed a slight change in mortality to distort the picture. From that time, the high infant death rate from diarrheal conditions in the warmer part of each year is visible.[69]

The same pattern is to be found in the United States. In the South, diarrhea was sometimes called "April–May disease" (spring in the Northern Hemisphere). Cheney, having analyzed monthly mortality for thirty-one cities in the United States in 1879–80, discovered that marked increases occurred in summer in all but two cities. In Philadelphia (which she studied in depth), the excess summer mortality during the last twenty-five years of the nineteenth century increased total infant mortality by 10–16 percent. For fifteen American cities, the summer mortality increased overall infant mortality by 25 percent. Seasonal levels began to decline in 1880–1900, but the major decline took place in the early twentieth century. In 1920, for the first time, the seasonal effect was absent.[70]

The burden of infant diarrheal disease fell disproportionately upon the working class. Newsholme, in 1899 medical officer of health for Brighton and from 1908 medical officer of the Local Government Board, presented three influential reports on infant mortality in England and Wales—the first in 1910, the second in 1913 and the third in 1914. He showed that the main source of infection was in the home, thus shifting attention from contamination of the milk supply. His work helped establish concern with promotion of breastfeeding and teaching of "mothercraft" as the central focus of infant welfare work. Newsholme pointed out that infant diarrhea was mainly an urban problem; "as a fatal disease," it was, he argued, "a disease of the artisan and still more of the lower laboring classes to a preponderant extent." In London, the poor districts had most epidemic diarrhea. In Birmingham, it was found that in the early 1900s, practically all the deaths occurred in houses occupied by the artisan classes. In Glasgow, diarrheal mortality varied according to economic class—from 1,698 per million in Dalmarnock Ward and 1,686 in the Calton Ward to 238 per million in the Park Ward and 201 in Kelvinside.[71]

Unsanitary domestic conditions, substandard housing and poor nutrition combined to make infant diarrheal disease in Australian, British and American cities mainly a health problem of the working classes. There is evidence from New South Wales that low incomes prevented working-class mothers from providing good substitute food for breast milk. In 1875, the *New South Wales Medical Gazette* claimed that the cost of milk prevented the poor from using it for feeding their children. Milk cost eight pence per quart, approximately the retail price in the early 1920s. In the early 1900s, it was again claimed that working-class mothers found milk too expensive to feed infants. In any case, they did not see it as nutritious. Instead, arrowroot and corn flour, nutritionally suspect, were widely employed. In the 1880s, a cooked flour preparation known as "tops and bottoms" was a popular alternative to milk for working-class infants.[72] Condensed milk was another popular infant food, because it kept well in a warm climate, whereas much fresh milk was contaminated. The cheaper brands purchased by poorer families in Australia and in Britain were very low in fat content. Indeed, widespread use of patent foods and condensed milk for infant feeding in late nineteenth-century Britain produced a good deal of infantile scurvy and rickets. During debate of the Pure Food Act of 1908 in the NSW parliament, a member for an inner-city electorate reminded his colleagues that "among the poorer classes, a mother, very frequently unable for want of sufficient nourishment to properly sustain her child, purchases condensed milk as a substitute for the food which should be provided by nature."[73]

Poor nutrition and poor housing together were responsible for an excess of infant mortality. But Newsholme and other investigators showed that while poverty was influential, the quality of maternal care could influence the baby's welfare. Chadwick and the sanitarians had earlier sought an answer to the high levels of death and disease among the lower classes in the engineering solution of drainage, not in an attack on poverty as such. The infant welfare movement sought to reduce infant mortality not by a call for income redistribution but by an individualistic and less radical demand for better mothercraft. Breastfeeding and mothercraft became the watchwords of organized infant-welfare work across the Western world. Even where, as in the United States, early work concentrated on the provision of clean milk through milk depots—Nathan Strauss, a philanthropic businessman, established depots in New York in 1893—the emphasis later shifted to the education of mothers in infant care.[74] Leading figures in infant and child welfare in England and Australia often pointed out that economic inequality per se was not responsible for high infant death rates. An English expert, Sir George Newman, wrote in 1906: "Poverty is not alone responsible, for in many poor communities the infant mortality is low. . . . [T]his loss of infant life is in some way intimately related to the social life of the people."[75] The eminent Australian physician Sir Charles Mackellar, who helped pioneer child-welfare measures in NSW, wrote in 1917, "Although history shows that in the older countries of the world poverty is often associated with infant mortality, yet even there it is not by any means the only, or even the chief cause."[76] Good mothercraft was the key factor he argued. In France, the pioneers of infant welfare stressed breastfeeding and quality of care. Professor Pierre Budin established an infant clinic at the Charité Hospital, Paris—the first "*consultation de nourrisons*"—in 1892. Breast-feeding was strongly promoted in the clinic, and only where this was impossible was a supply of sterilized milk provided.[77]

THE DEVELOPMENT OF PUBLIC HEALTH LEGISLATION

Epidemic disease, or the threat thereof, was a great stimulus to public health legislation in the United Kingdom, the United States and Australia. Between 1817 and 1902, there were eight global pandemics of cholera. Endemic in Bengal, it spread in 1817 from India to Arabia and via northern Europe to England in 1831. In 1831–32, Asiatic cholera took more than fifty thousand lives in Britain; the temporary Central Board of Health and the local health boards were ineffective against it. It spread to New York and the eastern seaboard of the United States in 1832 and thence to Latin America. Coming back into the southern United States, it later reached Canada. In 1848, a second epidemic of cholera in Britain caused fifty thousand deaths and prompted support for the first Public Health Act (the *Times* observed that "the Cholera is the best of all sanitary reformers").[78] The third epidemic, in 1854, caused twenty thousand deaths in Britain, but in Russia in 1847–61 cholera killed a million people. The final epidemic in Britain, in 1866, caused fourteen thousand deaths.[79]

Britain

After Chadwick's fall from power in 1854, John Simon, former medical officer of health for the city of London, became medical adviser to the General Board of Health. The work of the board was divided in 1858 between the Local Government Act Office, which now oversaw public works loans, and Simon's Privy Council Medical Department. Simon's powers were very limited, but he set out to use information to persuade government and public opinion of the need for public health reform. In the process, he introduced medicine and science into public health and established the medical expert's role in public administration.

In the period up to his resignation in 1876, a number of important pieces of legislation were passed. Nuisances Acts enabled local authorities to deal more vigorously with environmental hazards—rubbish, river pollution, slaughterhouses and industrial waste. The 1858 Local Government Act made possible compulsory purchase for sanitary reasons. The 1866 Sanitary Act empowered local authorities to establish clean water supplies and to set standards for tenements. The 1867 Vaccination Act introduced greater penalties for parents who did not have their babies vaccinated. The Public Health Act of 1875 consolidated public health legislation since 1848. For the first time every sanitary district in England and Wales had to have a medical officer of health. In 1868, Simon noted the growth of state interference in civil society in the interests of collective health: the state "has interfered between parent and child . . . [by] requiring that children should not be left unvaccinated[;] . . . between employer and employed . . . [by] insisting . . . that certain sanitary claims be fulfilled in all places of industrial occupation[;] . . . between vendor and purchaser . . . to put restrictions on the sale . . . of poisons[. I]t has prohibited . . . certain commercial supplies of water . . . adulterated food or drink or medicine or . . . meat unfit for human food. . . . [I]t has provided that in any sort of epidemic emergency organized medical assistance, not peculiarly for paupers, may be required of local authorities and in the same spirit it requires that vaccination . . . shall be given gratuitously to every claimant."[80]

In the early 1860s, Simon supported epidemiological inquiries into a range of public health problems, taking state medicine well beyond environmental sanitation. Reports were produced by his medical staff on nutrition, housing, infant diarrhea and occupational diseases. But in practical terms these led nowhere. From the late 1860s he sponsored research projects on areas from epidemiology to pathology, programs that had the effect of heading public health toward domination by the scientific expert. The 1875 Public Health Act represented the first stage of this progression to "government by experts" in that it made compulsory the appointment of medical officers of health to local government areas. But in the absorption of public health and local government administration into the new Local Government Board in 1872, public health had already been subordinated to administration of local government law. Simon, appreciating his loss of independence, resigned in 1876, but his successors—Edward Seaton, George Buchanan, Richard Thorne—did not speak out against their subordination.

While public health activism at the center died, activism at the local level by the new public health professionals, of which the most prominent were the medical officers of health, was very much alive. Public health initiatives were now based in local affairs. The new public health practice was more localized and professionalized than the earlier Chadwickian public health paradigm had envisaged. Politically, public health ceased to be the elite's answer to the ill health and poverty that might otherwise lead to working-class revolution; an enfranchised working class, through control of local government, now sought to influence the direction of public health policy.[81]

The United States

In the American Civil War, which resulted in six hundred thousand military deaths, sickness (mostly infections) killed twice as many men as injuries in battle. The U.S. Sanitary Commission, created in 1861, showed that proper sanitation, isolation of infected soldiers, personal hygiene, and the use of fruits and vegetables to prevent scurvy could much improve the health of troops. These lessons in public health subsequently influenced large numbers of the civilian population and promoted the cause of sanitary reform. At the same time, the concerns of doctors had been shifting from quarantine as the means to control infectious disease to sanitary improvement. New York, the largest city and destination of masses of poor immigrants, became the site of a sanitary crusade led by physicians J.H. Griscom, E. Harris, J.M. Smith and S. Smith. They formed in 1859 the New York Sanitary Association, which in turn supported the formation of the New York Citizens Association.

In 1864, the Citizens Association asked for medical support for new health legislation. Doctors formed a special council of hygiene and public health, which carried out a sanitary survey of New York City, like Shattuck's in Massachusetts. The report, intended to have a public educational effect, made clear that all classes were at risk from infectious diseases. Asiatic cholera flared up in late 1865, and early the next year, the Metropolitan Board of Health was created. The New York Metropolitan Health Act of 1866 brought into being the first modern health department in a large city. It became the benchmark for many other city health departments. The city council of Chicago, concerned about cholera and smallpox, in 1867 set up a permanent health board. The cholera epidemic of 1866 gave rise to health boards in Cincinnati and St. Louis. Enjoying wide powers, the boards were nonetheless dependent on city councils to endorse and enforce regulations; Pittsburgh's weak and lay-dominated board was typical of urban health authorities. In any case, since public health was an urban phenomenon, the majority of the population, located in rural areas, was untouched by these developments.[82]

The sanitary idea in Britain and the United States had used the generalized method of environmental sanitation to reduce mortality and advance the community's health. In the late nineteenth century, a new public health paradigm emerged. This identified "risk populations" and drew on bacteriology's principle of specificity to understand diseases—specific pathogens cause specific infections. In the process, scientific expertise rather than social reform came to be seen as the key to progress. As H.W. Hill, director of the Epidemiology Division of the Minnesota Board of Health, pointed out that concerning tuberculosis control the goal would be to prevent two hundred thousand active TB cases from spreading infection, not to better the living conditions of a hundred million Americans. In the light of the discoveries of Pasteur, Lister, Koch and other German bacteriologists, the bacteriological laboratory was seen as central to the new public health. The laboratories needed professionals trained in science, not reforming amateurs. Americans trained in bacteriology in Germany taught the new laboratory methods at home. The 1880s saw Charles Chapin's public health laboratory in place in Providence, Rhode Island; V.C. Vaughan's state hygienic laboratory in Michigan; and William Sedgwick's bacteriological studies of water supplies and sewage disposal at the Lawrence Experiment Station, Massachusetts.

The new epidemiology, concerned with control of specific diseases, taught that the health officer's main effort should go not into urban sanitation but into control of specific routes of infection. Indeed, the first handbook for health officers, J. Scott MacNutt's *Manual for Health Officers* (1915), contained six hundred pages on infectious diseases, four pages on industrial hygiene, and only a brief discussion of housing, water, environmental sanitation and public education. The conceptualization of public health in biological terms in the United States supported the medical profession's bid for dominance in public health. In Britain, where the dominance of the medical officer of health was already established, the emphasis on specificity of disease transmission mode gave rise to demands for notification, isolation and disinfection in policy and practice. In 1889 permissive legislation made most common infections reportable, but compulsory notification was introduced in 1899. Journals on prevention were full of material on control of infectious diseases. Further, since notified cases required confirmation by bacteriological analysis, medical officers of health pressed health authorities for laboratory facilities.[83]

In the 1870s in the United States, there was considerable advance in the institutionalization of public health. Where in 1872 health boards had existed in only six states, by 1878 sixteen had boards, and almost fifty cities possessed health departments.[84] The 1880s and 1890s saw the apogee of the sanitary revolution as water supply and sewerage, and garbage and refuse removal were introduced into urban areas. But population growth always outstripped sanitary facilities, and housing quality deteriorated as tenements, often poorly constructed, became more overcrowded. Horses, still widely used for transport, and urban dairies remained sources of ill health and mortality, because of the flies attracted to the ubiquitous manure heaps.

The political and administrative context of public health in the United States was different from those of the United Kingdom, France and Germany. In Britain, with its small land mass and unitary government, a national public health authority—the Central Board of Health—was established quickly, although strong local government traditions ensured a large role for local health authorities. In contrast, in France and Germany, a history of centralized, authoritarian government ensured that public health measures came from the central government. In contrast, the great geographical size of the

United States and the heritage of strong local government from Britain meant that in the United States local public health initiatives were very significant. Because of the federal structure of government and the value placed on local autonomy, when action was beyond the capacity of urban or county government, state, not national, authorities assumed responsibility.[85] Australia, as a federation of states from 1901, saw the same emphasis on state-level responsibility in public health, although the national government began to become significantly involved from the 1920s. But local government was never as strong in public health matters as in the United Kingdom and the United States.

As a very large country with considerable internal differences in culture and economy, climate and terrain, the United States experienced marked regional variations in disease prevalence and in other health problems. The sanitary revolution began in the cities of the East in the earlier nineteenth century and spread to the Midwest and South in the later years of the century, to arrive on the West Coast only in the 1900s. Corrupt city administration reduced the efficiency of the New York health department in the 1880s, but by the 1890s the organization was again at the forefront, acting as a model for many other departments. In the 1880s it already had sections for sanitary inspections, contagious diseases, plumbing and drainage, and food inspections and regulations on offensive trades. Legislation in the 1890s on tenements extended its concerns. This was also the era of departmental laboratories in city and state departments.

Other eastern city departments expanded at a slower rate than New York's. Newark, New Jersey, a city of moderate size, did not have an effective department until the early 1890s, when two competent officials were appointed. Cities of the Midwest were usually smaller and often had lower mortality. Chicago (undergoing rapid expansion as an industrial center) and Cincinnati had reasonably effective departments in the immediate post–Civil War period, but city governments failed to sustain the sanitary advance in following decades. In the aftermath of the Civil War, southern cities lagged well behind, and progress there was largely delayed until very late in the century. Memphis, Tennessee, was early to implement reforms; disastrous epidemics of yellow fever in the 1870s had shocked the city into action. A sanitary survey revealed appalling living conditions. By the 1880s, the city had been sewered, a new water supply provided, refuse disposal implemented, streets paved, and sanitary regulations enforced. Sanitary improvements came more slowly in Atlanta, Georgia, than did those of Memphis, because the stimulus of an epidemic was absent, but by the 1890s most of Atlanta was sewered and an adequate water supply was in place. Even in the cities, however, the areas occupied by African Americans to a large extent missed out on improved sanitation. Although San Francisco, like Seattle, had low death rates compared with the more densely populated eastern cities, this important

Californian city had by the 1870s more miles of sewers than most comparable eastern cities. Indeed, because it was so early into the field, it was forced to renovate its system in the light of engineering advances. It also had an effective health department from 1870.

Just as industrialization in Britain both helped create health problems and provided the wealth to finance sanitary improvement, so in an industrializing United States rising gross domestic product underwrote the capital and operating costs of sewerage and water systems and health departments. Australia's high gross domestic product in the later nineteenth century likewise financed urban sanitary improvements.

Although most states had health boards by the end of the century, most were ineffective and lacking in authority and funds. The first effective board had been set up in Massachusetts in 1869 after a very long political struggle. It quickly encouraged creation of local boards and carried out inquiries into a range of contemporary public health issues: slaughterhouses, tenements, vaccination, food adulteration, water quality, sewerage and ventilation. From the 1880s it became very concerned with water pollution and sewage disposal; a decade later the state was recognized as being at the forefront of sanitary engineering. For three decades from 1886, when it was reconstructed, the board was an example for boards in other states, even though it had to a large degree to employ education and persuasion to achieve its ends. It directly inspired establishment of the Michigan board in 1873; Michigan, like Massachusetts, requested health reports from cities and towns. In 1877 towns were required to appoint health officers. From 1870 California had an active board, which soon concerned itself with a range of matters from diseases in schools and tuberculosis to a national sanitary bureau and establishment of chairs of hygiene in medical schools. But ongoing community support was not forthcoming, and only in the 1890s did Californian towns and cities respond to Sacramento's call to create local boards.

By the end of the century few states had strong, well-funded boards. If anything, local health officers were in an even weaker position than state officers. The North Carolina board was so starved of funds that it had to wait more than thirty years after it was created, in 1877, before it could afford to employ a full-time health officer. In the mid-1880s, the Missouri board received no funding from the legislature; in the early 1890s the board complained that there were no local boards in existence and no vital statistics being reported.[86]

Australia

As we have seen, before the passing of public health legislation inspired by the sanitary idea in the middle of the nineteenth century, public health in Australia, as in Britain and the United States, was largely synonymous with quarantine and vaccination activities. As in the two other Anglophone countries, epidemic disease was a powerful spur to introduction of legislation, though smallpox in Australia usually played the part of cholera in Britain. Not surprisingly, given the colonial ties with Britain, Australian legislatures borrowed much from British law. The first public health act passed in Australia was modeled on the 1848 English act. It was passed in Victoria in 1854, and it created a Central Board of Health. Fear of infectious disease was a powerful influence. The overcrowding resulting from the inflow of immigrants attracted by gold produced very insanitary conditions in Melbourne and the towns of the goldfields. The Victorian authorities became concerned about the prevalence of typhoid and other bowel infections. Smallpox in New Zealand, Victoria and NSW pushed Queensland into action in 1872. Dr. Kevin O'Doherty introduced a brief health bill (which took as its model a Canadian act) allowing the government to create a temporary Central Health Board if a "formidable" epidemic threatened. He had failed as a private member to have a comprehensive bill enacted.

The next year South Australia produced an act providing for a range of measures to improve environmental sanitation and to prevent the spread of "epidemic, endemic or contagious disease." The South Australians had borrowed from both the English and Victorian acts. However, it was the example of the English Public Health Act of 1875 and the spur of smallpox epidemics affecting NSW, Victoria, South Australia and Tasmania in the 1880s that gave rise to a plethora of legislation: in NSW, the Infectious Diseases Supervision Act, 1881; the Dairies Supervision Act, 1886; and eventually a comprehensive Public Health Act, 1896. In Victoria, the existing act was amended in 1883 to provide for notification of "malignant, infectious or contagious disease," while the long-standing problem of excessive typhoid morbidity and mortality prompted legislators to enact the Public Health Act, 1889. In South Australia, an amending act was passed in 1884 providing for notification and isolation of cases of smallpox, cholera, plague, yellow fever and any other proclaimed disease. It drew on the 1875 English act and the 1883 Victorian act. Further legislation was enacted in 1898. Influenced by the 1875 English act, Queensland also passed new legislation in 1884. Western Australia escaped the smallpox visitations of the 1880s but passed a new act in 1886 as a result of an official inquiry into the sanitary conditions of Perth and the prevalence of typhoid in the colony. Tasmania enacted its main legislation of this era in 1885.[87]

By the end of the nineteenth century, all the Australian colonies had enacted public health legislation in the English style. One clear difference from the English system was the supervision exercised from the center because of the comparative weakness of local government in the colonies, a function of smallness and thinness of population and the colonial tradition, initiated in the convict era, of strong government from the capital. Lacking funds, administrative skill and often the resolve to act against local propertied and business interests, local government had to be subsidized and controlled by the central health authorities. The Victorian chief secretary (and future prime minister of Australia) Alfred Deakin observed in the debate on the 1889 Health Bill that "local authorities regard the health jurisdiction with which they have been entrusted as something ornamental . . . as something to which . . . to give only a small portion of their time and attention." Indeed, in some cases, local health officers had been rewarded for their vigilance with dismissal.[88] By the close of the nineteenth century, public health in Australia involved state-imposed prevention of disease through environmental sanitary regulation—reinforced by publicly run reticulated water and underground sewerage systems, at least in the larger colonial cities—and controls over infectious diseases through the practice of notification, inspection, disinfection and isolation.[89]

The parlous sanitary state of Melbourne was a concern well before the great inflow of immigrants in the early 1850s. The fear was that cholera would strike as savagely as it had in Britain in the 1830s and 1840s. Moreover, enteric fever became sharply more active in Victoria in 1850–54.[90] The *Argus* noted in January 1854 that "Melbourne is gradually acquiring the reputation of being the most unhealthy city in the Australian colonies. . . . Dysentery seems now to occupy the position here which plague does in Constantinople, and the yellow fever in New Orleans."[91] In August, it was learned that cholera had devastated Mauritius; the Melbourne City Council asked the legislature to establish a health board to eradicate the "filthy nuisances" of the city. The Medical Society of Victoria, like the other medical associations of the colony hitherto uninterested in sanitary reform, memorialized the lieutenant governor concerning the need to appoint "a Board of Health with a constitution and powers similar to those of the Board of Health of England to counter the threat of cholera's spread because of the appalling sanitary state of Melbourne."[92] No cholera epidemic transpired, but "An Act for promoting the Public Health in populous Places in the Colony of Victoria" was passed by the Legislative Council and assented to by the Crown in December 1854. Early the next year, the governor appointed a central board of health—Doctors William McCrea (chief medical officer of Victoria) and Richard Youl (coroner), and Capt. Andrew Clarke (surveyor-general)—to execute the act. The act was proclaimed to apply in the first place to Melbourne and also to Geelong, a port town forty miles from Melbourne. In its first report, the central board praised the local board at Geelong for improving the sanitary condition of the town by paving and "channelling" streets, removing "accumulations of filth," and ensuring inspectors of nuisances carried out their duties. It was, however, critical of the Melbourne City Council for being "tardy" in the pursuit of sanitary improvements and of the local board for failing to cooperate in the matters of sewerage, drainage and water supply. Only the "natural salubrity of the climate," in its view, had prevented "a vast amount of disease."[93]

The City Council and the central board were already in conflict over the board's refusal to approve the appointment of a city health officer, a progressive appointment very much the work of Richard Eades, a former lecturer at the Ledwich School of Medicine, Dublin, and now member of the council. Dr. McCrea, criticizing the City Council in the board's report, may well have wished to ram home the fact of Eades's subordinate position in the colonial health hierarchy. The council's Health Committee retaliated by decrying the central board's "overbearing spirit." In 1861, the board finally agreed to the appointment of John Macadam, a government analyst, as part-time health officer of the council. The problem was that both the central board and local boards (municipal councils) lacked power. The central board could publicly embarrass a local board and complain to the chief secretary, but its own orders were so weak that the City Council prosecuted sanitary transgressors under the Town and City Police Act, 1854. Like the board, the council did not have power over the police, and after the coming into being of new municipalities, it had no power over the wider city.[94]

By 1864 the Public Health Act had been extended to the whole colony. Yet the local boards were hampered by lack of capacity to pass by-laws on nuisances and other sanitary matters or to enter into contracts for scavenging services. The Victorian police, unlike the British but like the French, were under central control and were much involved in sanitation. By 1861 many local health inspectors were police sergeants. Throughout the colony the police had the power to prosecute individuals creating nuisances in relation to slaughterhouses, piggeries and privies, as well accumulations of rubbish, those polluting waterways, and those adulterating food or purveying damaged food. In the first thirteen years of its existence, the central board complained repeatedly about its lack of power over local boards. In its report for 1862, the board said that Melbourne was still without sewers and drains, and that the existence of a copious water supply only added to the dangers, because it resulted in over-full cesspools. Melbourne had a good water supply from the Yan Yean scheme of 1857, but it acquired a sewerage system only in 1897. In 1864 the board decried the "apathy and indifference" to sanitation and the inadequacy of the act to deal with the "opposition" to sanitary improvement.[95] In 1866 it complained that "the bench [judges] here do not view gross breaches of sanitary laws as serious offences" and that the courts were unwilling to accept the testimony of local board officers unless supported by that of neighbors, who too often were reluctant to testify against their fellows.[96]

The Public Health Amendment Act, 1867, did not outlaw cesspits, but it enabled local councils to deal with defective ones. T.M. Girdleston, the new, part-time health officer of the City Council (and a London-trained hospital consultant who believed that the high death rate was due to a filthy environment), pushed the corporation to act to abolish cesspits. In 1870–71, more than 4,800 tenements with leaking cesspits were required to have their pits filled. A weekly pan service removed the need for these and new buildings to use cesspits, and the night soil was buried in trenches in public parks. Outbreaks of measles, scarlet fever and diphtheria in the 1870s gave rise to a Melbourne-wide war on cesspits. From 1876, councils had the power to fill defective pits and stop construction of new ones. By the end of the 1870s, the City Council had eliminated six thousand cesspits attached to nine thousand tenements.[97] The central board complained in 1872 that too many country local boards failed to appoint health officers, and where they did too often paid them so little (as little as five pounds per year) that the part-time agents could not afford to take time away from private practice to the extent required to improve the sanitary condition of their areas. Moreover, some extrametropolitan local boards were ready to risk penalties under the amended act rather than deal with defective cesspits. In 1877 the Central Board recognised the great improvement resulting from the pan system but pointed to the need to do something about the "very offensive condition" in which emptied pans were returned to households.[98]

In the early 1860s, an act forbidding purveying of adulterated, mislabeled or unwholesome food, legislation that drew on a contemporary English act, had been passed; also, the 1883 Public Health Amendment Act dealt with what the member introducing the bill into the Assembly called this "crying evil." The Central Board noted in 1885 that while prosecutions for sale of adulterated milk and bread had in some districts been successful, too many local inspectors were slow in enforcing the law. Further legislation in the 1880s made it illegal to sell a food or drug carrying a false or deceptive description.[99] An 1888 public health act for the first time provided for doctors' reporting of infectious disease cases, although this was conditional on the central board's gazetting a particular area as being affected by disease. The 1883 act had simply obliged doctors to notify householders of infectious cases, and they in turn were to notify the local board.[100]

The 1883 act had reconstructed the central board. Richard Youl, who had become president of the board after the long-serving McCrea retired in 1879, had been seeking more power for the board in light of the deteriorating sanitary situation in Melbourne. In the 1880s a resident of Melbourne was more at risk of death from typhoid than was a resident of London. Conflict with Chief Secretary Berry led Youl (and academics James Robertson and H.B. Allen) to resign; A.P. Akehurst, a police magistrate, became president. But Akehurst also appreciated that the Central Board needed greater control over local authorities, especially concerning sanitation. The municipalities tried to bypass the board by seeking establishment of a central board of works that would take responsibility for sewerage. Akehurst, however, managed to get the colonial government to appoint a royal commission, chaired by Professor H.B. Allen, on the sanitary condition of Melbourne.

The focus of the sanitary debate was changing from sewerage and pollution of the Yarra River to the problem of pollution created by the City

Council's abattoirs and saleyards. The 1889 Public Health Amendment Act, following the royal commission's proposals, abolished the central board and established a Department of Health, responsible to a minister. It widened provisions on adulteration, introduced regulation of private hospitals, and defined more clearly requirements concerning nuisances and offensive trades. The passing of the long-anticipated consolidating Health Act of 1890 saw the creation of a new central board of public health.[101] The new board had seven representatives of local authorities and a chairman and medical inspector appointed by the government.[102]

The Public Health Act, 1889, was not a victory for sanitary reformers like Akehurst or Allen, who were seeking to locate the center of power for public health in the professionals and a minister of the Crown. Rather, the municipalities dominated the reformed board. The intention of the bill when introduced was to abolish the Central Board and the local boards, replacing them with a department of health responsible to a minister, and Akehurst was to be the secretary of the department. But the City Council and the municipalities outmaneuvred the proponents of this approach; Chief Secretary Deakin now said that the board, not the minister, would be the locus of power. The new medical inspector to the board, the English-born Dan Astley Gresswell, was not only a highly qualified public health professional but able, as it proved, to work very well with the municipal representatives. He became chairman of the board in 1894 and also head of the new health department.[103] In 1891 the Melbourne and Metropolitan Board of Works, which like London's Metropolitan Board of Works was intended to solve the problem caused by local-government fragmentation of authority, assumed control of Melbourne's water supply. It set about construction of an underground sewerage system. The first property was connected to the sewers in August 1897.[104]

Did the sewers have an appreciable effect on the health of Melbourne? Indeed, did the installation of sewerage systems in the six main cities of Australia markedly influence the course of the typhoid mortality rate in each colony? The typhoid death rate began to decline more than seven years before houses were first connected to the sewers in Melbourne, so that the fall in Victoria is not totally explained by the introduction of the Melbourne sewerage system. This was also the case for the other states. Moreover, the Victorian decline from about 1890 was occurring in extrametropolitan areas of the colony as well as in Melbourne. Thus Ballarat and Bendigo, unsewered regional cities, experienced a decline similar to Melbourne's, and at the same time. The construction of sewerage systems in Sydney in the 1880s and in Perth in the 1900s coincided with the beginning of the downward trend in each capital city. Adelaide obtained sewers in the early 1880s, but the death rate for typhoid is not available until the 1890s, so little can be said. In Hobart the decline began a few years before a sewerage system was constructed, in the second decade of the twentieth century.

In 1880–90, under the spur of smallpox outbreaks in three colonies, public health administration advanced, and sanitary improvement took place throughout Australia. As noted already, in Victoria the Public Health Acts of 1883 and 1889 were passed, and a royal commission on the sanitary state of Melbourne was established in 1888. In New South Wales, the work of pioneer epidemiologist John Ashburton Thompson on typhoid outbreaks associated with urban dairies led to the Dairies Supervision Act, 1886, which improved sanitation in Sydney and then in extrametropolitan dairies. In Queensland, five inquiries on typhoid and sanitation took place in 1884–89. Tasmania acquired its first comprehensive Public Health Act in 1885. In Western Australia, in 1884, a commission inquired into the sanitary state of its main urban areas, Perth and Fremantle. This progress in sanitation, particularly the spread of the pan system of human-waste disposal, better surface drainage and better water supplies, would seem to be the most likely factor causing the decline in typhoid mortality from about 1890 in all colonies but Western Australia (where because sanitation had not improved in the 1890s, typhoid manifested a pattern of activity like that in the other colonies at any earlier time). What sewerage did was to reinforce the existing downward trend in mortality, so that by the third decade of the twentieth century the typhoid death rate had become insignificant.[105]

In 1839 Governor Sir George Gipps had appointed a health officer for the port of Sydney, but this was an appointment purely related to quarantine, the officer's duties being inspection of suspect ships and (during quarantine) diagnosis, isolation and treatment. The 1848 English Public Health Act had direct reverberations in NSW. It led Governor Sir Charles Fitzroy in 1854 to propose the same system of a central board of health and local health authorities for the colony. However, the legislation was not passed.[106] The *Herald* had asked at the time, "If the inhabitants of the British Metropolis are so deeply sensible to the importance of sanitary progress as to employ 47 medical officers of health, cannot the wealthy prosperous city of Sydney afford to employ one?"[107] The newspaper offered to support even radical candidates for aldermanic positions if they were committed to sanitary reform. Henry Grattan Douglas, a leading doctor and member of the Legislative Council, had a strong interest in British "sanitary science," and he was able to secure (in the Sydney Corporation Restoration Act, 1857), in a climate of press support for sanitary reform, provision for appointment of a medically qualified city health officer.

The Sydney corporation had employed inspectors of nuisances since the 1840s, but they too often were unqualified and inexperienced. Isaac Aaron, the first health officer, appointed in 1857, was well qualified, having been a member of Birmingham's local health board before his emigration to Australia. Aaron enthusiastically pursued sanitary improvement, attacking problems of rubbish accumulation, defective cesspits, polluting trades, and overcrowded housing. He soon was in conflict with the City Council. The real cause of the council's opposition to Aaron was that he was too efficient; he resigned when his salary was reduced. During debate of the Municipalities Law Amendment Bill, 1867, Edward Deas Thomson suggested that appointment of health officers to municipalities with more than three thousand residents be made compulsory. The proposal was accepted by the Legislative Council but not by the Assembly, where there was concern about the capacity of municipalities, hampered by small rate revenues, to pay for health officers without cutting back markedly in other areas of activity. An 1873 inquiry into local government found that none of the twenty-four municipal districts presenting figures had a rate revenue larger than 450 pounds, while all except nine boroughs had revenues smaller than a thousand pounds. The 1858 and 1867 Municipalities Acts enabled all councils to appoint inspectors of nuisances, but apathy and lack of funds kept most from making appointments. It would be more than sixty years before formal qualifications were demanded of health inspectors.[108]

In the 1870s, sanitary reformers repeatedly pointed to the worsening condition of Sydney's environment. A local doctor in 1870 said that Sydney was subject to the same environmental evils as European cities of the same size. Professor Archibald Liversidge in 1874 analyzed water supplied to the Union Club in the city and described it as filthy and unfit for use. The *Sydney Morning Herald* publicized the unfitness of the Botany watershed for collection of the city's water.[109] In the 1860s, there had been official inquiries into the pollution of Sydney Harbor by sewerage, as well as into the quality of the water supply. But the resulting proposals (to construct ocean sewer outfalls at Bondi and Botany Bay or to carry sewerage to a distant treatment plant where it would be turned into fertilizer) were beyond the financial capacity of the City Council and required colonial government action. In the 1870s, the Royal Navy's Australian squadron complained about the very foul state of the harbor as a source of illness among naval personnel and pointed out that the governor's family was also at risk. Epidemics of measles and scarlet fever in 1875 finally prompted action, the still-strong miasmatic conception of disease causation linking (wrongly) filth and its effluvia to appearance of these infectious diseases. Premier John Robertson set up the Sydney City and Suburban Sewage and Health Board the same year. There was in any case a need to resolve a conflict with the City Council, which had rejected the previous Parkes government's proposal for a metropolitan board of works, modeled on that of London, to administer the city's water and sewerage systems. The council wanted to retain the profitable water supply.

The new expert board, composed of scientists, engineers, surveyors and doctors, and sitting between 1875 and 1877, produced twelve extensive reports covering a range of sanitary issues. The board recommended an interceptor system of sewers to divert flow from the city system to an ocean outfall at Ben Buckler, the north arm of Bondi Bay, and a south-flowing system for the southern suburbs to discharge onto a sewage farm at Botany

Bay. To solve the problem of pollution of the water supply, it proposed legislation to require flushing cisterns, and to grant councils power to deny water to lavatories liable to pollute the water system. A night-soil removal system to be run by local councils was recommended to remove the hazards presented by cesspits, still used extensively, especially outside the city area. Councils would also regulate cesspits and sewered lavatories. Tanneries and noxious trades, including the notorious Glebe Island abattoirs, were to be regulated better under the Nuisances Prevention Act, 1875. The board also extensively investigated substandard housing. It called for urgent action to implement strict inspection, adequate building regulations, efficient refuse removal, and a system of requiring landlords to keep properties in a good state of repair. Probably the board's main achievement, apart from documenting the very insanitary state of Sydney, was a much improved sewerage system.

In 1874, a search had been begun for an overseas engineer to evaluate the proposal for a new water supply drawing on the Nepean catchment area. William Clark, a distinguished hydraulic engineer, who had been responsible for Bristol's and Calcutta's sewerage systems, came to Sydney in 1876. Premier Robertson had looked to Britain "to mitigate greatly, if not wholly silence, any reasonable objections of our own engineers."[110] Clark approved in 1877 the proposed water and sewerage schemes for Sydney. The press and public opinion kept up pressure for construction of the new schemes. In 1877, 3,800 people petitioned for a comprehensive sewerage system, declaring that harbor pollution not only endangered health and life but discouraged the wealth-creating activities of immigration and trade. The colonial government's public works department carried out the construction of the schemes. The main southern sewer was finished in 1885, the Bondi outlet two years later. The Nepean water supply system was completed in 1888. Real estate advertisements now included the words "Nepean water laid on." In 1888, the Metropolitan Water and Sewerage Act created the Board of Water Supply and Sewerage, composed of the three interests historically concerned with water and sewerage: the colonial government (three members), the City Council (two members) and the suburban municipalities (two members). Between 1890 and 1914 the board achieved a great deal: average daily water supply increased from 8.4 to 36.5 million gallons; houses supplied with water, from 71,500 to 166,100; houses sewered, from 22,800 to 119,800; water mains, from 355 to 1,966 miles; and sewer mains from 70 to 930 miles.[111]

The 1875 board had recommended immediate creation of a central health authority, not democratically elected (because it had to be able to ignore intermittent unpopularity) and with power to compel action: "The disgraceful condition of the back yards and closets . . . should alone be sufficient to show the necessity for sanitary legislation."[112] As the *Sydney Morning Herald* observed, it was hopeless to leave reform to local government, with its ill-qualified inspectors and its aldermen so influenced by the "dictates of business" that they ignored vital public health concerns. An independent, expert and powerful authority was needed. But the colonial government continued to be inactive. A Health Society deputation in 1878 urgently pressed Premier James Farnell to introduce a public health bill. He replied that he could not guarantee it would pass.

Then, suddenly, apathy evaporated. What cholera did for England in 1848, smallpox did for NSW in 1881–82. A smallpox epidemic, the most serious to date, killed 26 percent of the 154 persons infected, although it did not spread beyond Sydney. Moreover, it quickly revealed the inadequacy of public health organization. The port health officer struggled with the emergency, and popular alarm mounted. About seven months from the start of the epidemic, the Parliament passed the Infectious Diseases Supervision Act of 1881, which created a Central Board of Health and required householders and doctors to report smallpox cases.[113] Since compulsory vaccination did not exist, the authorities instituted draconian isolation procedures. Ignorance and fear gave rise to scapegoating of the Chinese community. A ship carrying Chinese immigrants had been in quarantine because of a case of smallpox, and a child in a Chinese merchant family in the city was thought to have had smallpox, at the beginning of the epidemic. Popular racist feeling (buttressed by arguments about cheap Chinese labor taking jobs from Australian working men) was strongly reinforced, and Premier Henry Parkes lost no time in having the Influx of Chinese Restriction Act passed in December 1881.

On the face of it, the part-time board, born of crisis and lacking policy guidance as well as support staff, was doomed to oblivion once the emergency had passed. However, its president, the leading physician C.K. Mackellar, occupied two key medical positions—medical adviser to the government and port health officer. Further, board members were part of Sydney's small social elite and enjoyed some political influence. Even so, the board labored under the burden of divided ministerial responsibility, which reduced the board's effectiveness. While the board answered to the colonial treasurer, the colonial secretary usually dealt with public health policy matters.[114]

Sanitary reformers associated with the Board of Health, like Mackellar and H.N. MacLaurin, in the 1880s urged enactment of comprehensive public health legislation in the context of concern about the high prevalence of typhoid. In 1882 and again in 1884, Mackellar, president of the board (1882–85), told the medical section of the Royal Society of NSW that an act was greatly needed. A public meeting called by the mayor, Thomas Playfair, resolved that the meeting believed "it absolutely necessary" for the government to submit to Parliament "a comprehensive bill to provide for the public health." The resolution's seconder, Sir William Manning, had tried as early as 1854–55, when he was solicitor general, to have a public health bill enacted. The colonial secretary, Sir Alexander Stuart, told a deputation that a bill was being drafted but it faced obstacles: "The moment [a man's] . . . property was touched a serious difficulty was raised, and a measure of this kind could not be of service unless it interfered to a great extent with what men might call the liberty of property."[115] A comprehensive bill, modeled on the English Public Health Act, 1875, was introduced; Mackellar, having resigned as president of the board and become a member of the Legislative Council, strongly supported its enactment. The board had to have the power to force local authorities to act in the public interest, and the Victorian situation, where the public health bill had been "emasculated" in the interest of preserving local government powers, should not be repeated.[116] His successor as board president, MacLaurin, another leading medical practitioner, observed of a typhoid outbreak traced to a suburban dairy in 1886, "From the story of this outbreak we can all see the absolute necessity of some form of sanitary legislation."[117] The fall of the Stuart government and the dissolution of Parliament halted the bill's progress. The board, unable to obtain powers of compulsion, had to continue to rely on education and persuasion.

As early as the 1870s, a number of British epidemiological studies pointed to an association of typhoid epidemics with the milk supply. In 1877, the *Sydney Morning Herald* reported some of this work. The 1880s saw the identification of important bacterial pathogens associated with milk. Indeed, from the late 1880s medical and scientific publications on milk increased greatly in number, and this high interest was sustained until about 1915, after which there was a marked decline in concern.[118] In 1885, in Britain, the first of a series of "dairies, cowsheds and milkshops orders" was made by the Privy Council under the Contagious Diseases (Animals) Act, 1878. This law was concerned with cattle inspection, cleanliness of milk receptacles, and protection of milk from contamination.[119] In the United States, the first legislation dealing with milk was enacted by Massachusetts in the 1850s, and it prohibited adulteration. Bacterial standards were first proposed by New York in 1901; it set the standard (which was not implemented) at one million micro-organisms per cubic centimetre.

In 1860, following a parliamentary inquiry and in the face of rising public concern, the British Parliament had passed an Adulteration Act. When administration proved difficult, the Sale of Food and Drugs Act 1875 was passed; this allowed local authorities to appoint public analysts. Their appointment was made compulsory in 1879.[120] In NSW, the Adulteration of Food Prevention Act, 1879, was almost unused. In the first five years of its existence, only one prosecution was attempted, and it was dismissed. When the 1896 Public Health bill was being debated, D. Thomson, the member for Warringah in the Legislative Assembly, said that the act was "practically a dead letter."[121] The problem was that local authorities were notoriously reluctant to act against alleged adulterators; the lack of public analysts compounded difficulties.

In early 1886, John Ashburton Thompson, medical inspector to the Board of Health, was instructed by the president to inquire into the cause of a typhoid epidemic in Leichhardt, now an inner western suburb of Sydney. Thompson possessed a diploma of public health, virtually unknown in Australia at this time; he had gained it from Cambridge University in 1882. His report, the fruit of the first modern epidemiological inquiry in Australia, pinpointed milk from the insanitary Helsarmel dairy as the source of infection. It also revealed the poor sanitary state of the municipality and the negligence of the Leichhardt council, highlighting the need for the central control of local authorities that had been embodied in the failed 1885 Public Health Bill. In his report Thompson sounded a clarion call for further attempts at reform: "If it is clear that a people are exposed to a source of illness and death from which practically they cannot defend themselves, it becomes necessary for their Government to step in and set up a defence for them."[122] The Jennings government reacted quickly, with a Dairies Supervision Bill.

Mackellar, introducing the Dairies Supervision Bill, which was based on a section of the failed Public Health Bill, made clear the government's intention to leave regulation as far as possible to municipal councils. But in a shift toward central control, the act gave the board concurrent powers and capacity to compel compliance by local authorities. The four dairy inspectors originally appointed by the board had grown to fourteen by 1914. This was a first step toward a modern health bureaucracy. The act, which applied initially only to the metropolitan police district, was four years later in effect in the whole of the county of Cumberland, to the south in the Illawarra district, and to the west in Broken Hill. It was the first legislation to be influenced by the germ theory of infectious disease, still not universally accepted even in the local medical profession. It required human and some bovine infectious disease cases to be reported and forbade people infected or recently recovered to involve themselves in milk production. It also set strict standards of sanitation for dairies.[123] Although four further outbreaks of typhoid were traced to polluted wells on suburban dairies, by the mid-1890s, the board could report considerable sanitary improvement of metropolitan and country dairies.[124]

Calls from sanitary reformers and from doctors continued to be made for a general Public Health Act. In 1892–93, while in England, MacLaurin gathered information on legislation and administration; in his report to the Colonial Secretary he proposed a general health act. In 1895, the profession's journal, the *Australasian Medical Gazette,* made the same proposal, pointing out that such legislation had lowered the mortality rate in England and in Victoria.[125]

A comprehensive Public Health Act was finally put in place by the Reid government in 1896. Although G.R. Dibbs, leader of the Protectionist Party, had declared support for a bill while in opposition, in office he only went so far as to have passed the Noxious Trades and Cattle Slaughtering Act,

1894, which was modeled on the Dairies Supervision Act. It gave to the board general control over slaughterhouses and all noxious trades. When George Reid, the leader of the Free Trade Party, won the 1894 general election, he began to implement long-promised measures. His first reforms were economic: taxes on income and land, and universal local government taxes, along with lowering of customs duties and promotion of public service efficiency to reduce government spending. Reid observed, "Here are the people . . . paying over 2,000,000 pounds sterling through the Customs House; here are property and income paying nothing."[126] By the end of 1895, the colony's first Income and Land Tax Acts had been passed, and a Customs Act had got rid of Dibbs's tariff. Reid then embarked on social reform in a Public Service Act, a Factories and Shops Act, and a general Public Health Act.

In his second-reading speech, Reid pointed out that the bill was much briefer than Victoria's Act because the government wished to be cautious after the long delay in getting a Public Health Act; in any case, some matters were covered in existing legislation. The bill largely followed English acts, except where local conditions—such as the sparsely populated nature of rural areas—made this impossible; there, outside municipal areas, the police would administer the act. The number of preventable deaths was such that it was a "disgrace to our legislature" that legislation had not already been passed. While municipalities would execute the act, the Board of Health was given enough power to see that they did their duty. W.J. Lyne, the leader of the Protectionist opposition, said that having heard Dr. Ross, member for Molong (and sometime medical officer of health in Scotland and England) endorse the measure, the opposition would not obstruct it, although Parliament must not "take away any rights that exist." Dr. James Graham, well-known physician and member for Sydney, sympathized with the premier's difficulty in deciding the content of the bill inasmuch as public health embraced "a very great variety of subjects." He criticized the fragmented nature of administration and urged emulation of England, where the Local Government Board oversaw water supply and sewerage, factories and health care as well as general hygiene. The colony should follow England because "no nation in the world had a better health organisation" or "a better sanitary code."

The upper house also supported the bill. Mackellar noted that the legislation circumvented the situation where many local councillors had apparently sought election in fact to undermine the work of the health authorities. Other members, like Sir Arthur Renwick and R.E. O'Connor, were more sympathetic to the position of local councils, pointing out how lack of funds could hamstring effective execution of the act. O'Connor signaled the change in general attitudes since the 1880s when he observed that this interference with liberty and private rights would be intolerable but for the fact it was necessary for the public good.[127]

If appointment of dairy inspectors under the 1886 act and Ashburton Thompson's fine epidemiological work on typhoid outbreaks in the 1880s marked the beginning of professionalization of public health in NSW, the 1896 act represented another notable advance. Full-time medical officers of health were appointed to the two most populous urban centers in the colony, Sydney and Newcastle. W.G. Armstrong, appointed at Sydney, and Robert Dick at Newcastle, had been trained in the English school of public health, and they brought to bear the same skills and attitudes as those so effectively employed by their English counterparts. Armstrong was directly inspired by the efforts of leading English medical officers of health, like Arthur Newsholme, to reduce infant mortality. Soon after his appointment, Armstrong began the first systematic work in Australasia—three years before Truby King's more widely known work in New Zealand began—to reduce infant deaths from diarrheal and associated conditions. Inspectors of nuisances were transformed into sanitary inspectors under the 1896 act; soon after, courses of training were instituted for them, although it was only in 1933 that formal qualifications for health inspectors were required.[128]

Although a public health bill was debated in the Queensland Parliament not very long after the colony separated from NSW in 1859, many politicians failed to see sanitary reform as significant, let alone necessary. Even as late as 1919, a review of legislation placed the 1884 Health Act much lower in order of importance than the Crown Lands Act and the Defence Act. In 1865 an executive-order-in-council appointed a Central Board of Health, consisting of the colonial secretary, R.G.W. Herbert (president); the colonial architect, C. Tiffin; the harbors and rivers engineer, J. Brady; the police commissioner, D.T. Seymour; the Medical Board president, Dr. K. Cannan; and the health officer, Dr. W. Hobbs (secretary). The board drafted a bill, based wholly on the Victorian Public Health Act, to improve "the sanitary condition of towns and populous places within the colony."[129]

Introducing the bill to the Legislative Assembly in July 1865, Colonial Secretary Herbert said that it was needed to abate the nuisances prevalent in Brisbane and other large towns. But urban populations were too small to justify expensive sewerage systems; what was required were proper cesspits with an efficient night-soil disposal service. The bill received some support, but one member, a Mr. Taylor, opposed it as it benefited only insanitary towns like Brisbane and imposed additional municipal taxation on areas like his that were not insanitary. Herbert did not seem to value the measure much; at the committee stage he said it was not "immediately required," and at the end of the parliamentary session he allowed it to lapse. When the bill was reintroduced in 1866, it contained a new clause enabling the health officer to inquire into deaths where the person had been assisted by an unregistered practitioner, and then to launch prosecutions. At that time many in colonial parliaments and in the community resisted attempts by orthodox, registered doctors to have unregistered practitioners outlawed, and now a number of members of the Queensland parliament objected to this provision. The *Brisbane Courier* saw it as evidence of the registered practitioners' quest for a legal monopoly on medical care. The bill was, because of such objections, discharged from the paper. Moreover, some parliamentarians could not accept that the state should save individuals from the consequences of their insanitary habits. The Hon. W. Wood told the Legislative Council that he could not understand why, "if the inhabitants of a town chose to be dirty, the Ministry should step in to prevent them."[130]

Dr. K.O. O'Doherty, who was to become a great exponent of public health legislation, tried unsuccessfully to get health and hospital legislation through Parliament in 1871. However, the appearance of smallpox in New South Wales and Victoria had a facilitating effect when O'Doherty introduced another bill in July 1872. Based on a Canadian law, the legislation created a board of seven people. The appointees were H.G. Simpson MLC (Member of the Legislative Council), and Doctors W. Hobbs, K.I. O'Doherty, K. Cannan, and H. Bell, F. Rawkins and A.W. Manning (secretary). Dr. Hobbs, who had charge of the bill in the Legislative Council, emphasized that it was merely a temporary measure.[131] While the board was to advise on all sanitary concerns and issue regulations, and local boards were appointed, longer-term health advances were precluded by the fact that the measure applied only for six-month periods, although it could be reproclaimed. Local authorities, led by Brisbane Council, opposed proclamation. The Brisbane Council argued that its own by-laws were more effective but the real reason for its opposition was very likely reluctance to spend on local health boards.

Through the 1870s, attempts were made to improve the legislation. In 1874 the Central Board proposed a bill covering vaccination, regulation of boarding houses and adulteration of food, drinks and medicines. It also provided for compulsory creation of local boards. But some legislators saw the board members as legally unanswerable to voters whose taxes they could use for sanitary improvements. Its progress was halted when the colonial secretary had it removed from the paper. Another attempt to amend the act failed in the following year, and the same thing happened in 1877. An 1878 bill was introduced at a time of wide concern about Brisbane's excessive infant mortality rate: 245 per thousand births when that of England and Wales was 153. The bill covered quarantine, food adulteration, lodging houses, and the earth-closet system, and it ended the need to extend the legislation at six-month intervals. Yet, this bill too was defeated. Various factors account for this failure. The government health officer, Dr. Challinor, resented the board's interference in quarantine and its proposal to adopt the less restrictive British system of medical inspection of ships; he therefore lobbied the colonial secretary against the bill. Local authorities in that era of liberalism and strong belief in the sanctity of private property resented the board's desire to establish a clear right for inspectors to enter premises, and this resistance continued even beyond the 1884 Health Act.

Public health reformers, nonetheless, enjoyed some successes. In its 1877 report the board had urged control of adulteration, and here it made progress. The Sale of Food and Drugs Act of 1881 outlawed sale of goods "not being the article demanded" and containing substances injurious to health. The colonial government appointed Robert Mar government analyst, and the local authorities were entitled to appoint analysts as well.

As smallpox had hastened the birth of the 1872 act so typhoid smoothed the way for the 1884 act. The press and the public were concerned about both typhoid and the urban sanitary conditions. W.H. Groom, mayor of Toowoomba, told the colonial secretary in 1884 that earth closets were a disgrace and that typhoid was prevalent once more. Brisbane residents petitioned Colonial Secretary McIlwraith about the state of the sanitary depot on Ithaca Creek, itself so polluted and obnoxious some people in the vicinity had been forced to leave their homes. Creeks in other areas were polluted by slaughter yards, tanneries and other noxious establishments. With typhoid and dysentery very prevalent in 1884, and the press throughout the colony criticizing both the government and local authorities for failure to deal with insanitary conditions, the government introduced a new bill in August, just after news of cholera epidemics in Europe reached Brisbane. Based on the English Public Health Act, 1875, the 1884 bill was more comprehensive than that of 1872, and it was supported across the spectrum of politics. Dealing with the problem of inadequate funds for sanitary work, the act allowed the local authorities to levy a special health rate, while it required the government to pay the same endowment for this as for general rates. Premier Griffiths declared that in "every law relating to the public health[,] . . . the comfort of the individual must yield to the good of the public."[132] Even so, the 1884 measure very much needed to be supplemented by introduction of modern sewerage and drainage systems, as well as by a proper medical officer and department of health, as the *Colonist* wisely observed at the time.[133]

The corporation of the city of Adelaide had from the 1840s responsibility for control of infectious diseases and of public nuisances. During the 1850s and '60s, it continued to show its concern about disposal of liquid wastes and about infectious diseases. Indeed, in an era when the miasmatic conception of disease was still strong, the first problem was seen to be clearly related to the second.

There was considerable population growth in Adelaide in the 1860s and '70s. This, combined with the failure of local corporations to use their power under the municipal acts to abate nuisances and the lack of regulations in unincorporated areas, had the result that Adelaide had indeed become by the 1870s "a city of stenches" and foul airs. It was "impossible to walk through any of the streets . . . without being sickened by the smells from closets, stagnant water, and decomposing matters."[134] One of the key provisions of the 1873 public health bill was provision of a central board with capacity to do the work of recusant corporations, as one member fervently hoped would be the case: "District Councils and Corporations might not find it in their interests or inclination to stir up any matter to abate a nuisance. . . . [It was earnestly to be hoped] that if the bill became law it would not be allowed to remain a dead letter but that action would be taken to put down such nuisances as had been described."[135] Only the City Council Nuisance Committee had been actively concerned, and in 1865 the council offered a prize for the best essay on the subject of a sewerage system.[136] In 1870, under Mayor Judah Moss Solomon, the corporation had established a committee of inquiry and had taken evidence about a system of deep drainage, but when Solomon ceased to hold office, interest in the matter had died. Solomon had called a meeting in early 1871 after a deputation of leading colonists urged action to reduce nuisances, and the mayor of Kensington and Norwood as well as a number of district chairmen had attended. Sittings continued for well over two years, and a report was produced as well as interviews arranged with the chief secretary. The efforts of this local government group seem to have had an impact on the 1873 Public Health bill.[137]

The chief secretary, the Hon. A Blyth, introducing the 1873 bill, said that its intention was to create a central board of health with a paid chairman and local boards having the capacity to levy rates for public health work. The need for the legislation had become clear in the summer of 1870–71, when noxious smells, the "seeds of very dangerous maladies," had been especially prevalent. Existing sanitary provisions had proved inadequate, because the municipalities had been too susceptible to the influence of those employed in the noxious trades. There was always the danger of a cholera incursion and of epidemic under the sanitary conditions that existed.[138]

The 1873 Public Health Act established a central board and local boards, and it obliged the latter to appoint medically qualified health officers. It also provided for control of noxious trades, insanitary houses, drains and sewers, nuisances, and unwholesome food. The central board kept pressuring the local boards to be more active in sanitary reform, using the infant death rate and the infectious-disease death rates to show the need for a better water supply, sanitation and building regulations. From the late 1870s, two doctors at the Children's Hospital, S.J. Magarey and Allan Campbell (Campbell was a central board member), added their voices to the central board's campaign to reduce the infant mortality rate, particularly from diarrheal disease. Both stressed the critical role of the care provided by mothers in prevention of such deaths—a perspective on reduction of infant mortality that was common in Australia, as in the United Kingdom and United States in the late nineteenth and early twentieth century, as noted earlier.

In 1876, Parliament had appointed a commission composed of legislators, Doctors William Gosse and Allan Campbell of the central board, and J.M. Sinclair, mayor of Port Adelaide, to inquire into sanitary provisions within the colony. But the amending act of the same year was more limited than reformers wanted. This was because of the opposition of members from rural districts to provisions aimed at ensuring adequate water and sanitation for new houses: "A bad house was better than no house at all," asserted one member.[139] Dr. Horatio Whittell, president of the central board, 1883–99, reported in 1883 to the board and the chief secretary on the dreadful state of Adelaide and the legislative amendments needed to empower local boards to improve it. He wrote concerning Adelaide, "Sanitary conditions are either utterly disregarded, or are left to the caprice of the inhabitants."[140]

In 1884, an amending bill was introduced in reaction to an outbreak of smallpox at Border Town. The original intention was to provide for control of "exotic diseases" of this type, but its provisions were widened to cover more mundane infections like scarlet fever, diphtheria and typhoid.[141] The 1884 act empowered health authorities to isolate tenements and prevent access to premises in which infections had occurred. For the first time in Australian public health history, the law unambiguously required the attending doctor to report infectious diseases to the central health authority.[142] In 1891, the health officer for Kensington, Norwood, St. Peters and Burnside, Thomas Borthwick, drawing on the annual reports of the Central Board, observed that "throughout the colony hygienic conditions are bad—defective drainage, imperfect construction of cesspits, tainted water supply, and insufficient scavenging arrangements being perhaps the chief faults."[143] Sanitary legislation was too permissive, granting the Central Board only "limited and ill-defined powers." It allowed local boards to be too often full of men opposed to spending on sanitation, and to employ ill-paid health officers who were required not to carry out their duties too zealously.

From the late 1880s, influenced by the advent of a bacteriological approach to public health, the South Australian medical profession had been urging that notification of infectious diseases be extended. Allan Campbell spearheaded this campaign. In 1898, in an address to the South Australian Institute of Hygiene and Bacteriology, he proposed such measures as regulation of dairies and inspection of beef cattle carcasses to control the spread of tuberculosis. Even so, the 1898 Health Act did not create a powerful Central Board for metropolitan areas, as proponents had wanted. Indeed, opponents of the bill, as of earlier bills, did not want a strong health authority, acting from collective responsibility, to replace individual responsibility for health; governments "should not always be mollycoddling," nor should state legislation challenge the law of the survival of the fittest. Indeed, one indication of the value placed on the work of the central board is to be seen in the refusal of the government to accede to the request of the new president, William Ramsay Smith (who replaced Whittell in 1899), to publish its annual report. No report was published between 1891 and the mid-1930s.[144]

In July 1856, the *Tasmanian Daily News* initiated a series of pieces on public health in Hobart. Intended to arouse public awareness of the appalling state of the city, they were authored by Dr. E.S. Hall, Australia's first epidemiologist and a pioneer of public health reform. The newspaper introduced its educational campaign with an editorial on public health, pointing out that for reasons of humanity, self-preservation, community well-being, and financial stability, public health should be the concern of everyone. Yet collective fatalism reigned supreme, except for "a few ardent individuals—the medical practitioners . . . leading the van—perseveringly drawing public attention to the vast extent of remediable and preventable disease . . . inflicted upon us by neglect of the most simple laws of hygiene."[145] In 1855, it said, Hobart had a general death rate of almost thirty per thousand population, or 25 percent more than what was considered an excessive rate in London. Hall began another service to public health education in October 1856, when he wrote his first monthly statistical report on the health of Hobart (sent first to the Royal Society of Tasmania and then to the press). He identified the types of diseases prevalent and their causes as well as the number of deaths. He continued to furnish these reports without interruption for the next twenty-five years, until his death in 1881.[146]

With the coming of responsible government in 1856, Hobart and Launceston, the two major urban centers, were incorporated. The Hobart Town Improvement Act, 1857, and the Launceston Improvement Act, 1858, gave the two corporations power to pave, cleanse and drain as well as to appoint city surveyors and health officers. The Police Act of 1865 replaced the above acts, giving the councils control over everything to do with "the health and comfort" of residents. The act enabled the council to appoint "a legally qualified medical practitioner of competent skill and experience who shall be styled the Officer of Health."[147]

Hall believed that various measures taken by the two corporations had improved community health in the two cities. In 1872, using his statistical records, he concluded that "deaths in Tasmania have been undergoing a great reduction of late years."[148] A better water supply, a larger proportion of native-born citizens, and the decline in numbers of ex-convicts, "imported adults of originally depraved constitutions," all had contributed to this improvement. But Hobart still suffered from the effects of cesspools (which were rarely cleaned out), unremoved refuse, and badly built drains.[149] The government of W.R. Giblin showed that public health awareness was growing by having enacted three laws: the Sale of Food and Drugs Act, 1880, which enabled councils to appoint analysts to deal with adulteration or have the work done by the government analyst for a fixed charge; the Rivers Pollution Prevention Act of 1881 (drawing on the 1876 British act), which sought to prevent pollution by sawmills, sewers, factories and mines; and the Women and Children Employment Act, 1884, which aimed to improve sanitary facilities in establishments employing women and children.[150] In 1884 was also passed the Public Health (Hobart) Act, which required that cesspools be eradicated by 1887 and introduced penalties for public exposure of infected persons. In the following year the new Public Health Act was passed. This closely followed the Victorian Act of 1883. Amending acts dealing with details of administration were passed in 1887, 1889 and 1896. Premier Adye Douglas justified any "restriction of public liberty" in the 1885 act on the ground that "all knew that it was the duty of all Governments to protect as far as possible the public health." Since ratepayers' personal interests were not infrequently prejudicial to public health, the legislation created a Central Board of Health as "an independent body, apart from the municipal body [*sic*], who, perhaps, were prevented from taking action by dread of their constituents."[151] Both the Hobart and Launceston corporations opposed the bill, Launceston manifesting the typical nineteenth-century democratic suspicion of unelected and centralized boards. To place the local authorities elected by the people under a board nominated by the Crown was considered "a retrograde step subversive of the spirit which animates every British Constitution." Hobart corporation pointed out that it had a qualified health officer and "faithfully administered" the current sanitary legislation.[152] The opposition was fruitless. Central supervision of the sanitary activities of local authorities had arrived, and laissez faire principles gave way to more efficient pursuit of the people's health.

In Western Australia, while the Police Act of 1861 had included sections on nuisances, privies and night soil removal, only with the Municipal Institutions Act of 1871 were general sanitary powers instituted. The act empowered municipal councils to put down nuisances; prevent the sale of unwholesome meat, fish and vegetables; compel householders to cleanse premises of offensive matter; and restrain noisome trades. It also gave them responsibility for licensing slaughterhouses. The 1876 Municipal Institutions Act enlarged the powers of councils. It gave them control of drains and sewers and of the maintenance of privies, while providing for prevention of domestic overcrowding and for creation of sanitary depots. If the municipal councils had the means to advance sanitation, however, they failed to make much use of them, as the colonial surgeon, Alfred Waylen, noted in 1883: "I have for so many years past animadverted on the absence of some system of sewage disposal and the consequent contamination of drinking water not only in Perth and Fremantle but in other towns of the colony, that I only now refer to the subject in the hope that ere long, Municipal Councils will become alive to a sense of this duty."[153]

Governor Napier Broome decided that if the councils would not deal with the problem, the colonial government would. A royal commission on the sanitary condition of Perth and Fremantle, with Waylen as chairman, decided in 1885 that underground drainage was both expensive and unnecessary. The municipalities had ample powers, and to make sure they enforced regulations, the commission recommended establishment of a Central Board of Health, nominated by the governor. The Public Health Bill, 1886, provided for a Central Board and local boards answerable to it, all nominated by the governor. Some protest was expressed in the debate on the bill about this step away from representative government at the local level. The period 1883–89 was a difficult one for the governor, because of the impact of the early gold rushes and the growing demand for self-government.[154] But the acting attorney general, the Honorable S. Burt, defended the move by pointing to the elective principle as the enemy of local government efficiency in health. The 1871 Municipal Institutions Act was a dead letter; while it contained numerous provisions on public health, only in a few cases had these been enforced. Constant complaints had been made, and the medical profession had continued to warn about the need for enforcement of sanitary regulations. Moreover, the colony, being now in frequent communication with Singapore, Mauritius and other potential sources of epidemic disease, needed a body to deal with the threat of epidemics of cholera and smallpox.[155] Even Mayor George Shenton of Perth admitted that it was impossible for councils to deal properly with sanitation, because, elected only for short periods, "they did not care to take upon themselves the serious responsibilities of carrying out such a bill as this."[156]

The Public Health Act of 1886, the first general health code in Western Australia, was framed along the lines of the 1875 English act with modifications to allow for local conditions. Sections concerning reporting of infectious diseases and control of movements of contacts were drawn from the South Australian act. Amendments were made in the 1890s. The 1895 amendment included "low, Colonial, or Typhoid Fever" among the dangerous infectious diseases; it arose from the contemporary experience of high mortality from typhoid on the Coolgardie goldfields. Sanitary improvements were being made, but typhoid remained at the close of the century a serious health problem. Lacking adequate sanitation control, Western Australia experienced in 1890–1900 typhoid activity of a level seen in the other states only in earlier periods.[157]

THE RISE OF THE PUBLIC HEALTH PROFESSIONAL

Sociologists since Max Weber and Émile Durkheim in the nineteenth century have been concerned with the professions as central features of the organization of secular, scientific-industrial society. Weber saw professionalization as the process by which some occupations achieved monopolies in the market for their specialized labor. Contemporary sociologists of professions like Eliot Freidson have stressed the medical profession's control of its particular corpus of expert knowledge as a key to the maintenance of its monopoly. The licence to practice is the means by which control over the supply of expert knowledge is exercised, while state law lays down what the qualifications are to be. As Freidson has observed, special knowledge and state-conferred monopoly over practice are the two sources of professional power.[158]

Britain: The Medical Officer of Health

Parallel with the growth of modern public health administration in Britain from the mid-nineteenth century came the rise of the pivotal public health professional—the medical officer of health, or health officer. The 1848 Public Health Act empowered local health boards to appoint legally qualified medical practitioners as health officers. In 1855, it became compulsory for medical officers of health (MOHs) to be appointed to London sanitary districts, and in 1872 this requirement was extended to provincial sanitary districts in England and Wales, although the legislation laid down no special qualifications. The Local Government Act, 1888, which created a new tier of county authorities above that of local authorities, required health officers of districts with more than fifty thousand people to have a registered public health qualification, while the Public Health (London) Act of 1891 required all metropolitan appointees to have specialist qualifications. By 1900, the MOHs had not only achieved "closure" of their particular occupational market but used an ideology of prevention and community-oriented practice to differentiate their expertise from that of practitioners of curative medicine. Indeed, as early as 1851 the General Board of Health had defined their work as being different from that of private clinicians—"the detection . . . and . . . the removal and prevention of the common localising causes of disease. . . . This . . . forms no part of the ordinary duty of private medical practitioners."[159]

Henry Rumsey, general medical practitioner, supporter of state medicine and spokesman for the medical profession, told the Royal Sanitary Commission in 1868 that a physician or surgeon could become an MOH and even continue hospital work but that he should cease general practice. Rumsey, who published *Essays in State Medicine* in 1856, worked with William Stokes, Regius Professor of Physic in the University of Dublin, and George Paget, president of the British Medical Association (BMA), to obtain BMA support for postgraduate training in state medicine. The National Association for the Promotion of Social Science also supported the proposal. Despite a lack of regard for doctors and suspicion of their professional self-interest, Edwin Chadwick (with William Farr), representing the National Association, petitioned for a royal commission on state medicine, including training aspects. The BMA in early 1868 asked the General Medical Council to establish standards for a registrable state medicine qualification. When agreement on course content could not be reached, the universities went ahead on their own, developing a variety of curricula. In 1895, the General Medical Council finally imposed standardization.

Cambridge offered the first qualification, an M.D. in state medicine, in 1868, but this program was not to become a popular choice; the postgraduate certificates or diplomas of Trinity College, Dublin, Cambridge, Oxford, London and Edinburgh (degree) or the London Conjoint Board became the preferred qualifications in public health. By the close of 1886, fourteen licensing bodies were offering qualifications in sanitary science, state medicine and public health. In 1871–1973, when the diploma in public health (DPH) was required by law for public health practice, these five universities, together with the London Conjoint Board, were the major providers of training. In most years of that period, they awarded 50 percent of diplomas. Prior to 1900, Cambridge led in the award of certificates. Later, the London Conjoint Board and the London School of Hygiene and Tropical Medicine (University of London) became the leading bodies. The DPH carried considerable educational and professional weight, being equivalent to an M.D. or FRCS; unlike other postgraduate qualifications in medicine, it was an exclusive license to practice a particular discipline. The early 1890s saw two to three hundred doctors taking the DPH annually. Indeed, many more graduates were being produced than there were positions available.

Trinity College awarded its certificate in state medicine for the first time in mid-1871, but only one of the four graduates registered the qualification with the General Medical Council. The university did not teach students—this was common early on, and the situation changed only gradually—but it held examinations covering law, engineering, pathology, vital and sanitary statistics, chemistry, meteorology, state medicine, medical jurisprudence, and hygiene. Cambridge offered a certificate in sanitary science from 1875; Part 1 of the examination involved physics and chemistry and how they applied to sanitation, while Part 2 involved "the causes and prevention of epidemic and infectious diseases, the . . . conditions of life . . . injurious to health and the Laws of the Realm which relate to Public Health."[160] Edinburgh offered a B.Sc. in public health from 1874. It was the only degree registered until an M.D. in state medicine from London University was registered in 1892. Edinburgh's examination was practically oriented: Part 1 covered chemistry, sanitary law and physics; Part 2 was made up of two papers, one on medicine as applied to public health, the other on practical sanitation. At Oxford, until 1895 the certificate of public health and preventive medicine could be obtained only by graduates of the small preclinical school, so there was difficulty getting candidates—during the twenty-nine years this restriction applied, only two certificates were awarded. Oxford initiated the certificate in 1876, as did London its certificate in state medicine. In the 1870s and '80s the standards set by licensing bodies varied. But the 1886 Medical Act established a register for sanitary science qualifications.

In 1889, the surviving regional associations of MOHs (the North-Western, Yorkshire and Birmingham, and Midland, all formed in 1875) and the older Metropolitan Association (established in 1856) combined to form a national body, the Society of Medical Officers of Health, with aims both "academical" and "political." Organizational unity contrasted with divisions within the new profession: between full-time and part-time officers, between metropolitan and provincial, and between those with specialist qualifications and those without. When tenure was established in the metropolitan area in 1891, provincial officers became vocal about the failure of the society's London-dominated council to pursue the same for them. From the early 1880s the Local Government Board had been strongly pushing the local authorities to appoint full-time officers. The society was keen in its turn to persuade the board to support tenure for MOHs. Finally, in 1905, the president of the board, Gerald Balfour, declared that he could not support universal tenure, because it would entrench unqualified men, whereas the board wanted to replace them with full-time, qualified officers.[161]

With the passing of the 1872 Public Health Act, the Local Government Board had set out what was needed in inspectors of nuisances (as well as medical officers of health) by way of qualifications, tenure, and duties. Following a public meeting convened by Dr. Lory Marsh in London in mid-1876, the Sanitary Institute of Great Britain (later the Royal Sanitary Institute) was established. It had three objectives: to hold meetings for the purpose of hearing papers, to keep a watching brief on all public health bills, and to become chartered to examine and grant certificates to sanitary surveyors and inspectors of nuisances. The institute, supported by public health notables like Edwin Chadwick and William Farr, granted its first certificates to five of eight candidates in 1877. In 1894, examination of surveyors became the responsibility of the Institute of Municipal and County Engineers. Large numbers of women began to be trained for the certificate of the sanitary inspector, and they found ready employment as inspectors of factories and workshops having female employees. In 1908, the Sanitary Institute introduced examinations for health visitors and school nurses as public health services became involved with the health of particular population groups, like infants and school children. The conditions of appointment and duties of sanitary inspectors in the provinces were laid down in the Sanitary Officers (Outside London) Order of 1910. The Public Health (Officers) Act, 1921, conferred security of tenure on sanitary inspectors and MOHs employed by county boroughs and county districts; the minister of health had the final say in their removal from office.[162]

The United States: Schools of Public Health

Although many of the American states established boards of health in the 1870s and '80s, the United States was slower than Britain to create specific training and certification for public health professionals. When plans for educational programs were discussed in the early twentieth century, some wanted to follow the British model, which focused on imparting practical skills in public health administration, while others wanted the German model of research-oriented education, which enabled basic scientific approaches to be applied to changing problems. The University of Michigan awarded the first public health degree in 1910, but it was William Sedgwick (who had trained in biology at Johns Hopkins University) who organized the first school—at the Massachusetts Institute of Technology, where he had gone as assistant professor of biology in 1883. Sedgwick did not necessarily place the medically trained health officer at the apex, as chief executive, in the British tradition. Medicine might have spawned sanitary science, but the latter was now an independent discipline, focused on health, where medicine was concerned with disease. Sedgwick's Department of Biology produced the laboratory expert trained in chemistry, parasitology and bacteriology, and the Department of Sanitary Engineering the engineer, who dealt with removal of waste products from the environment (as well as with ventilation, heating, housing and industrial hygiene). The physician would diagnose infections, examine schoolchildren, and administer diphtheria antitoxin. Nonmedical laboratory workers or engineers, if they had the aptitude, could become health planners and administrators. Sedgwick saw his graduates assume posts as engineers, laboratory scientists and health officers in many municipal and state public health authorities, but he never managed to attract more than a few doctors into training.

In 1912, President A. Lawrence Lowell of Harvard asked Professor George Whipple to work toward connecting his Sanitary Engineering Department with MIT's program in sanitary science and engineering, in order to establish a course for health officers. Whipple, Sedgwick and Professor Milton Rosenau of Preventive Medicine and Hygiene at Harvard formed in 1913 the administrative board of the new joint School for Health Officers of Harvard and MIT. In 1914 the new school awarded its first certificates of public health. Admission standards were high, and while the M.D. was not necessary for admission, it was already clear that those having a medical degree had a better chance of gaining the higher administrative posts in public health. A doctor of public health degree was also available to nonmedical as well as medical graduates. Charles-Edward Amory Winslow, a biologist and former member of Sedgwick's department and the former director of publicity in the New York State Health Department, became in 1915 the first Anna M. Lauder Professor of Public Health at Yale University. Winslow's department was located within the Medical School, and although he lectured to medical students on public health, he was, like Sedgwick, not very successful in attracting them into public health careers. His main commitment was preparation of public health students for the Certificate in Public Health, Ph.D. and Doctorate of Public Health.

Despite efforts to encourage students to see medicine in its social context, as progress in basic and clinical sciences accelerated medicine returned to its reductionist path. It diverged from the population and from the preventive road of public health.[163] In the United Kingdom and countries, like Australia, that took over the British model of public health more or less complete, the dominance of the medically qualified public health professional was unchallenged by the end of the nineteenth century. But in the United States, public health leaders like Sedgwick and Winslow were biologists, coming out of the scientific research tradition pioneered by Germany, and departments of sanitary engineering were prominent parts of the university-based training of public health professionals. There in the early twentieth century the sanitary engineers, the only professional group significant enough to do so, challenged the growing influence of physicians. But while the model that set the trend in public health school development—the Johns Hopkins University School of Hygiene and Public Health—made training in public health institutionally separate from the medical school, medically trained public health workers continued to enjoy considerable standing, even if relatively few medical graduates forsook the income and status of private curative medicine for public health careers.

The Rockefeller Foundation formed in 1909 the Sanitary Commission to eradicate hookworm disease from the American South. This effort had inevitably led the commission into public health development, a concern that grew in scope when in 1914 the hookworm eradication program became international. Wickliffe Rose, the director of the commission, set out to promote university training for full-time public health professionals, believing that proper training of professionals had to be oriented toward community health rather than clinical medicine's individual patients.[164] In late 1914, Abraham Flexner—famous for his report on medical education in the United States and Canada (1910), which led to the modern organization of medical teaching in America—convened a conference of leading figures in public health and Rockefeller personnel under the auspices of the General Education Board. The conference explored issues relating to the future, including the difficult one of whether public health officials should be qualified in medicine. While some, like William H. Welch, dean of Johns Hopkins Medical School, were keen to take this path, others saw that medical graduates were overwhelmingly choosing the lucrative rewards of private clinical practice as the Flexner reforms led to higher incomes.

In 1915, the Welch-Rose report was accepted by the General Education Board. There were two drafts of the report—the first by Rose and the final text by Welch. Rose envisaged a national public health school connected to a network of state schools. The latter would spread public health education at the grassroots level through extension courses like the ones run successfully by state agricultural colleges under the Rockefeller plan to modernize agriculture in the South. Welch's emphasis was more on research than spread of existing knowledge and best practice, though he wanted ideally each to receive appropriate emphasis. He wanted more of the German emphasis on teaching and research in hygiene than the English concern with public health administration. Rose had been clear that the public health school should be separate from the medical school but cooperating with it, so that basic courses in medicine would not need to be taught in both schools. Welch played down the idea of the differences between medicine and public health, insisting that his independent public health institute should cooperate with a teaching hospital in the teaching of preventive medicine. Welch's insistence on easy access to medical education facilities proved to be vital in deciding where the new Rockefeller-supported public health school would be located. In the evaluation of universities (and cities), Columbia University in New York City and the University of Pennsylvania were found lacking, particularly because their professors of the medical schools were in many instances not outstanding researchers. Johns Hopkins won, essentially because of its medical school, which embodied Flexner's idea of proper medical education: "[Although the] general resources of the University and of the community are inferior . . . to those found in New York, Boston and Philadelphia[,] the Medical School fulfils the requisite conditions in the highest degree anywhere obtainable."[165]

In mid-1916, the Rockefeller Foundation provided initial funds for the new school at Johns Hopkins—"the School of Hygiene and Public Health," the title reflecting an attempted reconciliation of the English idea of "a school of public health" and the German one of "a research institute of hygiene." In the early life of the new institution, Welch promoted the latter model, while the Rockefeller Foundation wanted more emphasis on applied public health and community health education. The Hopkins model was soon taken up elsewhere in the country, even influencing the preexisting Harvard-MIT school. In 1922, having divorced itself from MIT, the new Harvard school (with funds from the Rockefeller Foundation) was opened near the Harvard Medical School, and its dean, D.L. Edsall, became dean of the School of Public Health as well. Public health programs in other important universities—Yale, Columbia and Michigan—copied the content and methods employed at Johns Hopkins and Harvard. The hope that medicine would be permeated by the public health approach was not realized, however, as high-technology medicine attracted superior resources, and medical graduates overwhelmingly chose careers in clinical research and practice. These leading schools of public health pursued the "medical model" of public health, producing a small flow of graduates into elite public health posts.[166]

Australia: The Medical Officer of Health

Australia did not acquire its national school of public health until 1930 (its establishment and growth will be discussed later). However, British-trained specialists in public health, at first British-born medical immigrants and then graduates of local medical schools of the British type, became more common. As might be expected, it was the larger colonies that tended to attract the first modern public health professionals. The first was John Ashburton Thompson (born 1846), who came to enjoy an international reputation for his epidemiological work on leprosy and plague. In 1872 he had become surgeon in London to the Great Northern Railway Company; thereafter he had practiced obstetrics, becoming a member of the council of the Obstetrical Society of London in 1877. A breakdown in health led to departure in 1878 from London for New Zealand, from where he soon went to Australia. Having obtained the M.D. of the University of Brussels with distinction in 1878, Thompson obtained the diploma of public health of Cambridge University in 1882. In 1884, he was appointed temporarily medical officer to the NSW Board of Health, and the next year he became medical inspector to the board and deputy medical adviser to the NSW government.

Thompson was the first public health doctor with modern qualifications in public health to be employed by that or any other colonial government in Australia. In 1896, he became chief medical officer and president of the Board of Health, embarking upon the construction of a public health service. He was much involved in the preparation of the 1896 public health bill. He had likewise been heavily involved in the drafting of the previous significant public health legislation, the Dairies Supervision Act of 1886. He was a key figure in a number of significant commissions of inquiry, some national in scope. These included, in the 1880s, one on a national quarantine system for the colonies, and in the 1890s, one on the causes and prevention of lead poisoning among miners and smelters in the colony's metals-mining center, Broken Hill. In the 1900s he formulated a model pure-food code that enabled the different states to produce individual acts similar enough in content to achieve national uniformity. Distinguished as his record in public health administration was, it was his achievements in epidemiology that had international significance. He won international recognition for his publications on leprosy and on the bubonic plague. In 1896 he visited Molokai, the leper settlement in Hawaii, to study the disease. He won the prize awarded by the National Leprosy Fund of Great Britain for the best history of leprosy. The coming of bubonic plague to Sydney in 1900 enabled Thompson to contribute very significantly to etiological knowledge, which was still incomplete. Moreover, his practical efforts were highly successful. His well-organized war on rats—tens of thousands were killed—denied them food, water and harborage. Although the bacillus remained deadly (thirty-three of every hundred cases died), the epidemic was contained effectively. In the worst year, 1900, only 303 cases were reported in the colony.

Several observers in the 1890s had suggested that plague in humans was dependent on plague in rats. Thompson was impressed by E.H. Hankin's suggestion that "the degree in which plague prevailed stood in relation to the accessibility of dwellings to rats"[167] and by P.L. Simond's belief that the flea acted as intermediary between rat and human. However, experiments failed to support Simond's claim. Indeed, the German Plague Commission of 1899 concluded that fleabites were probably not a route of transmission.

The first Indian Plague Commission, in 1901, declared the epidemiological significance of rats was limited to the first outbreak of disease in a place, and that when plague was established, human agency was more significant in diffusion than that of rats.

Thompson appreciated that epidemiological methods had been hitherto greatly overlooked and understood that Sydney conditions offered a fine opportunity to apply his epidemiology. As Thompson noted in his address to the American Medical Association in 1906, "At Sydney . . . the invaded population numbered about 500,000. It was not merely wholly white, of English extraction and speech, and fully civilised, but intelligent, instructed and orderly, accustomed to direction and amenable to it. Management of the outbreaks rested solely with the central Department of Public Health, which had not merely wide statutory powers, but in unforeseen contingencies had the practically unlimited authority which the Executive Government occasionally conferred upon it."[168] Thompson produced a series of official reports on plague in 1900–1907. His analysis of the epidemiological facts led him to conclude that plague was transferred from rat to rat, and from rat to human by the flea. The second Indian Plague Commission (from 1905) endorsed his findings through experiment and field and laboratory observation, quoting him freely in its reports. He also received further recognition. The American Medical Association invited him to address their meeting in Boston in 1906. He subsequently addressed the International Congress of Hygiene in Berlin and the Royal Society of Medicine in London. In 1912 he received an invitation, which he was unable to accept, from the committee organizing the International Congress of Hygiene meeting in Washington, D.C., to become an official referee on plague, along with Surgeon General Rupert Blue, head of the U.S. Public Health Service, and Professor Shibanuro Kitasato (who had been, with Alexandre Yersin, the discoverer of the plague bacillus in 1894) of Japan.

Thompson was himself one of the new breed of diplomates in public health, and he insisted that all medical staff members of his new public health service possess the diploma or an equivalent qualification. He had trained medical officers of health appointed to Sydney and Newcastle. W.G. Armstrong and Robert Dick, the new MOHs, conducted regular courses of lectures in sanitary law and practice for sanitary inspectors from 1898. Thompson, who was an honorary fellow of the Royal Sanitary Institute and was elected an honorary fellow of the Society of Medical Officers of Health of Great Britain in 1896, requested the institute to conduct examinations for local sanitary inspectors. The NSW board of examiners was the first to be established outside the United Kingdom, and the first examination was held at the close of 1900. By the mid-1920s more than four hundred trained sanitary inspectors were at work in NSW. Following the NSW lead, other Australian states and New Zealand instituted such examinations.[169]

Local textbooks for sanitary inspectors were soon being produced. In 1901, *The Australian Sanitary Inspector's Text Book* was published in Sydney. Its authors were J.L. Bruce, lecturer in charge of the Sanitation Department of Sydney Technical College, examiner for London Sanitary Institute Certificates in Australia, president of the Sanitary Department Examining Board, and formerly consulting engineer to the Glasgow corporation; and T.M. Kendall, medical adviser to the Metropolitan Board of Water Supply and Sewerage, Sydney. In his preface, D.A. Gresswell, chairman of the Victorian Board of Public Health, welcomed the book, because hitherto the sanitary inspector had lacked "a trustworthy, complete, and withal readily understood handbook." The coverage was certainly comprehensive and up to date, with chapters on climate, food, water, parasites, infectious diseases, disinfection (including vaccination, quarantine, compulsory notification, isolation and disinfection of the person), air, buildings, and sewage and refuse disposal.[170] As other states introduced modern public health services, some felt the need for locally produced books as well. Thus, J.S.C. Elkington, M.D., DPH, commissioner of public health for Queensland and later an important figure in the development of the Federal Health Department, published *The Queensland Sanitary Inspector's Guide* in Brisbane in 1911. Elkington wrote about half of it, but there were also contributions from senior sanitary inspectors, architects and lawyers.[171] By the 1920s, the sanitary inspector, now "the health inspector," could be sure that he had arrived as a public health professional. The Health Inspector's Association of Australia (NSW Branch) noted in 1923: "In years gone by the Local Health Inspector was regarded as an official of little account. All this has now changed, and the occupation is now coming to be regarded as an honourable profession."[172]

NSW might have employed the first public health doctor with postgraduate qualifications in public health, but Victoria, the other colony with a large urban population, was not far behind. The 1889 Victorian Health Act provided for a Department of Public Health and a medical inspector. Warmly recommended by Sir Richard Thorne, principal medical officer of the Local Government Board, Dan Astley Gresswell, M.A., M.D. (Oxon), MRCS, DPH, arrived in Melbourne in 1890 to become the first medical inspector. In 1894 he became chairman of the Board of Public Health and permanent head of the Department of Public Health. Soon after his arrival in the colony, Gresswell carried out an extensive and critical survey of sanitary conditions and administration in Melbourne. Between then and his premature death in 1904, he produced sixteen special reports important to public health progress in Victoria. The reports included one on isolation of persons with communicable diseases (1891), remediable conditions concerning typhoid (1892), disposal of liquid waste and human refuse (1892), smallpox (1892), Asiatic cholera (1892), dysentery and the water supply (1893), charitable institutions (1893), typhoid in the city of Ballarat (1896), diphtheria in the suburb of Hawthorn (1897), drinking water (1897), microorganisms in airborne dust (1897), a metropolitan fever hospital (1898), and prevention and cure of tuberculosis (1902). Among his contributions was a code of duties for health officers and sanitary inspectors.[173]

Victoria had been the first colony to introduce a public health act, as we have seen. It was also to have a professional association of health officers at an early stage. In 1872, when forty-nine health officers served the colony, an association was formed for the purpose of better carrying out the requirements of the Health Act and for the promotion of the interests of doctors who acted as health officers. One such interest was improvement of the poor salaries that most municipalities paid their part-time health officers. The association died after only a very brief life, meeting only a couple of times, but the issue of poor remuneration continued to irk health officers. In 1884, the *Australian Medical Journal*, the Victorian medical profession's journal, complained that salaries were kept to a minimum. Indeed, Parliament, which had recently contemplated a statutory minimum of fifty pounds per annum, had misguidedly opted for ten pounds a year as the minimum.[174] With the passing of modern legislation in 1889 and the creation of a modern administration under Gresswell in the 1890s, the health officers appear to have taken heart again. The Society of Health Officers of Victoria held its first general meeting in Melbourne in late 1896.[175]

The process of professionalization of public health continued in the smaller colonies and states. In South Australia, Thomas Borthwick, a fellow of the Society of Medical Officers of Health, London, and a fellow of the Royal Institute of Public Health, was appointed medical officer of health for the city of Adelaide in 1900. He was a keen exponent of the new bacteriologically based public health, being appointed honorary bacteriologist of Adelaide Children's Hospital in 1894. He also lectured on bacteriology at the University of Adelaide Medical School and was an examiner for the Royal Sanitary Institute. He might have become president of the Board of Health instead of William Ramsay Smith in 1899 but for the bitter political conflict between the local medical profession and the reforming premier of South Australia, the radical-liberal Charles Cameron Kingston. Smith and A.D.L. Napier, both well-qualified physicians, were recruited by the South Australian government in 1896 in Britain and were brought out to Adelaide to staff the Adelaide Hospital and so break the "strike" by the honorary (unremunerated) medical staff.[176]

Nathaniel ("Bertie") Burnett Ham, an Australian-born pharmacist from Victoria, graduated MRCS, England, and LRCP, London, in 1896. He received his DPH, Cambridge, in 1897 and was awarded his M.D. with distinction in 1900 by the Université Libre de Bruxelles. The Queensland Home Secretary, J.G. Foxton, stated in 1900 that Burnett Ham, "a medical practitioner experienced in sanitary science,"[177] would be appointed first commissioner of public health. When still at Guy's Hospital Medical School,

London, Ham had received in 1896 the Golding-Bird Gold Medal and Scholarship for Sanitary Science. His popular textbook on public health, *A Handbook of Sanitary Law for the Use of Candidates for Public Health Qualifications,* published in London in 1899, was "intended mainly for the use of medical students desirous of taking the Diploma of Public Health."[178] By 1938 it had gone through twelve editions. Elected a fellow of the Royal Sanitary Institute of Great Britain, he became a fellow of the Society of Tropical Medicine and Hygiene in 1909, the first Australian to be elected. In Queensland Ham focused on food adulteration (in 1905 he called for uniform food and drug laws across recently federated Australia); improved sanitation (during the plague outbreaks of the 1900s, he zealously pursued rat destruction, rectification of defective drains and sewers, and education of the community); and control of infectious diseases (he introduced compulsory reporting). He was the founder of a modern Department of Public Health and chairman of the Board of Public Health. He had enlightened views for the time on control of venereal disease. He had already worked for repeal of the coercive, discriminatory and ineffective Queensland Contagious Diseases Act, 1868, against the opinion of the majority of local doctors. He advocated later in Victoria prevention of venereal disease through education, compulsory but confidential reporting, mandatory treatment by doctors, free treatment, and legal penalties for individuals knowingly infecting others. Legal coercion would be used only when patients did not obtain treatment from a medical practitioner. He resigned from his public health posts in Victoria and went to England in 1913 after "differences of opinion between Dr. Ham and Mr. Edgar, the Minister of Health."[179]

Like Ashburton Thompson, Ham made important contributions to scientific knowledge about plague. His *Report on Plague in Queensland 1900–1907* received international recognition, and Ham provided some significant information: plague-infected fleas survived in food produce after departing from a host rat; the activity of fleas increased under favourable environmental conditions; and meteorological variations affected the survival, growth and virulence of the flea's bacterial flora, including the plague bacillus.

Public health and preventive medicine were taught from the outset at the University of Sydney Medical School. W.H. Goode, a graduate in medicine from Trinity College, Dublin, in the 1860s and a former assistant government health officer in Sydney, was appointed lecturer in public health and preventive medicine at Sydney in 1883. He was succeeded in the lectureship in 1904 by one of his first students at Sydney, William George Armstrong. Armstrong was one of the first of the new wave of medical officers of health in Australia, men who were graduates of local medical schools but still often obtained the diploma of public health in Britain. He was awarded the Cambridge DPH in 1895, having obtained the required practical experience doing outdoor public health work in the slums of London's Whitechapel. As noted earlier, he became first medical officer of health for

Sydney in 1898 and in 1900 also city health officer. Appointed deputy director general of public health in 1913, he became director in 1920. The pioneer of organized infant health work in Australasia, he published many papers on epidemiology and preventive medicine.[180] Harry Brookes Allen, professor of anatomy and pathology at Melbourne University, returned from a visit to Europe in 1890 impressed by the need to promote research and teaching in bacteriology. He proposed that the colonial government establish an Institute of Preventive Medicine along the lines of one recently established in Cambridge. Although the institute was to be independent of the university, the director would lecture to medical undergraduates and postgraduates. When the government failed to respond, Allen arranged for a recent Melbourne graduate, Thomas Cherry, to work with Professor D.J. Hamilton of Aberdeen and also on the Continent. In 1892, Cherry initiated practical instruction at Melbourne in pathological histology and bacteriology.[181]

The University of Melbourne Faculty of Medicine offered a postgraduate diploma of public health from 1906, and the first award was made in 1908. A course of instruction was not provided, however, and once the national School of Public Health and Tropical Medicine was established at Sydney University in 1930, few students sought the Melbourne diploma. Regulations governing the diploma were ultimately suspended. The University of Sydney also offered a diploma of public health, occasionally awarding it from about 1910.[182] The University of Adelaide Faculty of Medicine had begun teaching medical students in 1887. The final examinations at the end of fifth year included examination on the "Elements of Hygiene." In 1904, William Ramsay Smith, president of the Board of Health, was a candidate for doctoral degrees in both science and medicine. Awarded the degree in science, he failed to obtain the M.D., because under existing regulations the extensive examination was confined to purely medical subjects. As a result, the medical faculty amended the regulations to make the M.D. examination apply to one of five areas of medicine, and one of these was state medicine. Further, a thesis might be presented in lieu of an examination. In 1906, Western Australian health authorities requested establishment of a diploma in public health, but the Adelaide faculty, believing it could not provide the requisite teaching, did not accede to the request. However, teaching of tropical medicine and a course on vaccination were instituted. Adelaide decided not to join the Universities of Sydney and Melbourne in a scheme to establish a national Institute of Tropical Medicine in Sydney. This scheme ultimately led to the creation of the Australian Institute of Tropical Medicine in Townsville in tropical Queensland, which in turn was absorbed into the national School of Public Health and Tropical Medicine when it was set up at the University of Sydney in 1930. In 1929, the Adelaide Faculty of Medicine rejected a proposal for establishment of a Department of Public Health.[183]

PUBLIC HEALTH NURSING

The origins of public health nursing lie in traditional Christian charitable provision of medical and nursing assistance to the sick poor and, more latterly, the Enlightenment wish to educate the poor, who would then discover the rewards of self-help. The more proximate roots lie in mid-nineteenth-century England, when the Epidemiological Society of London devised a program under which pauper women would be trained to nurse the sick poor in the community. The society's program failed to develop, but in 1859 a Liverpool Quaker, William Rathbone, planned for a nurse and "lady visitor" to work in each of eighteen districts of the city. They together provided nursing, health education and social work services. Impressed by his achievements, the Manchester and Salford Association in 1864 began their own work. The Leicester Association followed in 1867, and the East London Nursing Society in 1868. Birmingham had a district nurse from 1870, and Glasgow from 1875, while the Metropolitan and National Nursing Association, which had the aim of training district nurses, came into being in 1874 in London. When an 1862 initiative of the Ladies Section of the Manchester and Salford Sanitary Association to distribute pamphlets on hygiene to poor homes had little effect, working-class women were employed to teach domestic hygiene to poor women in their homes. By 1900 health visitors worked in many urban centers. In the rigidly gendered and class division of labor in Victorian times, health education and surveillance of hygiene practices were accepted as an extension of the natural role of women, whether women of the middle classes who ran the voluntary associations or working-class health visitors who educated their "sisters" in the home.

By the 1900s, nurses were becoming health visitors, a trend promoted particularly by the growth of infant and child health services. In the 1890s Florence Nightingale had proposed that the district nurse should act as a "health missioner" or "health minister" as well as a caregiver to the sick—the term "health visitor" was not commonly employed before 1900. She was deeply committed to district nursing, the social mission of which was larger than that of hospital nursing. Indeed, for her the ultimate aim was to nurse all ill persons in their homes. Local government authorities began to collaborate with the voluntary agencies in the employment of home visitors. In 1890 Manchester corporation provided the salaries of six of fourteen visitors working for the Ladies Sanitary Association, and these were supervised by the medical officer of health. Soon after, Salford corporation and the association agreed to the same type of cooperation. By the early 1900s, fifty communities used a mixture of voluntary visitors and women sanitary inspectors or health visitors. The health visitors, who focused on domiciliary care of young children, were often designated "sanitary inspectors," because local authorities had no legal power to employ health visitors. In 1908 the London County Council obtained legislation allowing them to employ such people. The following year, Local Government Board regulations required the health visitor to be medically qualified, have full nursing training, and possess the Central Midwives Board certificate or have received some training in nursing plus a certificate from an approved society. No such requirements existed in extrametropolitan areas. However, certification and training facilities soon evolved. The Royal Sanitary Institute in 1908 instituted examination of health visitors and school nurses. School nurses came into being after medical examination of school children became mandatory in 1908. The Maternity and Child Welfare Act, 1918, required health visitors to have qualifications satisfactory to the Local Government Board. In 1928, full-time visitors had to possess the Royal Sanitary Institute certificate; a total of 2,938 health visitors were employed by local authorities, and 2,546 by voluntary bodies, by the early 1930s.[184]

District nursing and home visiting were the forerunners of public health nursing in the United States as well as in England. In the 1870s, the New York City Mission and the Society for Ethical Culture provided domiciliary nursing for the poor. District nursing societies were established in Buffalo, Boston, and Philadelphia in the 1880s. Indicating that education and care went hand in hand, the Boston body called itself the Instructive District Nursing Association. Around 1900 public health extended into personal health services in the United States, as in the United Kingdom and Australia, and health departments began to employ public health nurses. While the Los Angeles health department employed a nurse for domiciliary work with poor households as early as 1898, it did not create a bureau of nursing until fifteen years later. The New York City Health Department, in contrast, developed nursing services quickly once it entered the field. In 1902, a nurse from the Henry Street District Nursing Service, a voluntary organization established by Lillian Wald and Mary Brewster in 1893, was employed by the Health Department in school work. Employment of more school nurses quickly followed. In 1903 the department employed three nurses to instruct tuberculosis sufferers at home in personal hygiene. Local and state health departments across the country soon took up public health nursing. In the U.S. Public Health Service development was slower; although a public health nurse worked on a trachoma project in 1913, only in the 1930s did public health nursing become established in the service.

Public health nursing in the United States as in England—and as we shall see, in Australia—was originally specialized, focusing on particular areas, such as infant and maternal health, health of school children, and care of people with tuberculosis. This specialization was partly due to the tendency of voluntary bodies to be organized to work on particular diseases or assist particular subpopulations. The National Organization of Public Health Nursing, established in 1912, was devoted to advancing the educational status of, and the quality of services provided by, public health nurses. By the mid-twentieth century, more than twenty-five thousand public health nurses worked in the

United States and its territories, about half of them employed in local health activities.[185]

In Australia, local government health authorities employed the first official health visitors in the early 1900s. Registered nurses had come to dominate the work by 1920, and these public health nurses worked in a variety of settings—in infant health, health visiting, in school health, and in occupational health and safety in factories. Just as in hospitals, doctors (as medical officers of health) in these community health settings sat at the top of the occupational hierarchy, in accord with the medical model of health and disease.

Religious organizations were early involved in the work of district nursing. Thus, from the 1890s the Wesleyan Church's Perth Central Mission provided home visiting services, combining skilled nursing with material relief for needy cases. Even "secular" district nurses were expected to display Christian altruism and to promote morality as well as hygiene in the home. Although district nursing associations were created in Sydney, Melbourne and Adelaide in 1895–1900, they concentrated on domiciliary clinical nursing rather than public health.

By the 1900s, sanitation had spilt into various areas along gendered lines. Men were employed as sanitary inspectors in the surveillance of domestic buildings and commercial establishments, and of premises where food was processed or sold. With medical experts on the health of babies and young children arguing that reduction of unacceptable infant death rates was much dependent on the cleanliness of environments and the awareness by mothers of the importance of breast feeding, local health authorities began to employ women to carry out surveillance and education in the homes of the inner city poor.[186] Seen in a wider perspective, urban poverty lay behind the excessive infant mortality borne by the working classes. While the infant welfare movement, including public health nurses, helped to reduce mortality, it also softened the social and demographic consequences of undue economic inequality. Poor housing and lack of bathrooms and iceboxes, as well as recurrent pregnancies and large numbers of children, would not be whisked away by very limited contact with health visitors.

There are parallels between the infant welfare movement and the contemporary town planning movement. The latter suggested the physical solution of better housing, parks, playgrounds, and slum clearance for the social problem of crime, delinquency, overcrowding, and ill health and premature mortality. In Sydney, the town planning association, formed in 1913, was dominated by middle-class professionals and businessmen. The exception was R.F. Irvine, professor of economics at the University of Sydney, who understood that town planning had to be linked to macro-economic planning and income redistribution to achieve social reform. He withdrew from the movement in 1917, apparently because of its failure to accept the political nature of planning. Humanitarian concern for the poor motivated middle-class town planners, but self-interest was important as well. Slums reduced the heath and so the efficiency of the workforce, and they bred crime and even political discontent. They threatened social, economic and political stability.[187]

Australian health authorities adapted the health visitor model developed in Britain. The Australian health visitors later became specialist public health nurses in the fields of infant health, school health and tuberculosis. The Sydney City Council's first health visitor was Margaret Ferguson, a former British health visitor and graduate of the Royal Sanitary Institute, London. From 1902, she worked under the direction of W.G. Armstrong, the city health officer and metropolitan MOH, visiting homes in the inner city to advise mothers of newborn babies on infant feeding in an effort to combat the high diarrheal mortality. Armstrong was aware of the effects of poverty and deleterious environmental factors on infant mortality but pragmatically intervened at the level of behavior to persuade mothers to breast-feed, both to assist the nutrition of children and protect to them from pathogens in the domestic environment: "My aim was the visiting of every mother of a newborn child in the city . . . by the health visitor, who . . . talked to her confidentially on the management of the child, and advised her . . . as to cleanliness and the general sanitary state of the dwelling. . . . Full records were kept in each case, and . . . in cases of poverty, the household was referred to the appropriate charitable institutions."[188]

Women health visitors and sanitary inspectors had to respond to any public health problem encountered, whether infant and maternal issues, infectious diseases, hygiene or sanitation. Thus, the smallpox outbreak in 1912–13 in Sydney took them away from infant welfare work, halving the number of visits to new mothers. Domiciliary visits increased so much (from 781 to 1,554 in 1904–10) that the City Council health visitor, Miss Ferguson, required the help of nurses from the Alice Rawson School for Mothers. Opened in 1908, the school was supported by the National Council for Women, which had been established in the 1890s. The school worked for the welfare of infants of the poorer classes in Sydney. The cooperation of philanthropic voluntary bodies with local government or state personnel was also a feature of early organized infant health work in other parts of Australia, and health visiting quickly spread to other states.[189] But wide social acceptance of the idea of individual responsibility for health and well-being, and the opposition of a politically effective medical profession strongly committed to private practice, limited the extension of public health into infant and maternal and other personal service areas. This matter will be extensively discussed in the following chapter.

NOTES

1. T. McKeown and R.G. Record, "Reasons for the Decline of Mortality in England and Wales during the Nineteenth Century," *Population Studies* 16 (1962),

102, 104; T. McKeown, R.G. Record and R.D. Turner, "An Interpretation of the Decline of Mortality in England and Wales during the Twentieth Century," *Population Studies* 29 (1975), 395, 421; R.M. Smith, "Demography and Medicine," in *Companion Encyclopedia of the History of Medicine,* ed. W.F. Bynum and R. Porter (London: Routledge, 1993), vol. 2, 1665.

2. McKeown and Record, "Reasons for the Decline of Mortality in England and Wales during the Nineteenth Century," 120–21.

3. R. Schofield and D. Reher, "The Decline of Mortality in Europe," in *The Decline of Mortality in Europe,* ed. R. Schofield, D. Reher and A. Bideau (Oxford: Clarendon Press, 1991), 3–4; G. Caselli, "Health Transition and Cause-Specific Mortality," in *The Decline of Mortality in Europe,* ed. Schofield, Reher and Bideau, 68–69.

4. Schofield and Reher, "The Decline of Mortality in Europe," 9–15.

5. S. Szreter, "The Importance of Social Intervention in Britain's Mortality Decline c. 1850–1914: A Re-interpretation of the Role of Public Health," *Social History of Medicine* 1 (1988), 15–26.

6. Ibid., 27–37.

7. H.O. Lancaster, *Expectations of Life: A Study in the Demography, Statistics, and History of World Mortality* (New York: Springer-Verlag, 1990), 430–31.

8. R. Higgs, "Cycles and Trends of Mortality in 18 Large American Cities, 1871–1900," *Explorations in Economic History* 16 (1979), 382–402.

9. G.A. Condran and R.A. Cheney, "Mortality Trends in Philadelphia: Age- and Cause-Specific Death Rates 1870–1930," *Demography* 19(1) (1982), 119–20.

10. R. Higgs, "Mortality in Rural America, 1870–1920: Estimates and Conjectures," *Explorations in Economic History* 10 (1973), 177–92.

11. Lancaster, *Expectations of Life,* 423; G.W. Rice, "Public Health in Christchurch, 1875–1910: Mortality and Sanitation," in *A Healthy Country. Essays on the Social History of Medicine in New Zealand,* ed. L. Bryder (Wellington, N.Z.: Bridget Williams Books, 1991), 88–107. See M.J. Lewis, "'Populate or Perish': Aspects of Infant and Maternal Health in Sydney, 1870–1939" (Ph.D. dissertation, Australian National University, Canberra, 1976), 323.

12. P. Curson, "Spatial Therapy: Epidemics and Public Health in Australia," unpublished paper, Macquarie University, North Ryde, NSW, 1992, 1–4; J.H.L. Cumpston, *Health and Disease in Australia: A History,* ed. M.J. Lewis (Canberra: Australian Government Publishing Service [hereafter AGPS], 1989), 180–81.

13. R. Taylor, M. Lewis and J. Powles, "The Australian Mortality Decline: All-Cause Mortality 1788–1990," *Australian and New Zealand Journal of Public Health* 22(1) (1998), 27–32.

14. Quoted in D. Gordon, *Health, Sickness and Society* (St. Lucia: University of Queensland Press, 1976), 190.

15. R. Taylor, M. Lewis and J. Powles, "The Australian Mortality Decline: All-Cause Mortality 1788–1990," *Australian and New Zealand Journal of Public Health* 22(1) (1998), 33; Gordon, *Health, Sickness and Society,* 192; M.-F. Morel, "The Care of Children: The Influence of Medical Innovation and Medical Institutions on Infant Mortality 1750–1914," in *The Decline of Mortality in Europe* ed. Schofield, Reher and Bideau, 216–19.

16. Quoted in J.M. Powell, *Watering the Garden State: Water, Land and Community in Victoria 1834–1988* (Sydney: Allen and Unwin, 1989), 40.

17. Quoted in G. Reekie, "Nineteenth-Century Urbanization," in *Australian Studies: A Survey* ed. J. Walter (Melbourne: Oxford University Press, 1989), 86.

18. Quoted in ibid., 87.

19. N.G. Butlin, *Investment in Australian Economic Development 1861–1900* (Cambridge: Cambridge University Press, 1964), 6.

20. M. Lewis and R. MacLeod, "A Workingman's Paradise? Reflections on Urban Mortality in Colonial Australia 1860–1900," *Medical History* 31 (1987), 391–92.

21. N.G. Butlin, "Long-run Trends in Australian Per Capita Consumption," in *The National Income and Social Welfare*, ed. K. Hancock (Melbourne: F.W. Cheshire, 1967), 5–8; J. Lee and C. Fahey, "A Boom for Whom? Some Developments in the Australian Labour Market, 1870–1891," *Labour History* 50 (1986), 1.

22. Quoted in R. White, *Inventing Australia: Images and Identity 1688–1980* (Sydney: Allen and Unwin, 1981), 41.

23. T.A. Coghlan, *The Wealth and Progress of New South Wales 1886–87* (Sydney: Government Printer, 1887), 491.

24. T.A. Coghlan, *A Statistical Account of the Seven Colonies of Australasia 1901–1902* (Sydney: Government Printer, 1902), 367.

25. Lee and Fahey, "A Boom for Whom?" 1–2.

26. M. Kelly, "Picturesque and Pestilential: The Sydney Slum Observed 1860–1900," in *Nineteenth-Century Sydney: Essays in Urban History*, ed. M. Kelly (Sydney: Sydney University Press, 1978), 67.

27. S. Fisher, "The Family and the Sydney Economy in the Late Nineteenth Century," in *Families in Colonial Australia*, ed. P. Grimshaw, C. McConville and E. McEwen (Sydney: Allen and Unwin, 1985), 153–62; Lee and Fahey, "A Boom for Whom?" 3.

28. M.E. Pooley and C.G. Pooley, "Health, Society and Environment in Victorian Manchester," in *Urban Disease and Mortality in Nineteenth-Century England*, ed. R. Woods and J. Woodward (London: Batsford, 1984), 148, 175.

29. W.S. Jevons, "Remarks upon the Social Map of Sydney 1858," unpublished manuscript, Mitchell Library, Sydney.

30. Kelly, "Picturesque and Pestilential," 73.

31. *Report from Select Committee on Condition of Working Classes of Metropolis* (Sydney: Government Printer, 1860), 8–10, 32–38, 78, 95; D.L. Clark, "The Development of Sydney's Water Supply, 1842–1887" (honours dissertation, University of Sydney, Sydney, 1967), 136–37.

32. Sydney City and Suburban Sewage and Health Board, Progress Report, *Journal of Legislative Council of New South Wales* 25 (1875), 5.

33. Quoted in Kelly, "Picturesque and Pestilential," 78.

34. W.G. Armstrong, "Municipal Sanitation in the City," *Australasian Medical Gazette* 20 (1901), 462.

35. *Report of Commission of Inquiry into Question of Housing of Workmen in Europe and America* (Sydney: Government Printer, 1913), 16–17.

36. Quoted in D. Dunstan, *Governing the Metropolis: Melbourne 1850–1891* (Carlton, Australia: Melbourne University Press, 1984), 145.

37. D. Dunstan, "Dirt and Disease," in *The Outcasts of Melbourne. Essays in Social History*, eds. G Davison, D. Dunstan and C. McConville (Sydney: Allen and Unwin, 1985), 140–41.

38. Quoted in Dunstan, *Governing the Metropolis*, 13.

39. W.A. Sinclair, "Economic Growth and Well-being: Melbourne 1870–1914," *Economic Record* 51 (1975), 154.

40. Quoted in M. Cannon, *Life in the Cities: Australia in the Victorian Age* (South Yarra: Currey, O'Neil, Ross, 1983), 264.

41. D. Dunstan, "Dirt and Disease," in *The Outcasts of Melbourne. Essays in Social History* eds. G. Davison, D. Dunstan and C. McConville (Sydney: Allen and Unwin, 1985), 167–70.

42. Quoted in G. Greenwood and J. Laverty, *Brisbane 1859–1959: A History of Local Government* (Brisbane: Council of City of Brisbane, 1959), 81.

43. Quoted in J.M. Powell, *Plains of Promise and Rivers of Destiny. Water Management and the Development of Queensland, 1824–1990* (Bowen Hills: Boolarong Publications, 1991), 38.

44. R. Lawson, *Brisbane in the 1890s: A Study of an Australian Urban Society* (St. Lucia: University of Queensland Press, 1973), 63–74.

45. Quoted in P. Woodruff, *Two Million South Australians* (Kent Town: Peacock Publications, 1984), 31–32.

46. T. Stevenson, "Miasmas, Morbidity and Milieu: Mortality in Victorian South Australia," *Proceedings of Royal Geographical Society* (South Australian Branch) 81 (1980), 42.

47. Quoted in S.J. Hunt and G. Bolton, "Cleansing the Dunghill: Water Supply and Sanitation in Perth 1878–1912," *Studies in Western Australian History* 2 (1978), 2.

48. Quoted in S.J. Hunt and G. Bolton, "Cleansing the Dunghill: Water Supply and Sanitation in Perth 1878–1912," *Studies in Western Australian History* 2 (1978), 3.

49. S.J. Hunt and G. Bolton, "Cleansing the Dunghill: Water Supply and Sanitation in Perth 1878–1912," *Studies in Western Australian History* 2 (1978), 4–11.

50. Quoted in S. Petrow, *Sanatorium of the South? Public Health and Politics in Hobart and Launceston 1875–1914* (Hobart: Tasmanian Historical Research Association, 1995), 8.

51. Quoted in ibid., 156.

52. Quoted in ibid., 180.

53. Quoted in ibid., 185.

54. J. Lewis, *The Politics of Motherhood. Child and Maternal Welfare in England, 1900–1939* (London: Croom Helm, 1980), 13–21, 61–67, 165–67.

55. A. Newsholme, "On Child Mortality at the Ages 0–5 Years, in England and Wales," *Journal of Hygiene,* 16(1) (1917–18), 69–71.

56. M.B. Pell, "On the Rates of Mortality and Expectation of Life in New South Wales as Compared with England and Other Countries," *Transactions of Royal Society of NSW* 1 (1867), 69, 74.

57. W.G. Armstrong, "The Infant Welfare Movement in Australia," *Medical Journal of Australia* 2 (1939), 647.

58. T.L. Stevenson, "Light and Living Conditions: Mortality in Nineteenth-Century Adelaide," unpublished paper, 49th Australian and New Zealand Association for the Advancement of Science Conference, Adelaide, 1979, 9, 35.

59. Gordon, *Health, Sickness and Society,* 161.

60. B. Gandevia, *Tears Often Shed. Child Health and Welfare in Australia from 1788* (Sydney: Prince Henry and Prince of Wales Hospitals, 1978), 79; J. Leavesley, "Cholera," *Medical Journal of Australia,* 141 (1984), 660.

61. W.G. Armstrong, "Some Lessons from the Statistics of Infantile Mortality in Sydney," *Transactions of Australasian Medical Congress* (1905), 395; Central Board of Health, *Report of the Board for 1885* (Melbourne: Government Printer, 1885), 17; E.C. Meyer, *Infant Mortality in New York City* (New York: Rockefeller Foundation International Health Board, 1921), 19; Sir A. Newsholme, *Fifty Years in Public Health; A Personal Narrative with Comments* (London: Allen and Unwin, 1935), 351.

62. G.F. McCleary, *The Maternity and Child Welfare Movement* (London: King and Son, 1935), 6.

63. G.J. Cuthbert, "Infant Mortality in New South Wales," *Medical Journal of Australia* 1 (1950), 76.

64. Armstrong, "Some Lessons from the Statistics of Infantile Mortality in Sydney," 395; *New South Wales Vital Statistics,* 1901(Sydney: Government Printer, 1901); *Report of Medical Officer of Health to Metropolitan Combined Sanitary District,* 1911 (Sydney: Government Printer, 1911); *New South Wales Statistical Register,* 1933 (Sydney: Government Printer, 1933); *New South Wales Statistical Register,* 1947 (Sydney: Government Printer, 1947).

65. N.S. Scrimshaw, C.E. Taylor and J.E. Gordon, *Interactions of Nutrition and Infection* (Geneva: World Health Organization, 1968), 253.

66. W.F. Litchfield, "Summer Diarrhoea in Infants: From the Public Health Point of View," *Transactions of Australasian Medical Congress* (1905), 241; Armstrong, "Some Lessons from the Statistics of Infantile Mortality in Sydney," 386–88; R.R. Stawell, "Some Notes on the Aetiology and Pathological Anatomy of Summer Diarrhoea in Infants," *Australian Medical Journal* 17 (1895), 71–77; R.M. Woodbury, *Causal Factors in Infant Mortality: A Statistical Study* (Washington, D.C.: U.S. Children's Bureau, 1925), 6.

67. C.D. Hunter, *What Kills Our Babies* (Melbourne: Australian Health Society, 1878), 10.

68. T. Stevenson, "Miasmas, Morbidity and Milieu: Mortality in Victorian South Australia," *Proceedings of Royal Geographical Society* (South Australian Branch) 81 (1980), 50.

69. M. Durey, "Infant Mortality in Perth, Western Australia, 1870–1914: A Preliminary Analysis," *Studies in Western Australian History* 5 (1982), 65.

70. R.A. Cheney, "Seasonal Aspects of Infant and Childhood Mortality: Philadelphia, 1865–1920," *Journal of Interdisciplinary History* 14(3) (1984), 563–69.

71. A. Newsholme, "Domestic Infection in Relation to Epidemic Diarrhoea," *Journal of Hygiene* 6(2) (1906), 139–46; W.M. Frazer, *A History of English Public Health, 1834–1939* (London: Ballière, Tindall and Cox, 1950), 331–32; G. Newman, *Infant Mortality: A Social Problem* (London: Methuen, 1906), 150–51, 174–76.

72. "Impure Milk," *New South Wales Medical Gazette* 5 (1875), 304; T.M. Kendall, "On the Preservation of Infant Life," *Australasian Medical Gazette* 4 (1885), 229.

73. J.C. Drummond and A. Wilbraham, *The Englishman's Food: A History of Five Centuries of English Diet* (London: Cape, 1939), 449–51. *New South Wales Parliamentary Debates* 30 (5 August 1908), 400; and 31 (12 November 1908), 2441.

74. P. Van Ingen, "The History of Child Welfare Work in the United States," in *A Half Century of Public Health: Jubilee Historical Volume of American Public*

Health Association ed. M.P. Ravenel (New York: American Public Health Association, 1921), 307.

75. G. Newman, *Infant Mortality: A Social Problem* (London: Methuen, 1906), vi.

76. C.K. Mackellar, *The Mother, the Baby and the State* (Sydney: Government Printer, 1917), 5.

77. W.G. Armstrong, "The Infant Welfare Movement in Australia," 642.

78. Quoted in R. Porter, *The Greatest Benefit to Mankind: A Medical History of Humanity from Antiquity to the Present* (London: HarperCollins, 1997), 412.

79. J. Leavesley, "Cholera," *Medical Journal of Australia* 141 (1984), 660; *Public Health in the Victorian Age: Debates on the Issue from 19th Century Critical Journals* (London: Gregg International Publishers, 1973), n.p.; Porter, *The Greatest Benefit to Mankind,* 403–4.

80. Quoted in Porter, *The Greatest Benefit to Mankind,* 414–15.

81. C. Hamlin, "State Medicine in Great Britain," in *The History of Public Health and the Modern State,* ed. D. Porter (Amsterdam, Atlanta: Editions Rodopi B.V., 1994), 148–52.

82. J. Duffy, *The Sanitarians: A History of American Public Health* (Urbana: University of Illinois Press, 1990), 110–23.

83. E. Fee and D. Porter, "Public Health, Preventive Medicine, and Professionalization: Britain and the United States in the Nineteenth Century," in *A History of Education in Public Health,* ed. E. Fee and R.M. Acheson (Oxford: Oxford University Press, 1991), 32–38.

84. Duffy, *The Sanitarians,* 131.

85. Ibid., 138.

86. Ibid., 139–54.

87. See M.J. Lewis, "Editor's Introduction," in Cumpston, *Health and Disease in Australia,* ed. Lewis, 6.

88. *Victoria Parliamentary Debates* 62 (22 October 1889), 1986.

89. See Lewis, "Editor's Introduction," 7.

90. Cumpston, *Health and Disease in Australia,* 231.

91. Quoted in Dunstan, *Governing the Metropolis,* 124.

92. D.J. Dyason, "The Police and Public Health Acts in the Early Years of the Colony of Victoria," *Proceedings of Australasian Association for History and Philosophy of Science Conference,* 1975, n.p.

93. Central Board of Health, *Report for 1856* (Melbourne: Government Printer, 1856), 5–7.

94. D. Dunstan, "Health Officers of the City of Melbourne," in *Patients, Practitioners and Techniques,* ed. H. Attwood and R.W. Home (Melbourne: Medical History Unit, University of Melbourne, 1984), 134–35.

95. Central Board of Health, *Report for 1862* (Melbourne: Government Printer, 1862), 11, 16; Central Board of Health, *Report for 1864* (Melbourne: Government Printer, 1864), 8–9.

96. Dyason, "The Police and Public Health Acts in the Early Years of the Colony of Victoria."

97. Dunstan, *Governing the Metropolis,* 246–47.

98. Central Board of Health, *Report for 1872* (Melbourne: Government Printer, 1872), 4–7; Central Board of Health, *Report for 1877* (Melbourne: Government Printer, 1877), 6.

99. Cumpston, *Health and Disease in Australia*, 386–87; *Victoria Parliamentary Debates* 44 (16 October 1883), 1462; Central Board of Health, *Report for 1885* (Melbourne: Government Printer, 1885), 8.

100. Cumpston, *Health and Disease in Australia*, 386–87.

101. Dunstan, *Governing the Metropolis*, 273–75; Cumpston, *Health and Disease in Australia*, 387.

102. "Public Health in Victoria," *Health Bulletin* 112 (1954), 16–17.

103. Dunstan, *Governing the Metropolis*, 278–81; *Victoria Parliamentary Debates* 60 (1889), 196–203; "Public Health in Victoria," 17.

104. T. Dingle and C. Rasmussen, *Vital Connections: Melbourne and Its Board of Works, 1891–1991* (Ringwood, Victoria, Australia: McPhee Gribble, 1991), 17–19, 79.

105. Cumpston, *Health and Disease in Australia*, 234–37.

106. C.J. Cummins, *A History of Medical Administration in New South Wales, 1788–1973* (Sydney: Government Printer, 1979), 64; F.A. Larcombe, *The Stabilization of Local Government in New South Wales 1858–1906* (Sydney: Sydney University Press, 1976), 117.

107. Quoted in F.A. Larcombe, *The Development of Local Government in New South Wales* (Melbourne: F.W. Cheshire, 1961), 57.

108. Larcombe, *The Stabilization of Local Government in New South Wales 1858–1906*, 118–24.

109. A.M. Brown, "Medical Reform in Relation to Public Health," *New South Wales Medical Gazette* 1 (1870), 33–40; "The Water Supply of Sydney," *New South Wales Medical Gazette* 4 (1874), 160, 219.

110. Quoted in D. Coward, *Out of Sight: Sydney's Environmental History 1851–1981* (Canberra: Department of Economic History, Research School of Social Sciences, Australian National University, 1988), 106.

111. Larcombe, *The Stabilization of Local Government in New South Wales 1858–1906*, 124–33; Coward, *Out of Sight*, 101–109; F.J.J. Henry, *The Water Supply and Sewerage of Sydney* (Sydney: Halstead Press, 1939), 54–55; D.L. Clark, "The Development of Sydney's Water Supply, 1842–1887" (honours dissertation, University of Sydney, Sydney, 1967), 227.

112. Sydney City and Suburban Sewage and Health Board, Eleventh Progress Report, *Journal of Legislative Council of New South Wales* 26(2) (1875–76), 11.

113. W.G. Armstrong, "The Establishment of a Central Health Authority in New South Wales," *Medical Journal of Australia* 1 (1937) 401; Cumpston, *Health and Disease in Australia*, 384–85; Larcombe, *The Stabilization of Local Government in New South Wales 1858–1906*, 134.

114. Coward, *Out of Sight*, 141–46.

115. Quoted in ibid., 147.

116. Ibid., 146–48.

117. "Report on Outbreak of Typhoid Fever in Municipal District of Leichhardt due to Polluted Milk, 1886," *Journal of Legislative Council of New South Wales* 40(1) (1885–86), 5.

118. Coward, *Out of Sight*, 149; C.E. North, "Milk and Its Relation to Public Health," in *A Half Century of Public Health*, ed. Ravenel, 237–38.

119. Frazer, *A History of English Public Health, 1834–1939*, 463–66.

120. Ibid., 226.

121. *Votes and Proceedings of Legislative Assembly of New South Wales* 11 (1883–84), 977; *New South Wales Parliamentary Debates* 85 (6 October 1896), 3, 757.

122. Quoted in Coward, *Out of Sight,* 150.

123. Ibid., 151–54.

124. See Lewis, "'Populate or Perish,'" 57.

125. "The Necessity for a Public Health Act for New South Wales," *Australasian Medical Gazette* 14 (1895), 167–68.

126. Quoted in Coward, *Out of Sight,* 182.

127. *New South Wales Parliamentary Debates* 85 (6 October 1896), 3, 752–63; and 86 (27 October 1896), 4, 362–64, 371–74. Coward, *Out of Sight,* 183–85.

128. Larcombe, *The Development of Local Government in New South Wales,* 59.

129. E. Barclay, "Fevers and Stinks: Some Problems of Public Health in the 1870s and 1880s," *Queensland Heritage* 2(4) (1971), 3; Cumpston, *Health and Disease in Australia,* 387; R. Patrick, *A History of Health and Medicine in Queensland* (St. Lucia: University of Queensland Press, 1987), 50–51.

130. Quoted in Barclay, "Fevers and Stinks," 3. *Queensland Parliamentary Debates* 2 (7 July 1865), 378–81; 3 (23 May 1866), 294–96. R. Patrick, *A History of Health and Medicine in Queensland* (St. Lucia: University of Queensland Press, 1987), 51.

131. *Queensland Parliamentary Debates* 14 (11 July 1872), 595–97, 610; 14 (23 July 1872), 694–96.

132. Quoted in Barclay, "Fevers and Stinks," 11.

133. Ibid., 5–11; Patrick, *A History of Health and Medicine in Queensland,* 54–57.

134. *South Australia Parliamentary Debates* (14 September 1873), 752.

135. *South Australia Parliamentary Debates* (12 December 1873), 1480.

136. S. Holton, "Social Medicine in Nineteenth Century South Australia," *Community Health Studies* 7(2) (1983), 127.

137. *South Australia Parliamentary Debates* (28 August 1873), 252; and (9 October 1873), 708.

138. *South Australia Parliamentary Debates* (28 August 1873), 252; and (11 September 1873), 402–405.

139. Quoted in S. Holton, "Social Medicine in Nineteenth Century South Australia," *Community Health Studies* 7(2) (1983), 129.

140. Quoted in ibid., 129.

141. *South Australia Parliamentary Debates* (13 August 1884), 607–608.

142. Cumpston, *Health and Disease in Australia,* 388.

143. Quoted in Holton, "Social Medicine in Nineteenth Century South Australia," 129.

144. Ibid., 129–32.

145. Quoted in E.F. Haynes, "Edward Swarbreck Hall, Medical Scientist and Social Reformer in Colonial Tasmania" (M.A. dissertation, University of Tasmania, Hobart, 1976), 163.

146. E.F. Haynes, "Edward Swarbreck Hall, Medical Scientist and Social Reformer in Colonial Tasmania," 163–71.

147. Petrow, *Sanatorium of the South?* 390–91.

148. Quoted in ibid., 10.

149. Ibid., 10–11.

150. Ibid., 22–23.
151. Quoted in ibid., 23.
152. Quoted in ibid., 24.
153. N.P. Clapham, "The Development of Local Government in Western Australia, 1838–1906" (M.A. dissertation, University of Western Australia, Perth, 1949), 94.
154. B.K. de Garis, "Self-Government and the Evolution of Party Politics 1871–1911," in *A New History of Western Australia,* ed. C.T. Stannage (Perth: University of Western Australia Press, 1981), 328.
155. *Western Australia Parliamentary Debates* 11 (12 July 1886), 111.
156. Ibid., 115.
157. Cumpston, *Health and Disease in Australia,* 236.
158. D. Porter, "Stratification and Its Discontents: Professionalization and Conflict in the British Public Health Service, 1848–1914," in *A History of Education in Public Health,* ed. Fee and Acheson, 84–86; M. Lewis and R. MacLeod, "Medical Politics and the Professionalisation of Medicine in New South Wales, 1850–1901," *Journal of Australian Studies* 22 (1988), 69.
159. Quoted in R. Acheson, "The British Diploma in Public Health: Birth and Adolescence," in *A History of Education in Public Health,* ed. Fee and Acheson, 47.
160. Quoted in Acheson, "The British Diploma in Public Health," 61–62.
161. Ibid., 44–82; D. Porter, "Stratification and Its Discontents: Professionalization and Conflict in the British Public Health Service, 1848–1914," in *A History of Education in Public Health,* ed. Fee and Acheson, 83–113; Frazer, *A History of English Public Health, 1834–1939,* 235–36.
162. Frazer, *A History of English Public Health, 1834–1939,* 123–24, 232–36.
163. A.J. Viseltear, "The Emergence of Pioneering Public Health Education Programmes in the United States," in *A History of Education in Public Health,* ed. Fee and Acheson, 114–42.
164. E. Fee, "Designing Schools of Public Health for the United States," in *A History of Education in Public Health,* ed. Fee and Acheson, 157–60.
165. Quoted in ibid., 179.
166. Ibid., 163–68.
167. Quoted in B. Rosen, "Australia's Contribution to the Conquest of Plague," *Journal of Royal Australian Historical Society* 63(1) (1977), 66.
168. Quoted in ibid.
169. W.G. Armstrong, "An Eminent Epidemiologist," *Health* 3(4) (1925), 97–100; Rosen, "Australia's Contribution to the Conquest of Plague," 60–61; *Report of Medical Officer of Health to Metropolitan Combined Sanitary Districts, 1900* (Sydney: Government Printer, 1900), 9; "Public Health," *Australasian Medical Gazette* 16 (1897), 359.
170. J.L. Bruce and T.M. Kendall, *The Australian Sanitary Inspector's Text Book* (Sydney: William Brooks, 1901), n.p.
171. J.S.C. Elkington, ed., *The Queensland Sanitary Inspector's Guide* (Brisbane: Government Printer, 1911), n.p.
172. Health Inspectors' Association of Australia, New South Wales Branch, *Official Report of Lectures and Proceedings at Twelfth Annual Conference* (Sydney: Standard Publishing House, [1924]), 6.

173. W. Trathen, "A Distinguished Public Health Administrator," *Health* 2(1) (1924), 1–10.

174. "Association of Health Officers," *Australian Medical Journal* 17 (1872), 49; "A Little about Health Officers," *Australian Medical Journal* 18 (1873), 89–90; "Association of Health Officers," *Australian Medical Journal* 23 (1878), 177; "Health Officers and Their Duties," *Australian Medical Journal* 6 (1884), 167–69.

175. "Public Health," *Australasian Medical Gazette* 15 (1896), 496.

176. R. Jennings, "The Medical Profession and the State in South Australia 1836–1975" (M.D. dissertation, University of Adelaide, Adelaide, 1998), 160, 192–201.

177. Quoted in M.J. Thearle, "Dr. B. Burnett Ham. Father of Queensland's Department of Health," *Medical Journal of Australia* 161 (1994), 55.

178. Quoted in ibid., 56.

179. Quoted in ibid., 57.

180. H.M. Keleher, "Australian Nursing: For the Health of Medicare or the Health of the Public?" (Ph.D. dissertation, La Trobe University, Bundoora, 1999), 80–83; J.A. Young, A.J. Sefton and N. Webb, eds., *Centenary Book of the University of Sydney Faculty of Medicine* (Sydney: Sydney University Press, 1984), 121–22, 139–40.

181. K.F. Russell, *The Melbourne Medical School 1862–1962* (Carlton: Melbourne University Press, 1977), 80.

182. Ibid., 103, 162; Young, Sefton and Webb, eds., *Centenary Book of the University of Sydney Faculty of Medicine,* 401.

183. V.A. Edgeloe, *The Medical School of the University of Adelaide: A Brief History from an Administrative Viewpoint* (Adelaide: University of Adelaide Postgraduate Committee in Medicine, 1991), 5, 12–13, 20.

184. G. Rosen, *A History of Public Health* (Baltimore: Johns Hopkins University Press, 1993), 350–54; Keleher, "Australian Nursing," 26–27.

185. Rosen, *A History of Public Health,* 355–57.

186. Keleher, "Australian Nursing," 15–19.

187. See Lewis, "'Populate or Perish,'" 19–20.

188. Quoted in Keleher, "Australian Nursing," 85.

189. See Lewis, "'Populate or Perish,'" 134–35; Keleher, "Australian Nursing," 84–87.

Chapter 4

New Directions in Public Health?

THE EPIDEMIOLOGICAL TRANSITION AND CAUSE-SPECIFIC MORTALITY IN THE TWENTIETH CENTURY

In the last chapter we looked at the trends in mortality rates and life expectancy in Australia in the nineteenth and twentieth centuries, and we noted a decline in age-standardized death rates for both sexes from about 1860. The decline in significant infectious diseases like tuberculosis was the main contributor to the nineteenth-century fall in mortality rates. The secular decline in mortality from infections continued for both sexes in the new century as an epidemiological or health transition in which noncommunicable ("lifestyle") diseases replaced communicable diseases as the leading causes of death took place in Australia. The impact of the influenza pandemic in 1919 was so great that it temporarily reversed the downward trend, raising male mortality by more than 100 percent and female by more than 50 percent. But apart from that major obstacle, a progressive decline occurs between 1907 and the mid-1940s. Indeed, about 50 percent of the decline in infectious disease mortality between 1907 and 1990 happens in that period, before the introduction of penicillin and other widely effective antibiotics greatly increased the curative capacity of medicine. The decline becomes more precipitous between World War II and 1960, with a less steep decline in the 1960s and '70s and a plateau at a very low level from about 1980. The prewar decline is probably explainable by a combination of social and economic progress (widespread availability of nutritious food, widespread provision of primary and postprimary education and better housing) and public health advances (effective urban water and waste disposal systems, infectious disease control, food hygiene, and health education). The steeper decline from the mid-1940s very likely reflects the continuing effects of these two types of factors, and in addition the effects of antimicrobials and mass antituberculosis and immunization campaigns.

Australia seems to have experienced a cause-specific mortality decline similar to that of Western Europe. Between the 1870s and 1950s, in England and Wales (and in Italy), 40 to 43 percent of the decline is attributable to lower infectious disease mortality (25 to 33 percent of the reduction was due to lower tuberculosis mortality); 13 to 16 percent resulted from reduced mortality from bronchitis, pneumonia and influenza; and 7 to 11 percent from lower diarrheal mortality. The major, "lifestyle" or chronic "degenerative" diseases become more important as contributors to mortality with the decline in infectious disease mortality. What can only be called an epidemic of cardiovascular disease begins in Australia in about the mid-1920s. Cardiovascular mortality increases quickly up to the mid-1950s. Then in the period to 1970 growth slackens. A slow rise in males is offset by a slow fall in females. Both sexes experience a speedy decline from 1970, so that age-standardized death rates by 1990 are around the level existing at the beginning of the epidemic.

The decline, one of the speediest in the world, reflects both public health and treatment interventions, and cultural change, although the weight to be attached to each category of factor is uncertain. Certainly, less consumption of animal fat, salt, and tobacco, better medical control of hypertension and better treatment of cardiovascular disease are implicated. But the comparative importance of risk factor interventions, health promotion and general cuisine changes resulting from large-scale immigration from southern Europe, the Middle East and Asia is unclear. Trends in coronary heart disease mortality in Australia resemble those in Western Europe, North America and New Zealand. Age-standardized male death rates (forty-five to sixty years) rose in the period 1950–69 but declined subsequently. Female rates behaved in Australia in a way similar to that observed in other Western countries. However, the situation in Eastern Europe (and the successor states to the Soviet Union) is different. There, the epidemic of coronary heart disease (and lung cancer) rages on unchecked. Where mortality from coronary heart disease has been reduced, experts tend to give greater weight to the influence of prevention, while still allowing that lower case fatality rates and better long-term survival rates have contributed something to the reduction.

The story of cancer mortality is not so reassuring. While female death rates from stomach and uterine (including cervical) cancer fell in 1907–90, mortality from lung, colon, pancreas and ovarian cancer rose, so that overall cancer death rates hardly changed. Male cancer mortality grew slowly to 1950 and then increased more notably to the mid-1980s. It plateaued until the late 1980s. The increase is virtually entirely due to greater lung cancer mortality; changes in cancers of other sites tended to cancel each other out. Stomach and mouth cancer mortality fell, but that from cancer of the colon, rectum, pancreas and prostate (and leukemia) grew. Indeed, in developed countries, generally, cancer mortality not related to smoking was static from the 1950s to the 1990s. The growth and decline of male lung cancer mortality is very probably related to shifts in the prevalence of tobacco smoking, themselves much influenced by preventive campaigns. Likewise, the decline in mouth cancer is the result of reduced use of tobacco as well as better oral hygiene, whereas the decline in stomach cancer results from less harmful food preservation methods. The growth of colon cancer may be related to diet changes like reduced fiber intake.

For males, general mortality falls up to the 1930s, mainly because of a drop in the death rate from infections. There is no real advance in the 1930s, because further falls in mortality from infections are countered by increased cardiovascular death rates. Male mortality flattens again in the twenty-five years from 1945. The plateau effect resulted from the fact that decreasing mortality from infections and "other" causes were balanced by increasing mortality from cardiovascular disease and cancer. To about 1960, female mortality declined because of lower death rates from infections and from "other" and ill-defined causes. But for an increase in cardiovascular mortality between the 1930s and 1950s, the fall would have been more marked. In the decade from 1960, the female mortality trend flattened as movement in significant causes of death ceased. Males and females both experienced notable falls in mortality from cardiovascular disease (and females falls in "other" and external causes as well) after 1970; as a result, overall mortality for both sexes declined. Life expectancy at birth increased from fifty-seven years for males in 1910 to seventy-four years in 1990, and for females, from sixty-one years to seventy-nine years. The Australian evidence (and that from Pacific countries) seems to indicate that the replacement of communicable by chronic noncommunicable disease in a population as the primary cause of mortality is associated with achievement of an average life expectancy at birth of sixty years.[1]

THE COURSE OF INFANT MORTALITY TO 1930

As observed in chapter 3, and as can be seen clearly in table 4.1, all Australian states experienced a very marked fall in the infant mortality rate in the early 1900s, after which rates declined continuously.

Examination of cause-specific infant mortality for the period 1907–30 reveals that diarrhea and enteritis were the largest causes of death. A fall in these causes accounted for a major part of the improvement in the overall infant mortality rate from just over seventy-six to just under fifty-two per thousand births in that period. Other causes showing considerable falls were tuberculosis (from 0.92 to 0.32), syphilis (0.99 to 0.26), convulsions (3.65 to 1.23), and meningitis (1.67 to 0.56). Respiratory infections and influenza mortality remained virtually static. The high death rate for whooping cough in 1907–10 resulted from a severe epidemic in New South Wales, and

Table 4.1
Infant Deaths per 1,000 Live Births in States and in Australia, 1871–75 to 1926–30

YEARS	NSW	VIC.	QLD.	S.A.	W.A.	TAS.	AUSTRALIA
1871–75	104	125	123	158	121	102	119
1876–80	115	120	135	141	107	106	121
1881–85	124	122	137	134	107	109	125
1886–90	115	131	119	105	109	103	118
1891–95	111	112	103	99	130	94	108
1896–1900	113	111	103	112	156	98	112
1901–5	97	96	94	87	125	90	97
1906–10	77	80	71	68	90	83	78
1911–15	71	72	66	67	72	71	70
1916–20	65	67	63	62	62	64	65
1921–25	58	62	51	54	59	60	58
1926–30	55	52	47	47	49	53	52

Source: H.J. Exley, "Infantile Mortality in Australia, 1906–1930," *Journal of Royal Statistical Society*, 95 (4) (1932): 685. Figures have been rounded off.

the high rate in 1916–20 for influenza reflected the impact of the influenza pandemic of 1918–19, while the elevated rate from measles in 1911–15 probably reflected exceptional prevalence in New South Wales in 1912 and 1915.[2] Bronchitis, broncho-pneumonia and pneumonia remained fairly stable, falling only from a total of 6.64 to 5.98 per thousand births. Convulsions declined substantially, very probably because the diarrheal death rate was falling markedly, and as we have seen, mortality attributed to convulsions was often closely linked to movement in the diarrheal rate. Meningitis was falling in 1907–30, except in 1911–15, when it rose slightly. The history of the disease in Australia reveals that normally there was a small number of cases but that in 1915 in Victoria and South Australia there was an epidemic outbreak. The epidemic became acute in all states in 1916 but ended in 1918. This Australian upsurge was related to the epidemic wave that swept through European countries in 1896–1920.[3]

Syphilis mortality in infants declined considerably, and this may have been an effect of the venereal disease control legislation in 1915–18. Typically, the new laws required adult sufferers to obtain treatment from qualified medical practitioners until pronounced cured. There is some doubt about the effectiveness of the legislation in relation to infant health, because mortality from congenital malformations and debility, both of which might be expected to reflect greater control over syphilis, had not declined by a decade to a decade and a half after its introduction. Even so, the availability of the arsenical drug Salvarsan (Paul Ehrlich's "magic bullet") from 1910 or so meant unprecedented capacity to cure syphilis, providing that patients complied with the long and unpleasant course of therapy. It is noteworthy that in 1925–30, where syphilis mortality in legitimate babies was only 0.21 per thousand births, in the illegitimate it was 1.37. The unmarried mother's experience of deprivation put her baby at much greater risk generally; in this period illegitimate babies suffered an infant mortality rate of 92.64 per thousand, compared with 50.23 for legitimate children.[4]

Infant mortality from tuberculosis was of about the same order as that from syphilis in 1907–30, and it declined at about the same rate (see table 4.2). The course of the general death rate from nonpulmonary tuberculosis in Australia and that from pulmonary tuberculosis, after each began to decline in the 1880s, were so nearly parallel that it is not unreasonable to assume the same factors affected both. The bovine form of tuberculosis probably contributed much to the mortality from nonpulmonary tuberculosis. It was usually communicated through contaminated meat and milk.

Infants would, of course, have been particularly at risk from contaminated milk. The trend for nonpulmonary tuberculosis in New South Wales and Victoria reached a notable turning point in 1886–88 and 1889–91, respectively. These were the years when legislative and administrative control intended to reduce tuberculosis were introduced over dairies and abattoirs. Moreover, the number of tuberculous animals in metropolitan dairy herds

Table 4.2
Cause-Specific Infant Mortality, Australia, 1907–30 (per 1,000 births)

Cause	1907–10	1911–15	1916–20	1921–25	1926–30
Measles	0.23	0.41	0.22	0.16	0.22
Whooping cough	2.91	1.61	1.59	1.50	1.53
Diphtheria/croup	0.28	0.29	0.37	0.35	0.27
Influenza	0.34	0.24	0.42	0.25	0.24
Erysipelas	0.15	0.19	0.18	0.19	0.19
Tuberculosis	0.92	0.55	0.40	0.31	0.32
Syphilis	0.99	0.77	0.57	0.36	0.26
Meningitis	1.67	1.80	1.08	0.98	0.56
Convulsions	3.65	2.31	1.74	1.23	0.72
Acute bronchitis	2.27	1.81	1.48	1.05	0.65
Broncho-pneumonia	2.56	2.58	2.71	3.12	3.30
Pneumonia	1.81	1.78	1.74	1.93	2.03
Diarrhoea/enteritis	21.70	18.87	14.25	11.31	7.68
Total digestive	**22.92**	**20.44**	**15.83**	**12.57**	**8.64**
Malformations	2.77	3.37	3.85	3.99	4.44
Congenital debility/prematurity	23.76	24.01	24.48	21.74	19.84
Other diseases of early infancy (birth injury)	1.76	4.24	4.76	5.22	5.53
Total	**28.29**	**31.62**	**33.09**	**30.95**	**29.81**
All other causes	6.68	3.43	2.88	2.48	2.73
TOTAL (all causes)	76.24	70.32	64.57	57.88	51.99

Source: H.J. Exley, "Infantile Mortality in Australia, 1906–1930," *Journal of Royal Statistical Society* 95 (4) (1932): 689.

Table 4.3
Mortality in Periods of the First Year of Life, Australia, 1906–10 to 1926–30

Years	Under One Week	1 Week and Under 1 Month	Total Under 1 Month	1 Month and Under 12 Months	Total Under 1 Year
1906–10	21.19	10.16	31.35	46.25	77.60
1911–15	22.18	9.51	31.69	38.63	70.32
1916–20	23.10	8.59	31.69	32.98	64.67
1921–25	22.04	7.87	29.91	28.97	57.88
1926–30	22.39	6.56	28.95	23.04	51.99

Source: H.J. Exley, "Infantile Mortality in Australia, 1906–1930," *Journal of Royal Statistical Society* 95 (4) (1932): 688.

in New South Wales destroyed in 1901–13 perhaps indicates a declining incidence of diseased beasts in urban dairies. The risk of infection from milk from urban dairies was high because the milk was sold raw and unpasteurized. Investigations of raw milk from dairies in Sydney in 1921–23 seemed to show that it was virtually free of tuberculosis. Tests done in 1925–26 showed milk from only one of twenty-three dairies was infected. In 1927, milk from 127 dairies was examined, and no evidence of the tuberculosis pathogen was found. After the establishment of a Milk Board in 1930, regular testing was carried out, and from 1938 a dairyman-vendor's registration was made conditional on his herd's being certified free of tuberculosis.[5]

In the period to 1930, the death rate in Australia in the first week of life remained unchanged, although there was some improvement in the rate of babies one to four weeks old (see table 4.3). The greatest gains were made in the postneonatal rate, which halved from 46.25 per thousand births in 1906–10 to 23.04 in 1926–30.

There seem to have been three distinct patterns in the secular decline of infant mortality in Western Europe. The first, found in France, Belgium and possibly Italy, points to some decline from 1890, followed by a temporary rise in the late 1890s. The second, found in Sweden, indicates a decline from at least 1881, interrupted by a late peak in 1900. The Netherlands follows this pattern, as does Prussia, albeit not so closely. A third pattern can be seen in Britain, where the infant death rate increased in the 1880s and '90s but fell markedly from 1899. There an underlying gradual downward trend from causes other than diarrhea existed from the late 1880s or early '90s. However, working against this was the "urban-sanitary diarrheal effect," causing a rise in infant mortality in the 1890s. But as it began to work with, not against, the basic trend, it produced a rapid decline after the peak of 1899–1900.[6] A number of factors have been suggested as working to reduce infant mortality in Britain in the late nineteenth and early twentieth centuries. First, a decline in fertility from the 1870s meant that women were having fewer pregnancies and were experiencing longer intervals between births. Second, because of improvement in women's access to education there was a stronger likelihood that family limitation would be practiced and that better care of infants and more self-care would be pursued. Third, there was the impact of improved sanitation and cleaner water supplies—the fruits of the public health movement. Fourth, there were improvements in infant and maternal health services (and in the quality of milk in particular and food in general), although these reinforced the established trend by drawing attention to children most at risk in areas of the highest infant death rates.[7]

In Australia, the "urban-sanitary diarrheal effect," as we have noted previously, was at work, especially in Sydney and Melbourne. But the high infant death rates of Sydney began to decline from the late 1880s, while those of Melbourne fell after 1890. Unlike in Britain, the "urban-sanitary diarrheal effect" seems not to have worked against the general decline in Australia from about 1890, except in Perth, where the infant death rate soared in the late 1890s, and in Adelaide, where some high rates were recorded in the 1890s. It was declining infectious disease mortality that brought down the urban infant mortality rate from the late 1880s, as the case of Sydney shows (see table 4.4). Deaths from tuberculosis began to fall from 1887. "Zymotic" diseases (mainly whooping cough and measles), while fluctuating, fell to new lower levels in the 1880s. Both pneumonia and bronchitis mortality and mortality from prematurity and congenital defects remained stable. Likewise, deaths reported under the heading of diarrheal diseases remained more or less constant, expect for a marked fall in 1904. Indeed, historical epidemiologist J.H.L. Cumpston stated that diarrheal mortality nationally showed wide fluctuations from 1870 but no evidence of a real decline until after 1903.[8] But as we have seen, contemporary infant health experts like W.G. Armstrong and W.F. Litchfield in Sydney and their colleagues in Melbourne and Brisbane pointed out that to the mortality directly reported as diarrheal should be added that reported as due to associated conditions—"convulsions," "dentition," and "atrophy," "debility" and "inanition." If we take that path, mortality from diarrheal (and associated) conditions began to fall in 1886 in Sydney, and the "urban-sanitary diarrheal effect" can be seen to have worked with the decline in infant mortality from other causes from the 1880s, not against it as it did in Britain.

If we take Cumpston's path and see no decline in diarrheal mortality until after 1903, the course of infant mortality in Australia is not unlike that in Britain, with a modest decline due to falling infectious disease (other than diarrhea) mortality beginning in the cities in the 1880s. But diarrheal mortality holds back a major fall in infant mortality until the early 1900s. However, if we follow Armstrong and include convulsions and other inadequately defined classes of cause under diarrheal disease—and what else are we to do with that extensive but misleadingly labeled mortality?—a declining urban-sanitary diarrheal mortality from 1886–89 reinforced the slightly earlier trend downward in infant mortality.

SANITARY REFORM AND PUBLIC HEALTH ADMINISTRATION IN AUSTRALIA TO WORLD WAR I

The coming of bubonic plague, the ancient scourge, to Australia in 1900 promoted sanitary reform in a number of states. An epidemic in Hong Kong in 1894 marked the beginning of a new historical cycle of plague. By 1896 it was in Bombay; it caused almost thirteen million deaths in India in 1898–1948. In the first decades of the twentieth century it spread to Europe and, for the first time, to Japan, Madagascar, South Africa, North America, South America, and Australia.[9] New Caledonia, located in the Pacific a thousand miles northeast of Sydney, suffered plague in 1899. It is believed the disease traveled in shipboard rats from there to Sydney and ports in Victoria, Queensland, South Australia and Western Australia in 1900. It survived in Australia to 1909 and returned in 1921–23. In the first period, there were 443 deaths in a total of 1,212 cases (a case mortality of 37 percent), and in the second, 67 deaths in 153 cases (a case mortality of 44 percent). In the first period, all states except Tasmania were affected. But NSW and Queensland, with total cases of 570 and 318 respectively, were the most burdened. At the other end of the spectrum, Victoria suffered only twelve cases and South Australia only seven.[10]

In Sydney most of the plague cases in 1900 were traced to the Darling Harbor area, and the colonial government assumed control of the district from the City Council under the 1897 Quarantine Act. In what the *Sydney Morning Herald* called "a great crusade of cleanliness," cleaning gangs under the direction of Department of Public Health personnel removed thousands of tons of garbage, dead animals, sewage and silt from the wharves and adjacent areas between late March and early June. They killed forty-five thousand rats as well. The critical role of the rat flea not having yet been fully demonstrated, thousands of gallons of disinfectants were washed over wharves, streets and drains, while householders were encouraged to disinfect their houses. Even omnibuses, trams and cabs were disinfected. Disinfectants had killed tons of fish in Darling Harbor by mid-March. A number of municipal councils cleaned lanes and roads and disinfected gutters and drains, while also sending inspectors of nuisances on searches for sanitation problems on private premises.

Ashburton Thompson, believing in the importance of the rat flea as the vector of infection, strongly urged that the focus of effort be shifted to destruction of rats. Programs offering a capitation fee for dead rats and issuing free rat poison to municipalities were introduced by the Lyne government. The Darling Harbor Wharves Resumption Act of 1900 empowered

Table 4.4
Infant Mortality in Sydney and Suburbs, 1875–1904 (per 1,000 births)

1	2	3	4	5	6	7	8	9	10	11	12
Years	Zymotic (except Diarrhoea/ Dysentery)	Pneumonia and Bronchitis	Diarrhoeal Diseases	Convulsion	Dentition	Atrophy, Debility and Inanition	Prematurity	Congenital Defects	Tubercular Diseases	All Causes	Combined Mortality from 4, 5, 6 and 7
1875	22.0	14.1	24.7	18.6	8.4	43.5	15.0	2.6	10.9	176	95.3
1876	19.0	12.2	26.1	20.1	5.2	40.7	13.0	3.1	13.2	169	92.1
1877	15.9	10.8	32.5	16.6	7.4	28.4	11.9	3.6	10.5	156	84.9
1878	25.8	13.1	29.6	19.8	5.0	32.5	11.9	3.6	9.5	173	86.9
1879	9.5	11.5	36.3	20.6	5.1	30.8	10.4	1.8	9.8	153	92.8
1880	18.4	21.1	32.2	24.2	5.6	43.2	13.6	3.2	7.5	192	105.2
1881	12.1	14.8	32.1	22.8	4.3	35.5	8.9	2.5	9.2	162	94.7
1882	12.7	17.1	42.0	20.6	5.9	36.9	12.1	3.6	9.3	183	105.4
1883	10.3	13.8	31.9	19.0	4.6	38.8	12.9	2.7	9.2	163	94.3
1884	12.3	15.7	36.1	21.3	3.4	40.5	10.3	4.1	9.7	172	101.3
1885	10.9	14.5	39.9	22.3	6.8	42.2	13.3	2.5	11.1	186	111.2
1886	11.3	14.5	37.3	17.4	5.9	37.2	12.4	4.6	11.3	173	97.8
1887	6.3	10.5	34.6	14.2	6.3	22.1	12.6	3.4	9.5	140	77.2
1888	6.9	12.3	39.0	14.5	5.2	30.9	14.3	2.9	9.3	152	89.6
1889	14.8	16.2	44.4	14.0	6.6	25.5	13.6	4.3	8.7	172	90.5

1890	6.2	14.6	31.2	13.3	3.9	20.0	15.9	3.1	6.2	135	68.4
1891	8.7	17.7	34.5	13.6	4.0	23.9	14.8	3.8	5.1	148	76.0
1892	7.8	11.0	30.5	10.4	5.0	23.7	14.4	2.5	5.5	130	69.6
1893	12.6	11.7	37.9	13.5	1.6	25.7	13.9	4.5	5.8	147	78.7
1894	10.0	10.6	35.4	10.9	0.2	23.7	14.7	4.5	5.4	134	70.2
1895	7.0	10.1	39.2	9.0	0.7	21.7	15.1	3.8	5.4	130	70.6
1896	3.7	9.7	45.4	9.5	0.4	24.5	14.4	4.2	5.4	139	79.8
1897	3.5	12.8	43.4	8.9	0.4	21.2	17.1	3.7	3.9	129	73.9
1898	14.7	17.9	46.1	9.5	0.3	22.8	15.9	5.0	5.5	154	78.7
1899	9.2	10.7	33.6	6.1	0.2	16.8	17.1	4.6	4.7	120	56.7
1900	2.8	8.3	36.4	7.6	0.3	16.0	15.4	4.2	3.6	109	60.3
1901	10.3	11.8	37.4	5.5	1.4	17.1	15.5	4.2	2.9	120	61.4
1902	5.8	10.7	39.0	2.7	1.5	12.5	16.4	4.6	3.8	112	55.7
1903	6.7	12.5	44.2	3.9	0.8	12.5	14.5	5.4	2.3	116	61.4
1904	5.1	8.4	31.0	3.2	0.7	11.4	18.8	6.5	2.0	98	46.3

Source: W.G. Armstrong, "Some Lessons from the Statistics of Infantile Mortality in Sydney," *Transactions of Australasian Medical Congress* (1905): 395.

the colonial government to rebuild the notorious slums of the Rocks district, abutting the harbor at the north end of the city. The Sydney Corporation Amendment Act abolished multiple voting, which allegedly gave inordinate control of City Council policy to owners of unsanitary premises. The government made more secure the tenure of the city's sanitary inspectors by paying half their salaries, while the long-established post of city health officer was made full-time.

Epidemic measles and scarlet fever in the 1870s and typhoid in the 1880s had focused attention on the problem of human excreta disposal and had eventually led to construction of an underground sewerage scheme; plague now focused it on domestic garbage disposal. Although the plague epidemic induced the city to acquire an incinerator in 1902—the inner western municipalities of Petersham, Leichhardt and Annandale had acquired incinerators as early as 1899—most councils were not persuaded to change from use of infill tips, because the economics of incinerating did not seem attractive when so much vacant land remained available. When the city incinerator could not cope with the volume of garbage, the excess was dumped at sea. When in 1914 the city was blamed for garbage washed back onto beaches, it pointed out that other bodies, like suburban councils and the Harbor Trust, dumped their garbage much closer to shore. In the same year, the Department of Public Health lamented the fact that few of the many garbage tips in Sydney were properly covered. It suggested that garbage destruction by fire or other approved means was becoming a pressing need as population growth reduced the amount of land suitable for tips. By the mid-1930s, twenty-three councils used twenty incinerators in the metropolitan combined sanitary district (which had by then fifty-one local government authorities).[11]

In 1914, the Holman Labor government raised the status of public health in government by making Fred Flowers the first minister for public health. Labor had come to power in 1910 committed to state provision of a number of health services. In 1911, a deputation from the Labor Party Conference had urged the chief secretary to create a ministerial-level Department of Public Health.[12] The post of director general of public health (who was also president of the long-established Board of Health) was created in 1914 to replace the post of chief medical officer, which Ashburton Thompson had occupied until his retirement in 1913. Between 1898 and 1914, the central public health administration increased its inspectorial and professional staff from fifteen to eighty-six (see table 4.5).

At the 1908 Australasian Medical Congress, Ashburton Thompson had stated that "care for the public health . . . can be successfully managed locally only under conditions of strict control by a central authority." Public health administration was "very much a police duty."[13] The Department of Public Health in this era used its superior powers under various acts to try to counter local political pressures on councils to evade their duties. The

Table 4.5
Inspectors and Professionals, Central Public Health Administration, New South Wales, 1898 and 1914

Inspectors			Professionals		
	1898	1914		1898	1914
Pure food	–	9	Chemical analysts	2	4
Dairy and meat	–	16	Microbiologists	1	3
Glebe Island Abattoirs	4	15	Veterinary Surgeons	4	4
Export meat	–	13	Medical administrators	3	6
Bacon factory	–	12			
Sanitary	1	4			
Total	5	69	Total	10	17

Source: D. Coward, *Out of Sight: Sydney's Environmental History 1851–1981* (Canberra: Department of Economic History, Research School of Social Sciences, Australian National University, 1988), 186.

Sydney and Newcastle medical officers of health (MOH) drew the attention of local authorities to sanitary problems. The central authorities paid half the salary of municipal inspectors and set the conditions of their work. By 1914, 75 percent of metropolitan inspectors possessed the certificate of the Royal Sanitary Institute. On the eve of World War I, the metropolitan MOH, W.G. Armstrong, told an inquiry into the government of Sydney that there was still too many recusant municipalities but that while there were insanitary parts of the metropolis, there were no slums.[14]

Like NSW, Queensland was badly affected by plague. In Brisbane, as in Sydney, gangs were organized to exterminate rats and to disinfect and clean premises. Although plague died out in 1909, the Health Department continued its examination of rats for plague bacilli until 1916, after which it became the duty of local authorities. But surveillance appears to have been defective, because in 1921, although there was no evidence of plague in rodents, there was a death from plague in Brisbane. In his 1907 report on the plague epidemic, Burnett Ham, commissioner of public health, wrote that "the scare, alarm and excitement of the populace were at a name whose association conjured up fearful visions of the 'Black Death' of the Middle Ages [and] led to an urgent demand for sanitary reform."[15] The builders and laborers constructing the isolation hospital were ready to flee on the arrival of the first patient, but a medical officer persuaded most to stay. While visiting consultants did not hesitate to attend the sick, it was only upon the third funeral that a clergyman could be found to officiate at the burial service. Representatives of the Central Health Board, the Vigilance Committee and the joint Epidemic Boards (created from local authorities) had urged the home secretary to bring in a new Health Act to centralize control of public health matters. The *Brisbane Courier* carried the campaign farther in its editorials.

The Health Act of 1900 provided for a full-time commissioner of public health. The post was filled by Burnett Ham at the beginning of 1901. Ham dealt firmly with municipal councils, requiring the Brisbane City Council in 1902 to clear the city of waste—50 men over two months removed three thousand loads of filth and rubbish. The new act also required local authorities to provide isolation-hospital facilities for cases of infection. The 1900 act was amended in 1911, and the debate in Parliament on that occasion revealed an increase in concern with adulterants and harmful additives in food and drugs, an anxiety that was shared in other states in this period. This concern about harmful substances extended to control of the use of lead and arsenic antimony in cooking utensils, paints, wallpapers, "soft drinks" and other everyday articles.[16]

Although plague did not reach Tasmania, public and press fear of it in 1900 pushed the Hobart City Council into a short-lived burst of sanitary endeavour; houses were inspected and rubbish removal was ordered. However, regular weekly removal services were considered too costly for ratepayers, and the whole antirubbish crusade petered out by 1901. The colonial government, the City Council and the Marine Board shared the cost of systematic rat extermination; in addition, a capitation fee of two pence was paid to private hunters. The suburbs saw no need to participate in the campaign. The city corporation continued to exterminate rats until 1914, although the bacteriological laboratory set up at Hobart Hospital in 1897 detected no cases of suspected plague in this period.[17]

It was smallpox, not plague, that promoted modernization of Tasmania's public health administration. An outbreak in Launceston, the state's second city, in 1903 revealed that the Central Board of Health lacked power and knowledge adequate to the emergency, so an expert from outside the state, J.S.C. Elkington, was placed in charge of the effort to contain the disease. The emergency speeded the advent of the Public Health Act, 1903, which put a Department of Public Health in the place of the Central Health Board. The new department, headed by the new chief health officer, Elkington, focused on prevention of infectious disease and purity of food. He enjoyed wide powers, but he lacked the staff to properly carry out his responsibilities.

The 1906 Local Government Act reduced local authorities from seventy-three to fifty-one and endowed them with greater rating capacity for public health ends. But while the department now had a full-time sanitary inspector and three part-time assistants, the inspectorial staff was too small to supervise adequately all local authorities, even in the primary task of investigating disease outbreaks in local government areas. Moreover, the department soon acquired other responsibilities: school health from 1907, factory inspections from 1910, infant welfare from 1917, and public hospitals and the licensing of private hospitals from 1918. While from 1918 the department had a second sanitary inspector, two child welfare nurses, and an assistant health officer, the responsibility for curative as well as preventative services was in the longer term not only to burden the chief health officer with extra work but set up a potential for conflict with clinicians and hospital administrators. It directed the department's efforts away from its core commitment to prevention, much as the clinical responsibilities of English MOHs did in the interwar period. For over a decade after the resignation of the director of public health at the end of 1924, the post of director was left vacant, the running of the department being entrusted to the lay secretary. Moreover, when the post was filled in 1935, it was by the superintendent of the Lachlan Park Mental Hospital at New Norfolk, who had no specialist qualifications in public health. The department's responsibility for curative services increased with acquisition of control of the Psychiatric Institution at New Norfolk and another at Milbrook Rise. Governments of the interwar period seem not to have appreciated the difficulties faced by the understaffed department in effectively carrying out its public health functions while also meeting large responsibilities for curative services.[18]

Plague in Western Australia in 1900 set in train improvement in public health administration. The Central Board of Health acquired two permanent inspectors. In 1902, two inspectors were appointed to inspect meat at Fremantle abattoirs; one went to do the same work in Kalgoorlie two years later. G.H.S. Blackburne was appointed bacteriologist in 1902. The first medical laboratory opened in 1903 to deal with plague and other microbiological problems. The principal medical officer (and president of the Board of Health), T.H. Lovegrove, commented in 1908 that "the work of the laboratory . . . has increased phenomenally in extent, importance and usefulness."[19] Medical inspections of school children got off to a false start in 1906, but activities started again in 1910. As in Tasmania, the board became responsible for inspection of factories, starting this task in 1908.

Like Queensland and Tasmania, Western Australia centralized public health administration in a commissioner of public health under a minister of the Crown. In this was revealed the importance now placed by government on expertise in public health. This change was provided for in the 1911 Health Act, which also reflected the growing concern with adulterated food and drugs. James Hope, last president of the Central Board of Health, became first commissioner of public health in 1911, only to resign in 1915 over a salary dispute. Everett Atkinson, who had obtained his Cambridge diploma in public health (DPH) in 1907 and had joined the Health Department as bacteriologist in 1911, succeeded Hope and remained in charge until the 1940s. While the early twentieth century saw, in the Australian public health world, acceptance of the need to employ experts in the central administration—whether as commissioner of public health, bacteriologist, chemical analyst or trained sanitary inspector—the older idea of a central health authority offering leadership, with a multiplicity of local health authorities having responsibility at the grassroots level, continued.[20]

Plague in the early 1900s hardly affected Victoria and South Australia. As we have seen earlier, Victoria began to modernize its public health administration before the turn of the century. The Public Health Act, 1889, had abolished the existing Central Board of Health, composed of nominees of the colonial government. It had created a new board comprising representatives of the municipalities and two appointees of the government—the chairman and the medical inspector. A Department of Health had been established under a minister and a permanent bureaucratic head.

It was not until 1919 that the next major revision of the health code was made. The Health Act of 1919 got rid of the Central Health Board, replacing it with the Commission of Public Health, the chairman of which was the chief health officer. The commission's membership included a representative of the metropolitan municipalities, a representative of provincial cities, towns and boroughs, and a representative of country shires. Each local health authority was called upon to appoint a medical practitioner as a medical officer of health and a health inspector who had been certified by the commission as competent. However, by the mid-1930s only the city of Melbourne had a full-time medical officer of health; all other local authorities made do with the part-time services of local doctors.[21]

Victoria shared with other states a number of emergent public health concerns. As elsewhere in the Western world, Victoria set up machinery to apply the advances in bacteriological knowledge in order to control infectious diseases. The Victorian health authorities established a reference public health laboratory (now the Microbiological Diagnostic Unit) in the University of Melbourne's Department of Bacteriology in mid-1897, after negotiations with Professor H.B. Allen of the Pathology Department led to the university's agreeing, in return for 150 pounds per annum, to do bacteriological analysis of cases of diphtheria, typhoid and tuberculosis; provide a quarterly report on "colon bacilli" in the Melbourne water supply; carry out occasional analysis of any suspect water supply; and provide other occasional services. The Pasteur Institute in Paris had been established only in 1887, and the Royal Prussian Institute for Infectious Diseases (later the Robert Koch Institute) only in 1891. A Microbiological Laboratory was also established by the NSW health authorities in 1897, and a Bacteriological Institute was set up in Queensland in 1899. Similar facilities were created in the other Australian states early in the new century.[22] To add to its defenses against infectious disease, Victoria established in Melbourne the Queen's Memorial Infectious Diseases Hospital at Fairfield in 1904. In line with contemporary thinking, the hospital was intended primarily as an isolation facility, but it soon became a center for specialist treatment and training of nurses and medical students in the therapy of infections.

South Australia had been the first colony to make tuberculosis reporting compulsory, doing so in 1898. Victoria made the disease reportable in metropolitan municipalities in 1903 and in country municipalities progressively thereafter. NSW, Queensland and Western Australia introduced notification at about the same time, and Tasmania within a few years. Gresswell in Victoria, eager to begin to contain tuberculosis, had in 1899 prepared a report on the prevention of the disease. The health authorities entered upon other initiatives: supervision of the metropolitan meat supply by qualified inspectors from 1900, and provision of additional beds in country hospitals and special institutions in the Melbourne area for patients unable to afford private care.[23] (The Victorian story will be related in more detail when the history of control of tuberculosis is discussed at length in volume 2 of this history of public health.)

Like Victoria, South Australia had modernized its public health administration before the turn of the century. From the late 1880s, the medical profession had been pressing for reporting of infectious disease cases, and this demand became caught up in the 1890s with a campaign led by Dr. Allan Campbell to increase the powers of the central health authority, especially in relation to the containment of tuberculosis. The 1898 Health Act did not create a strong metropolitan board in place of the many local boards (as reformers wanted), although amending legislation in 1911 established a Metropolitan County Health District. It did, however, require reporting of a wide range of communicable diseases, including, as we have noted, tuberculosis. It also sought tighter control of noxious trades and water pollution, and extended inspection of factories, dwellings and lodging houses. Like modernizing legislation in other states, the South Australian bill concerned itself with surveillance of meat and milk to prevent the conveyance of infectious diseases, in particular tuberculosis. Parliamentary opponents of the measure focused to a great extent on the issue of individual responsibility for health and well-being, reflecting the still considerable influence of laissez-faire ideas in late Victorian times. They disliked the proposal for centralization of health administration. The longevity of the notion of individual responsibility significantly influenced the development not only of public health but also of health care, culminating in the 1940s in the epic struggle between the reforming federal Labour government and a conservative medical profession over the former's intention to introduce a state-funded national health service—the high point, in the period covered in this volume, of attempts to establish collective responsibility for the people's health in Australia.

The 1898 act was not superseded for almost forty years. A certain inertia marked public health in South Australia throughout this period.[24] Municipal and district authorities remained significant players in public health administration, and some continued to avoid their responsibilities. As president of the Central Board of Health, William Ramsay Smith, observed in 1910 in a publication on control of communicable diseases, "No local board has an officer of health devoting his whole time to public health work, unless he be a retired tradesman. Very few have a trained sanitary inspector. . . . Another difficulty . . . is that . . . while one board may exercise its powers actively and intelligently, its efforts . . . are frustrated or nullified by the apathy or the ignorantly-directed efforts . . . of the neighbouring local boards."[25]

CONTROL OF FOOD

Surveillance by the state of food supplies in the nineteenth and early twentieth centuries in Australia had two aspects: promotion of cleanliness of the product, and guarantee of purity to an established standard so that purchasers received full food value. Meat and milk, the former a large part of adult colonial diets and the latter important in the diets of many babies and children, were the primary focus of efforts to regulate production and distribution of food to minimize the chances of pathogens being communicated to the consumer and to ensure that adulterants (like preservatives in milk) did not compromise purity. Large-scale marketing and production made better food surveillance necessary as the chain grew longer between point of production and that of consumption and the potential for contamination increased thereby. Scientific and technological developments in the long run made more effective surveillance more feasible. As early as 1820, an analytical chemist named Frederick Accum had published *A Treatise of Adulterations of Food and Culinary Poisons.* This work showed that widespread adulteration occurred in Britain in common foods and beverages like bread, tea, confectionery, wines and spirits.[26] In the 1850s, A.H. Hassall's *Food and Its Adulterations* promoted public discussion of the issue in Britain.

In 1850, the *Lancet* appointed a commission of inquiry into adulteration of food. Public opinion was roused, and a Parliamentary investigation ensued. The result was the Adulteration Act of 1860, amended in 1872; adulteration of food or drugs, or the addition of injurious substances, thus became illegal. But administration proved difficult. New legislation, the Sale of Food and Drugs Act of 1875, permitting local authorities to appoint public analysts was passed. Appointment was made compulsory under an act of 1879.[27] Legislation on adulteration was introduced in the Australian colonies at an early date, as we have noted previously. An act relating to food and drugs, modeled on English legislation, was passed in the 1870s. But as in England, the law proved difficult to administer. It fell quickly into disuse.

The warm climate in much of Australia caused meat to putrefy quickly. Moreover, butchers too often were careless about pollution arising at the slaughtering stage and about the cleanliness of premises. In Sydney in the late 1840s, only twelve of the seventy-eight butchers had decent shops. Even after legislation in 1849–50 created a central abattoir on Glebe Island and a Cattle Slaughtering Act in 1851 penalized slaughter of diseased animals and sale of diseased meat, abuses continued. Indeed, in 1875 the *Sydney Morning Herald* identified three factors encouraging malpractice among butchers—the difficulty of getting a conviction, the slight penalties, and the collusion of pig-keeping aldermen. In country areas, the 1851 act was administered by the police, the competence of whom in this task is doubtful. Inspection of cattle and carcasses in the country remained limited even following the Noxious Trades and Cattle Slaughtering Act, 1894, and the percentage of unacceptable cattle culled was considerably lower than that at Glebe Island abattoirs.

Part of the problem was that many people were accustomed to eating meat that had "gone off" and that might be made more palatable by washing and dipping in vinegar to take away the smell. Commercial refrigeration in the later nineteenth century not only enabled the longer storage of meat and its transport over great distances but prevented contamination leading to food poisoning, although butchers were slower to install cool rooms than was desirable. Sydney entrepreneur T.S. Mort, one of the great early businessmen of the city, supported E.D. Nicolle's experiments with refrigeration in the 1860s. In 1877 Mort, who foresaw a vast overseas and local trade in fresh food based on refrigeration, made an attempt to ship a consignment of frozen meat to England; that undertaking was unsuccessful, but by 1880 frozen beef and mutton from Australia were being sold in London. In 1875, Mort established an abattoir at Lithgow, a town some distance west of Sydney, to supply the metropolis with meat. It was carried to Sydney by cool railway vans. Soon after, he brought cooled country milk to Sydney by the same means.[28]

In Australia, as in other parts of the Western world, in the later nineteenth century, the supply of milk to city dwellers was transformed into a large-scale industry, and milk from urban dairies was replaced by supplies brought from distant country centers. Thus, central London—London was one of the first great cities to experience this change—received milk from centers located thirty to fifty miles away.[29] By 1903, country milk accounted for 55 percent of the total Sydney supply, and by 1912, 69 percent.[30] Although some of this country milk was pasteurized from 1901, it seems unlikely that pasteurization ensured clean, pathogen-free milk at this time, because the methods used were unreliable, and milk, even if safe on departure to the consumer, was vulnerable en route, given careless retail handling methods. A safe and clean milk supply was not available in Sydney and other urban parts of Australia until well into the twentieth century.

From the 1890s, many studies in Europe and the United States were carried out in the bacteriology of milk, but even before modern germ theory, milk was being empirically identified as a means by which typhoid, scarlet fever and diphtheria could be spread. Although the eminent German bacteriologist Robert Koch publicly said in 1901 that he doubted milk from tuberculous cows was a danger to humans, in the early 1890s various researchers showed that the bovine form of tuberculosis is transmissible to humans. In 1886 F. von Soxhlet of Munich advised that cows' milk intended for babies be boiled for thirty-five minutes to destroy pathogens; Dr. A. Caillé of New York publicized his methods in the United States. In 1907, the American C.E. North showed that commercially viable quantities of milk could be heated to temperatures high enough to destroy pathogens without distorting the taste. Pasteurization traveled to England from the United States, where the practice had spread quickly, at least in the large cities. In the United States, the first legislation concerning milk—it prohibited adulteration—had been enacted in Massachusetts in the 1850s, and bacterial limits were first proposed by New York in 1901. As in Australia, official regulation of pasteurization was somewhat slow in coming in England; the first regulations were introduced there only in 1922.

Health authorities in Australia preferred to try to make the urban supply cleaner and safer by attention to the hygiene of dairies and retailers and to the health of dairy cattle. Thus, in Sydney, the metropolitan medical officer of health, W.G. Armstrong, waged a campaign to improve hygiene. Where in 1901, 12 percent of 537 urban diaries were classified as in bad condition, in 1910 about 1 percent of 339 were so classified. In 1904, Armstrong reported that shopkeepers were now storing milk in ice chests or in clean, soundly constructed boxes instead of in open buckets exposed to dust and flies. At least the more responsible municipalities prosecuted adulterators. The common adulterant was water, which was too often contaminated by pathogens. In NSW, from 1903 the use of chemical preservatives like boracic acid was regulated. Indeed, one large Sydney distributor of country milk admitted that it had been forced to introduce pasteurization because of vigorous regulation of the use of chemical preservatives. Under the 1886 Dairies Supervision Act, the NSW Board of Health tried to deal with milk-borne tuberculosis by inspection of dairy herds. The board promoted use of the tuberculin test once it became available in the later 1890s. Declining numbers of tuberculous animals from metropolitan herds destroyed between 1901 and 1913 indicate, prima facie, a declining incidence of dubious beasts supplying milk. The risk from urban herds was of course considerable, because urban dairies sold raw, untreated milk. Tests of urban dairy milk for mycobacteria tuberculosis over three periods in the 1920s indicated that this source of milk was almost totally free of the danger. However, there must be some doubt about the safety of the milk supply before the 1930s.

In 1913, T.B. Bavin, president of a royal commission established by the McGowen Labor government to inquire into food supplies and prices in NSW, produced a report on the milk supply in which he recommended that a central authority to control the metropolitan supply be created and that milk grades be introduced. In 1923, the NSW Board of Trade, reporting on the Sydney supply, supported introduction of a bacteriological standard and establishment of a milk authority. It said that there was no need for concern except about the needs of babies—indeed, baby health clinics at this time routinely advised against the use of fresh milk for infant feeding, recommending instead dried milk supplemented by fresh fruit juice. The 1929 Metropolitan Milk Act gave the new Milk Board the task of registering all dairymen and vendors, fixing prices, supervising the production and distribution of milk and establishing grades of milk. Unable to stabilize prices against the opposition of distributors, the board was dissolved, but a reconstituted board from 1931 exercised complete control over the supply. Only in the period after these changes did the metropolitan supply achieve modern standards of hygiene.[31]

As early as 1838 the colony of NSW had an Adulteration of Bread Act, which specified the ingredients of bread and punished anyone adding alum to the flour. The following year, a Markets Act made provision for inspectors of provisions with the authority to destroy unwholesome products. The Cattle Slaughtering Act, 1851, outlawed the butchering practice of "blowing" meat (improving the appearance by forcing air into it) and "spouting" it (spraying fat over it). The fact that legislation continued to be passed well after this period indicates that the effectiveness of these early acts in suppressing malpractices was very limited. British concern about adulteration in the 1850s stirred the NSW Legislative Council into setting up a select committee to look at bread, tea and coffee. The committee revealed that local authorities were not controlling adulteration, and it proposed that investigation of the abuses continue; this did not take place, and an Articles of Food Inspection Bill, then before the legislature, lapsed in 1858. Eighteen years later a bill aimed at preventing use of additives to increase the weight or volume of food (like water in milk) was passed by the Assembly but then lapsed. Finally, in 1879, the Adulteration of Food Prevention Act was passed. However, as noted earlier, it was hardly used. Up to 1884, only one prosecution was attempted, and that resulted in a dismissal.

The 1896 Public Health Act provided for penalties for adulteration practices intended to increase weight or volume. These penalties were increased fivefold if the additive was considered to be a threat to health. The Board of Health was to establish food standards. In 1897 it set a standard of 12.5 percent solids (including 3.25 percent fats) for milk. The metropolitan MOH was critical of the local authorities' failure to put down abuses. In 1901, of 212 samples of milk analyzed, he reported that over 60 percent were adulterated, more than 40 percent with preservatives. Ten years later the proportion of samples containing preservatives had fallen to 2 percent, and the City Council was taking the lead in acting against adulterators. The battle to improve the quality and safety of the milk supply was a long one. Even in 1917–21, 5.5 percent of metropolitan and 9.3 percent of country-origin milk were below standard.[32]

Victoria began to legislate about food quality at an early date. The 1854 Public Health Act and the 1855 Public Abattoirs Act together required local authorities to regulate the meat trade. The Central Board of Health complained in 1859 that councils failed to ensure "even a tolerable degree of cleanliness" in butchers' establishments. In 1864, Victoria enacted the first Australian legislation to prevent adulteration of eatables and drinkables. The Victorian Act followed the 1860 English act, and Victoria continued to copy the mother country: its 1873 act following the 1872 English act; its 1878 act, the 1875 act; its 1879 act, the act of 1879; and its Pure Food Act, the English act of 1899. The general health acts of 1883 and 1889 addressed regulation of abattoirs, butcher shops, dairy farms and milk shops. Yet throughout the 1880s, the Central Health Board complained of the apathy of local authorities in formulating regulations. In the 1890s instead of, as hitherto, proscribing adulteration and putting the onus on the prosecutor to prove such, authorities decided that it was better to define the composition of food. The 1899 English act had provided for establishment of standards. Moreover, it was now clear that veterinary aspects of the meat and milk trades needed to be better organized. In Victoria, the Meat Supervision Act of 1900, the Milk and Dairy Supervision Act, 1905, and the Pure Food Act, 1905, all reflected this shift in thinking about food control. The first introduced expert inspection of the whole beast at slaughter; only inspected and branded meat might be sold. The second transferred regulations of dairies from local councils to a special branch of the Agriculture Department; one indicator of improvement is that the proportion of udder tuberculosis to total tuberculosis fell from almost 72 percent in 1906–1907 to just over 6 percent in 1913–14. The Pure Food Act not only continued the general administrative provisions concerning purity and cleanliness but set up a Food Standards Committee to advise on the standards required for the composition of an extensive range of commonly used foods and drugs.

Victoria's transition from dealing with the problem of food quality in general adulteration sections of health legislation to passing specific legislation concerning food purity was followed in a number of other states. In NSW, the Wade government had a Pure Food Act passed in 1908. This strengthened the hand of the Board of Health in its efforts to put down adulteration. The central health authorities carried out the administration, whereas in the other states local authorities were primarily responsible. South Australia's Food and Drugs Act, 1908, like NSW's act, came into operation in 1909, while Tasmania followed with a Food and Drugs Act in 1910. Western Australia's Health Act, 1911, included relevant clauses and established an advisory committee. Similarly, Queensland relied on provisions in its general Health Act, 1911, to control the quality and purity of food.[33]

Interstate trade in food and drugs required some uniformity in standards, and the NSW government in May–June 1910 convened a meeting on the subject of chief medical officers, government analysts and representatives of commercial interests. The conference agreed on a code of definition and standards. Conferences were held in 1911, 1913, 1922 and 1927, where standards were revised. While a considerable degree of uniformity was attained, participants in the 1927 conference accepted that each state (and the Commonwealth of Australia) should be free to decide whether preservatives were to be permitted in cream and concentrated milk, and to set its own standard for fresh milk.[34]

The 1890s and the first two decades of this century saw considerable growth in the range of public health activities in Australia. There was, as we have seen, intensification of traditional concern with environmental sanitation and with pure food and drink. This may be explained in part by the rise of bacteriology, which heightened community consciousness of threats to health as well as provided doctors with unprecedented knowledge of many major diseases. Reliable knowledge and increasingly effective practice helped raise the influence and standing of the medical profession as a whole, and this growing prestige of medicine itself supported the advance of public health, especially as public health became a medical specialty. A corps of specially trained public health "subprofessionals"—nurses and sanitary inspectors—emerged in this period and were placed under the control of public health doctors. But the underlying trend was broader than the advance of specialist knowledge in an increasingly educated and science-oriented society, or the professionalization of public health (along with the larger process of the professionalization of medicine). Growing intervention in public health was part of an expansion of state involvement in civil society; interventions also occurred in education, social services, regulation of industry, and labor relations.

THE INTERVENTIONIST STATE

From the beginning of settlement, Australia, as a penal colony, had strong state governance. The governors dispensed justice, legislated like parliament, disposed of land, and generally supervised economic development. After a couple of decades they began to share their autocratic power. In 1814, three courts of civil justice were established, and in 1823 trial by jury and a legislative council were introduced. Yet by the time responsible government came in the 1850s, the state in the Australian colonies was "inevitably a strong, more intrusive, legitimately interventionist instrument than Victoria's Britain."[35] Even so, belief in laissez-faire and individual responsibility in social matters was strong before 1890, and very little social legislation existed. Then an avalanche of social reform occurred. Between 1894 and 1900, all colonies except Tasmania regulated working conditions in factories. The 1896 Factories and Shops Act in Victoria even created wage boards to establish minimum wages. Premier Charles Kingston of South Australia tried to introduce compulsory arbitration for industrial disputes. But Western Australia was the first to bring in an Arbitration Act, while NSW in its 1901 act created an arbitration court.

Such state intervention in industrial relations continued to be a feature of Australian capitalism. The 1890s also saw taxation of land and incomes in most colonies, which both Liberals and Labor supporters endorsed as a means by which the state could redistribute wealth. NSW and Victoria enacted in 1900 provision for old-age pensions for poorer members of the community, although the racism of the time was manifest in the exclusion of Aborigines and Asians from receipt of pensions. The vision of state intervention in industrial and social matters might have been born in the optimism of the expansive years of the long economic boom, but it took the serious economic depression and the great strikes of the early 1890s to bring middle-class Liberal reformers and the Labor party into a pragmatic alliance to achieve social justice through such intervention.[36] The concerns of fin-de-siècle liberalism are well expressed in the list of measures put forward by Alfred Deakin, a future Australian prime minister: "land legislation; [tariff] protection; free, compulsory and secular education; payment of members of Parliament; factory acts; early closing [of shops]; anti-sweating legislation."[37]

At the beginning of 1901, the six Australian colonies came together as the Commonwealth of Australia, a federated, self-governing member of the British Empire. Under the federal division of powers, the six states continued to have control over lands, railways, roads, schools, most industrial matters and health (except for quarantine). In the first decade of the commonwealth, at the end of which Labor began to enjoy great electoral success at state and federal level, the Liberals pursued a comprehensive national policy of protection of the European nature of the population, industries and the standard of living. The Liberals were more attractive to the Labor party in the federal parliament than the third party grouping, the loosely allied free-trade group, which contained more social conservatives than the Deakinite Liberals. The Liberal policy of protection emphasized maintenance of the British nature of the population by exclusion of Asians and Africans, who were seen, whether on grounds of race or cheap labor, to threaten wages and living standards. It was the Monroe Doctrine of the Commonwealth of Australia, said Deakin. For more than six decades, all political parties accepted an immigration policy based on the principle of a white Australia. Buttressing the policy of exclusion was another policy important to protectionist Liberals and Labor alike—the national customs tariff of 1902, behind which local industry could develop. Deakin believed that the existing level of protection was inadequate to the task of sheltering industry. After great debate, a strongly protective tariff was enacted in mid-1908. Industry received protection in return for providing a reasonable standard of living for workers.

A third pillar of national policy, which marked the establishment of substantial state intervention at the federal level, was industrial arbitration. In 1904, legislation created a federal tribunal and provision for compulsory conciliation and arbitration in interstate disputes. Its long-run importance was the way it promoted trade unionism and offered leadership to state authorities. In the years immediately prior to World War I, Labor's success in winning government at state and federal levels brought further development of intervention. At the federal level, Labor essentially extended Deakinite Liberal nation-building and industrial and social welfare measures, although distinctive Labor contributions were made, such as the creation in 1911 of the Commonwealth Bank. This institution was to act as a trading and savings bank, competitive with private banks and capitalized by the federal government. The Deakin government's 1909 national old-age pensions scheme was extended to women of sixty years and other categories of persons, and an invalid pension was introduced. From 1912, five pounds was paid as a "baby bonus" to mothers. The reach of the Federal Arbitration Court was extended to include new groups of workers.[38]

IDEOLOGICAL INFLUENCES ON PUBLIC HEALTH

Although state intervention in a broad sense dates from Australia's penal origins, and though the further development of state intervention in the late nineteenth and early twentieth centuries was driven by a pragmatic quest for social justice, both reforming Liberals and Labor were influenced by larger ideological currents. British theory and practice were influential with Australian Liberals and Labor (although the American philosopher Josiah Royce was a friend of Alfred Deakin and shared the ethical idealism of the Australian political leader). The British philosopher T.H. Green had modified liberalism's traditional emphasis on the primacy of individual freedom by incorporating a quasi-paternalism that allowed the state to intervene to protect the freedom of individuals unable to protect themselves, or to make better the life conditions of those who had through no fault of their own lacked the means to provide for themselves. Although Labor's was a pragmatic populism, Fabian ideas of state socialism had some influence in Australian Labor circles. In the 1890s, Bernard Shaw, the great Fabian ideologue, had, in combatting the anarchist opposition to the state as centralized coercive power and the Marxist theory of the state as an organ of class oppression, urged use of democratic means to capture the state in order to promote social justice.[39] If the Australian Labor party needed theoretical justification for using the state as a tool of social and economic reform, the Fabian conception of the state was ready to hand. Labor was basically pragmatic, seeking a greater share of the increasing product of a capitalist economy for workers, not fundamental social reorganization: "Socialist doctrine came to be employed less and less to justify complete social reconstruction and more and more to support . . . demands for land, banking and currency reform, control of monopolies, and public welfare measures."[40]

Progressivism, National Efficiency and Race Degeneration

The new liberalism of T.H. Green was shared by a number of leading politicians in the Australian colonies, men like B.R. Wise, QC (Queen's Counsel) of NSW, who had been a student of Green at Oxford; A.I. Clarke of Tasmania and C.C. Kingston of South Australia, who independently moved beyond the earlier liberalism of J.S. Mill; and C.H. Pearson and Alfred Deakin of Victoria. Pearson left academic life in Britain to farm in South Australia and then became involved in radical politics in Victoria, where he was a minister in the colonial government, 1878–81 and 1886–90. Pearson's book *National Life and Character: A Forecast* (1894) became well known in Britain and America. It was sympathetically reviewed by Theodore Roosevelt (who stated in 1905 that next to his own country he was most interested in the progress of Australia, the great island-continental democracy). The book forecast the emergence of the welfare state, which would also be the well-armed state in a world divided along racial lines.

Deakin as a Victorian colonial politician pursued protection, welfare, irrigation (influenced here by the Californian experience) and federation of the Australian colonies. After federation, Deakin was a key figure, as we have seen, in the creation of basic national economic and social policies.[41] But what this fin-de-siècle political figure represented was more than the new liberalism. In a broader perspective his program can be seen as part of a set of ideas and a program of action that emerged in the 1890s in Britain and the United States as well as Australia. It held sway until the pervasive disillusionment with moral and social improvement that World War I produced. The mainly middle-class reformers who spearheaded the reformist programs were supported by a larger constituency of professionals and other educated men who reached maturity in this period. They were reacting to the myriad of social problems created by late-nineteenth-century liberal capitalism as well as to the growing insecurity of a world comprising increasingly competitive and fast-arming national states and empires.

Michael Roe has suggested that American progressivism as espoused by Roosevelt best exemplifies the ideas and programs typifying this reformist, modernist politics and that therefore we should use progressivism to describe similar movements in Britain and Australia. Moreover, he argues, progressivism differed from earlier reform movements, whether those of utilitarians in Britain or transcendental moralists in the United States, in its prescribed approach to social problems rather than the social problems addressed—health, housing, education, industrial conditions and alleviation of poverty. Key concepts in progressivism were leadership, the state, efficiency, and nationalism. It advocated leadership by a meritocracy altruistically pursuing the common good, whether in the form of high-level political leadership, as typified by Roosevelt, or the professional, expert leadership of bureaucrats or city managers. It repudiated government by corrupt party politicians or by greedy, self-interested businessmen. Because laissez-faire had failed, positive government was needed, although action at the personal and communal levels was also required. Capitalism, while in need of civilizing, was not to be abandoned. Efficiency—purposefulness and skill in the pursuit of a good or a task—was a key objective. Efficiency involved application of science (or any special knowledge) to the solving of common problems; it contrasted with waste and mindless adherence to tradition. Nationalism at home meant in the United States the Americanization of immigrants from southern and Eastern Europe, their conversion to Anglo-Saxon (Protestant) values. Nationalism in the external environment meant wielding "the big stick"—sending in 1908 the American fleet through the Pacific as a warning to Japan—or shouldering "the white man's burden" in the Philippines as an imperial responsibility incumbent on a superior Anglo-Saxon race.

Health was a primary concern, because it was essential to national efficiency. The contemporary application of bacteriology to prevention of disease was a marvelous justification for the Progressives' faith in applied science in action. With their belief in the superiority of Anglo-Saxons, they were devoted to promotion of "racial health," which paralleled their commitment to education. They were supporters of eugenics, another international ideological movement in its own right. They agreed with the eugenists' advocacy of selective breeding—encouragement of reproduction by the healthy, educated and responsible, and the prevention of reproduction by the physically and mentally unfit. With their concern about vigor and virility and their desire to shape the future of the race, Progressives were particularly keen to advance the health of infants, mothers and children. They identified (and honored) women as mothers and so called for efficient mothering—which, like any other expertise, required special training.[42]

Progressive ideas influenced not only political leaders but influential figures in public health in Australia. The most important was J.H.L Cumpston, first commonwealth director general of health (1921–45) and a historical epidemiologist and historian of public health, who told a Western Australian audience in 1910, at the start of his career, that urgent action was needed to raise the birthrate and that the rapidly developing science of public health was a significant source of the power of the modern state. Moreover, as a eugenist, Cumpston believed that Darwin's struggle for existence and survival of the fittest applied as much to society as to nature. Two contemporaries, who were, like Cumpston, especially significant in the early development of the Federal Health Department were J.S.C. Elkington and R.W. (later Sir Raphael) Cilento. Like an army, the public health service had to be well equipped, well trained and effective in crises, Elkington believed. Two older doctors who made major contributions to public health at the state level were J.W. (later Sir James) Barrett of Victoria and Richard Arthur of New South Wales. Both were concerned with classic Progressive health issues: control of venereal disease, prevention of "race degeneration," the falling birthrate, and promotion of eugenics. Both had a strong interest in town planning, a contemporary international set of ideas that influenced thinking about the relationship between cities and health in Britain and the United States as well as in Australia. They were also involved in traditional public health matters like pure milk for infants, pure food, smoke abatement, and housing.[43]

Rosen identified what he saw as a resurgence of mercantilist ideas and policies in the United States in the 1890s and early 1900s—in the acquisition of colonies, the securing of markets and supplies of raw materials, and the promotion of fit and growing populations. A healthy population was an essential resource for the defense and economic development of the country. Where Britain was to receive a rude shock about the unfitness of her people from the number of recruits rejected in the Boer War (1899), the United States had a similar experience during World War I. In both instances the importance of the national fitness issue raised by Progressives seemed confirmed.[44]

The decline in the birthrate that began in the nineteenth century continued in most Western countries into the 1930s. There was intensification of political and economic competition among European and other Western nations; Japan became a significant competitor after its naval defeat of Russia in 1905. The quantity and quality of population came to be seen as fundamental. Infant and, to a lesser extent, maternal health became a primary public health concern in part because of this larger context. The infant lives lost no longer appeared inevitable, the consequences of a Malthusian world of scarcity; healthy babies were basic assets in the emerging "Darwinian" struggle among nations and races. In Australia, the widely read radical, republican *Bulletin* welcomed in the 1880s Thomas Huxley's argument that the struggle had progressed from the level of the individual to that of the nation and race. C.H. Pearson forecast that "inferior" coloured races would come to dominate the white race and that humankind would slip back to a lower evolutionary level.

In Britain, Joseph Chamberlain, while still a member of the government, publicly canvassed in 1899 the idea of an alliance of Britain, the United States and Germany on the ground of racial affinity, not the traditional ground of commonality of material interests. A eugenist, Professor Karl Pearson of University College, London, advanced a "scientific theory" of race conflict wherein efficient races would crush those that had fallen behind in the evolutionary struggle. Racist assumptions became part of the vocabulary of British imperialism. Warfare was viewed as inevitable and even desirable.[45]

The question troubling contemporary statesmen was how to obtain, from a working class riddled with physical defects, the many thousands of healthy and loyal recruits needed for the mass armies of the future.[46] The condition of the people was for social-imperialists now closely linked with the maintenance of empire. Social-imperialism transcended party political lines. Unionist social-imperialists had objectives in common with Fabian socialists, while the Liberal program of the years before World War I represented a rival form of social-imperialism. Social-imperialism in Germany and Italy also used social reforms to win the loyalty of a marginalized and disaffected working class, giving this class a stake in the future of the nation and so reducing the appeal of socialist internationalism.

The coming of the Boer War not only revealed the British army's poor organization but the widespread ill health and disabilities of its working-class recruits. Seebohm Rowntree's study of poverty in York had showed that more than 26 percent of applicants at York, Leeds and Sheffield depots in 1897–1900 were rejected as unfit, and that another 29 percent were accepted only provisionally. But it was a 1902 article by Gen. J.F. Maurice that particularly drew public attention to national physical deterioration. This, in the face of a vigorous and assertive Germany, became the aspect of national efficiency requiring most urgent action. The inspector general of recruiting soon confirmed Rowntree's claims. In 1903, the Balfour government appointed an interdepartmental committee on physical deterioration. In its 1904 report, the committee recommended extension of traditional public health measures, instruction in child care to mothers and domestic arts to girls, encouragement of physical training, provision of regular meals for needy state-school children, and creation of a school medical inspection system.[47]

Two viewpoints on the problem of physical deterioration emerged among the experts. Those convinced by eugenics urged that the birthrate of the gifted be promoted; the extremists among the eugenists also wanted sterilization of "failures." The medical profession, on the whole, favored state intervention of an educational kind—the teaching of hygiene and domestic science to the children of the poor in state schools. The British Medical Association called for medical inspection and physical training in schools.

The *British Medical Journal* in 1903–1904 concerned itself with "deterioration." Leaders of the increasingly influential public health lobby, like Arthur (later Sir Arthur) Newsholme, saw that eugenics in its pure form, as expounded by hereditarians like biometrician Karl Pearson, threatened preventive public health policies. Political and professional interest tended to polarize the issue of the causes of deterioration (and so its remedies) into nature versus nurture. Newsholme would recall in his memoirs, "Biometrical investigations . . . appear . . . to throw doubt on the value of many public health activities. The usefulness of not a few medical officers of health has been dulled by these doubts . . . and their too ready belief that pontifical statements based on (to them) incomprehensible statistics must be accepted implicitly."[48] Newsholme, who published, as chief medical officer to the Local Government Board, a number of influential reports on infant mortality from 1910, argued against the eugenists' interpretation of infant and child mortality statistics, engaging Pearson specifically in debate. More generally, he suggested that competition for survival in nature had been replaced in modern society by cooperation and mutuality.[49]

The Australian medical profession, like the British, was not enthusiastic about eugenics as a primary way of promoting the health of the population, although many of its members used the language of eugenics, and some individuals (like Dr. Richard Arthur, who founded the Eugenics Society of NSW in 1912) were strongly committed to that view. Although there was a good deal of public discussion of the desirability of fitness certificates as a condition of marriage (fear of venereal disease being an important motive) and some concern about procreation by criminals and the mentally defective, the *Medical Journal of Australia*, the profession's national journal, published only a few articles in the 1920s concerned with "scientific improvement of the race." However, on the specific issue of sterilization of mental defectives, the Federal Health Council, the national body representing federal and state health authorities, 1927–36, proposed in 1933 to make sterilization of mental defectives a condition of their discharge from institutions. Neither at the federal nor state level was legislation enacted, however, and the idea fell into disfavor.[50]

The debate over national efficiency and the wide influence of progressivist ideas made infant welfare an integral part of the general problem of physical deterioration and gave the long-standing concern of social reformers and public health doctors with infant death rates a new national importance and political urgency. The awareness of sanitarians like Newsholme in the 1890s that the urban improvement achieved by sanitation had had little impact on the infant mortality rate was now becoming a national awareness that public health had to address the specific health problems of special populations like infants and children.[51]

Eugenics and Hereditarianism

Francis Galton, fellow of the Royal Society and a well-to-do member of the English middle class, was the "father" of eugenics, a specially influential stream of thought within the broad flow of hereditarian ideas. From Darwinian evolution Galton took certain concepts to fashion eugenics: hereditary variation in domestic breeding, the survival of the fittest in the struggle for life, and the parallel between domestic breeding and natural selection. He applied these to human society in *Hereditary Genius* (1869), which argued that mental and moral qualities were as much the product of heredity as physical characteristics, with cultural processes (education) not significant. Darwin himself was reluctant to accept eugenic control of reproduction. But by the 1890s, deliberate selection to discourage reproduction by the unfit was beginning to be accepted for social as well as scientific reasons, and in the first three decades of this century hereditarianism gained in strength. Powerful social-change movements—working-class and suffragette movements particularly—were in the ascendant. Mid-Victorian optimism about social progress was replaced by pessimism about modernity. Serious diseases like tuberculosis, syphilis, alcoholism, and psychiatric illness were seen as hereditary, not environmental.

Science began to explain how heredity functioned. August Weismann in the 1890s offered evidence that the "germ plasm" was passed on impervious to external influences; he thus refuted the Lamarckian explanation of heredity as the inheritance of acquired characteristics. In 1900 Gregor Mendel's laws of the assortment and recombination of inherited characters in plants seemed to promise that the numerical ratios in plants might apply in humans. In a short time, the basic content of modern genetics was established—chromosome theory, the concept of the gene, and the employment of statistical and biometric techniques of analysis. An optimistic interpretation of Weismann saw good genetic qualities in all social classes, but a pessimistic one saw them concentrated in the upper strata of society, and the second view predominated. In the period from the 1900s to the 1930s, in the United Kingdom and the United States, eugenists advanced a two-prong policy: "negative eugenics," or the discouraging through marriage bans, sterilization and permanent institutionalization of defectives (the mentally ill, alcoholics, criminals, the feebleminded and prostitutes) of reproduction by the "unfit"; and "positive eugenics," or encouragement of "superior" people to have more offspring. In fact, little beyond education seemed practical in positive eugenics, whereas negative eugenic measures of the type noted above appeared quite achievable.[52]

Eugenic societies, of which some focused on the science and others on the development of public policy and legislation, were established in a number of Western countries: the German Society for Race Hygiene in 1905; the Eugenics Education Society in England in 1907–1908; the Eugenics Record Office in the United States in 1910; and the French Eugenics Society in 1912. Moreover, eugenic ideas influenced anthropology, psychiatry and sociology. As we have seen, the more extreme eugenists urged compulsory sterilization or euthanasia, but the more commonly recommended policies included child and family payments for "superior" couples, institutional segregation of defectives, and eugenically determined immigration. From the end of the 1920s, however, the emphasis was put more on "negative" eugenics, and sterilization became a prominent proposal. This shift represented a very notable attempt to restrict the traditional right of the individual to reproduce.

Sterilization laws first appeared in Europe, in Switzerland in 1928, and in Denmark in 1929. The Danes did not hold with the "Nordic" racism of German eugenics, seeing their 1929 measure instead as scientific and socially progressive; sterilization was carried out on more than 8,500 sexually and psychologically aberrant Danes in 1930–49. Sweden created an Institute for Race Biology in 1921, and fifteen thousand or more psychiatric patients were sterilized between 1934, when legislation authorized the practice, and the immediate postwar period. The Swedish law, while talking about voluntary sterilization, appears in practice often to have involved compulsion. In the United States, twenty-four states had compulsory sterilization legislation in place by the end of the 1920s; those sterilized were to a large extent the institutionalized intellectually handicapped from poor backgrounds. The period from 1907 to World War II saw about seventy thousand people sterilized.

By the early twentieth century, eugenics was an established part of social medicine and social hygiene in Germany. Among public health professionals of the Weimar Republic, eugenics was common to those on the political Right and Left. In the prominence given to eugenics in German medicine, the potential for authoritarian abuse was considerable. The Nazi sterilization law of 1933 was the most extreme of any Western country, visiting compulsory sterilization on those suffering from feeblemindedness, schizophrenia, manic depression, epilepsy, Huntington's chorea, heredity blindness and deafness, significant physical deformity and alcoholism—and subsequently, on individuals of "mixed race." Appeal was in principle possible. However, only 3 percent of appeals were upheld, and an estimated 1 percent of the German people had been sterilized by the end of World War II.[53]

The organized eugenics movement in Australia never had the impact on public policy that it had in the United States. In 1912, Richard Arthur, a well-known Sydney doctor and Liberal member of the NSW Parliament, founded the Eugenics Society of NSW. In 1930 as state minister of health, he introduced a bill providing for sterilization of mental defectives, but it was not enacted. Early in its life, at a Sydney health conference, the NSW Eugenics Society had sponsored a resolution calling for prevention of any increase in feeblemindedness by segregation of defectives. Segregation in institutions rather than sterilization became the preferred means of dealing with intellectual handicap. In 1936, Victor Wallace founded the Eugenics Society of Victoria, which had the aim of encouraging a higher birthrate among those of "superior natural endowments" and prevention of reproduction by those with inheritable "gross defects of mind and body." The society sponsored public lectures on subjects such as heredity, mental deficiency, sterilization of the unfit, and race and intelligence. It pressed for provision in a Victorian mental health bill of the 1930s for voluntary sterilization of the intellectually handicapped and psychiatrically ill. The chief secretary rejected the proposal, declaring that the files of the Victorian Department of Mental Hygiene contained no record of even a single request for such action.

Karl Pearson and others at the Galton Eugenics Laboratory had employed the statistics of state school populations to demonstrate that heredity was very much more important than environment in improving the quality of the "race." Alan Carroll, founder of the Australian Anthropological Society and president of the Child Study Association, sought but failed to establish an anthropometric laboratory to do similar work in Sydney. Carroll campaigned, again unsuccessfully, for state control of mental and physical standards for all seeking to marry. In the 1900s the state Education Departments began to carry out anthropometric surveys of school populations (where the British work tended to show the influence of heredity, the Australian work often stressed the effects of the environment). Harvey Sutton, Director of School Medical Services in Victoria and, later, foundation director of the School of Public Health at Sydney University, was concerned that the "intellectual classes" had a low birthrate; accordingly he supported the introduction of eugenic marriage laws.

In 1912, the chairman of the South Australian Board of Health, William Ramsay Smith, argued that the "race" could be improved by social legislation. Acknowledging the force of Mendelian genetics, he nevertheless showed a public health professional's faith in the power of environmental improvement.[54] Some psychiatrists were public exponents of eugenics. M.H. Downey, head of the South Australian psychiatric services and lecturer in psychological medicine at Adelaide University, told the Australasian Medical Congress in 1924 that mental defectives were a serious threat to national efficiency. Segregation, sterilization and prohibition of marriage would be needed if prevention of propagation by the criminal and the mentally defective was to be achieved. A national mental hygiene association such as existed in England and the United States might educate the community to accept such controls.

In 1911, W.E. Jones, Victorian inspector general of the insane, had urged an attack upon intemperance, venereal disease, and the "evil of defective inheritance" so that the "imbecile," "inebriate" and "degenerate ne'er-do-well" would be banished from the community. In the same year, the *Australasian Medical Gazette* proposed legislation to confine the intellectually handicapped to special colonies for life. The next year it welcomed the increasing international influence of the eugenics movement. Victoria's *Australian Medical Journal*, however, argued in 1913 that the compulsory aspects of eugenic proposals alienated observers otherwise keen to contain any increase in the number of mental defectives. The journal opposed legal prohibition of marriage by defectives, because it involved compulsion and because it was supported by fallacious ideas about the inheritance of defects. The successor to these two periodicals, the *Medical Journal of Australia*, was asserting in the 1920s that a substantial proportion of criminals were of low intelligence, and it advocated routine testing of jail populations in order that the mentally deficient criminal might be identified and segregated. By 1931 it believed that voluntary sterilization of the mentally retarded would be accepted once the community understood the issues involved. Compulsory sterilization of psychotics was needed, the *Medical Journal* held, because so many relapsed after discharge from hospital and permanent cures were elusive. Four years later it pointed out that two British committees of inquiry had come to conflicting conclusions about the significance of heredity and mental deficiency. Paul Dane, a Melbourne psychiatrist, argued before the Victorian Council for Mental Hygiene against sterilization of the "unfit" on the grounds, first, that the unfit were largely defined socially; second, that the part played by heredity in mental deficiency was unclear, and even if significant, could be eradicated by sterilization only if it were applied on a very considerable scale; and third, that poverty and other social causes were probably more important and their alleviation certainly more feasible.[55]

NEW DIRECTIONS IN PUBLIC HEALTH

If concern about national efficiency and quantity and quality of population was a powerful ideological and political influence pushing public health toward offering services for infants, mothers and schoolchildren, so was professional awareness that these subpopulations needed special attention if death rates were to be lowered further. Sir George Newman, chief medical officer of the Ministry of Health in England and an expert on infant health, wrote in the late 1930s that in 1900–1914 there took place a shift in public health toward "personal and positive hygiene." The listed objectives of the new Ministry of Health (1919) reflected the expansion of public health's interests. The objectives included the traditional ones of sanitation, food supply, research, education and prevention of infectious diseases. Now added were: a sound foundation of physique (eugenics, heredity and race, and "racial poisons" like venereal disease); maternity and the protection of the function of motherhood (maternity and child welfare); and infant welfare and the reduction of infant mortality.[56] In England and Wales, between 1841–50 and 1891–1900, mortality rates for all age groups except infants declined notably: 12 percent for zero to four years; more than 50 percent for five to twenty-four years; almost 38 percent for twenty-five to thirty-four years; and almost 19 percent for thirty-five to forty-four years.[57] Arthur Newsholme, chief medical officer of the Local Government Board noted in 1910 "the widespread awakening to the national importance of child mortality."[58] In 1891–1900, the infant death rate was 154 per thousand, precisely what it had been in 1851–60.[59] As noted earlier, Newsholme and other sanitarians were already conscious in the 1890s that improvement of the environment by sanitary methods had had little impact on the infant mortality rate. Concern about physical deterioration and about promoting the growth of a vigorous population as an essential source of national (and imperial) power conferred on the long-standing concern about excessive infant mortality evinced by public health doctors and social welfare workers a new national significance in the early 1900s.

Infant Welfare

Early infant health interventions in Britain, as in Australia, typically involved voluntary or local government programs. Moreover, the aims of health professionals and voluntary welfare associations alike focused on reducing mortality rates rather than poverty. As discussed already, maternal efficiency in the home came to be seen as the key influence, while poverty and sanitation were seen as indirect influences on infant health. The target of concern of the infant welfare movement thus fitted well with that of eugenics "to move the focus of preventative medicine . . . towards the individual, from whom more immediate changes could be expected."[60] Moreover, the middle-class organizers of voluntary infant welfare initiatives, as well as the public health professionals, acted as if their clients—mostly working-class mothers—existed in a social vacuum and as if health status and the client's capacity to carry out advice were unaffected by class and income.[61]

State concern for infants in Britain until the close of the nineteenth century had been focused on shelter for unwanted babies and on their protection from physical abuse and neglect. The Infant Life Protection Society was founded in 1870. Soon after, a Commons select committee had reported that "baby farming"—paid fostering of babies—involved widespread abuse and premature deaths. The 1872 Infant Life Protection Act proved to be less than perfect in the protection it offered. The execution in 1896 of a notorious "foster mother" for the murder of her charges led in 1897 to a new act that allowed local authorities to remove children when inspection was denied. As we have seen, the Manchester and Salford Sanitary Association had been employing working-class women to give health advice in poorer homes since the 1860s. But it was not until the 1890s that local authorities in Manchester, Liverpool and Birmingham began to employ lady health visitors for this purpose. In the 1900s infant milk centers and, soon after, advice clinics for mothers were opened by local authorities and in some cases by voluntary bodies.[62]

Collective concern in Australia also focused at first on protection of illegitimate babies from abuse. Thus, in Sydney a Foundling Hospital had been established in 1874, and the Benevolent Society's Asylum had been providing refuge for unmarried mothers and abandoned babies for a long time before that. J.M. Creed, a senior medical man, in 1886 persuaded the NSW Legislative Council to establish a select committee on abuse of infant life. Creed, like C.K. Mackellar, was publicly vocal about the need to arrest the declining birthrate so that population would increase in a British Australia. Creed's bill, based on the committee's findings, failed. Adverse publicity about baby farming in Sydney led in 1892 to the passing of the Children's Protection Act, which outlawed lump-sum payments to those fostering children, obliged them to notify deaths of infants, and required private maternity homes to provide lists of births.

In Australia, the event that more than any other heightened public and political awareness of infant health was the convening of the Royal Commission on the Birth-rate and on Infant Mortality of 1903–1904, which was a New South Wales inquiry but commanded national and even international attention. Mackellar, who had persuaded the state government to set up the inquiry and who became its president, was a pronatalist and social and political conservative like his fellow members of the commission, although concern about a declining birthrate was common on the Left and Right of politics in Australia.

The average size of completed families began to decline in most Western European countries—the decline began earliest in France—and in English-speaking communities overseas from the 1870s, and the decline continued in the twentieth century. The process commenced in Australia in the 1880s, a decade after it had in England. However, the economic depression of the 1890s saw marital fertility fall by 20 percent, a more substantial fall than that experienced in England and the United States in the early parts of their modern fertility transitions. So concerned about population growth was the British government that the Imperial Conference of self-governing members of the British Empire in 1907 was told the mother country would have to set a limit of three hundred thousand emigrants per year to the overseas dominions. This anxiety about British population was expressed at almost all official inquiries into emigration up to World War II.[63]

The NSW birthrate commission linked both maintenance of the European character of the population and Australia's future as a significant power in the Pacific to population growth: "The future of the Commonwealth, and especially the possibility of maintaining a 'white Australia,' depends on the question whether we shall be able to people the vast areas of the continent. . . . [T]his can only be done by restoring . . . a high rate of natural increase or by immigration. . . . With the maintenance of a high rate of natural increase is inseparably connected the preservation of infant life."[64] Japan's naval victory over Russia in 1905 reinforced concern about the flood of Japanese immigration into California and British Columbia in the 1890s and reactivated old anxieties about the "yellow peril," once focused only on China. Concern about population growth was strong among leaders of the infant welfare movement. Mackellar expressed this clearly in his work on the birthrate commission. Neville Mayman, president of the Benevolent Society, a long-established charitable provider of social welfare and health services in NSW, expressed, in a report on infant welfare in New Zealand presented to the Holman Nationalist government in 1918, concern for population growth in the interests of economic development.[65] The loss of young men in World War I became another reason—in addition to "white Australia," economic development, and the continuing growth of Japanese power—that interest in population and infant health remained live topics in the interwar years. In 1925, St. Margaret's Hospital, a leading Sydney maternity hospital, warned in an appeal for donations, "In the last few years, 122,990 infants have died[,] . . . more than twice the number of Australian soldiers killed during the war. . . . Just as surely as the white races took Australia by force from the aboriginals, so surely will the coloured races take Australia . . . unless something is done towards self-preservation."[66]

Other major Western nations demonstrated the link between concern for population and infant welfare initiatives. In France, fear of German power fed concern about both. In 1896, the Alliance National pour l'Accroissement de la Population Française came into being, and in 1902 an extra-parliamentary commission on population decline was established. Pronatalism advanced farther when the Conseil Supérieur de la Natalité was brought into being, with the broad responsibility to inquire into matters relating to fertility and mortality. From 1902, the Ligue Contre la Mortalité Infantile was focused on the particular issue of infant mortality. In Germany, a variety of policies were aimed at promoting population expansion—allowances for families with three or more healthy children, suppression of information about contraception, additional taxes to be paid by the childless, and severe punishment of those inducing abortions. Infant health promotion came under imperial patronage. The Kaiserin Auguste Victoria Haus in Berlin was set up to be a model institution devoted to research on infant health, the training of nurses, and the first-class care of women giving birth and of sick babies. In the United States, "race suicide," a synonym for the declining birthrate, was the subject of national debate in the years before World War I. A Yale economist, Irving Fisher, drew up for Theodore Roosevelt's Commission on the Conservation of Natural Resources a report on national vitality in which he urged warmly introduction of measures to promote the health of mothers and children. The American Academy of Medicine in 1909 sponsored a conference out of which grew the American Association for the Study and Prevention of Infant Mortality. In 1912, the federal government created the Federal Children's Bureau, with the wide-ranging task of inquiring into all things relating to the welfare of children and infant life.[67]

Knowing that America had one of the highest infant mortality rates among Western countries, the Children's Bureau—the first federal agency to be led by women—pushed for federal funding to promote "baby saving." By 1918, when the Sheppard-Towner Bill was introduced to Congress, over eleven million women were the subject of baby-saving efforts. Women's associations and well-known women reformers across the nation publicly supported the bill. The Children's Bureau believed that educating mothers about child care would in turn encourage them to call for state-subsidized health services. In deference, however, to powerful collective attachment to individual responsibility and states rights, and to the opposition of the American Medical Association to state support for health care, the Sheppard-Towner Act as passed was a limited exercise in federal intervention, providing a mere $1.48 million in 1921–22 and $1.24 million for the following five years.

These federal funds went to the states on a matching basis (Massachusetts, Connecticut and Illinois refused to participate) for education on hygiene and nutrition, for nursing aid for pregnant women and recent mothers, and for infant and child health conferences. But an alliance of medical and conservative groups accused people working under the act of promoting the three evils of birth control, Bolshevism, and state medicine; it waged so strong a campaign against the legislation that the act was repealed in 1929. The Social Security Act, 1935, again provided federal money for maternal and child health services, but unlike the earlier act, which saw such services as a right of all, the 1935 legislation provided assistance only to those lacking means to pay for private medical care.[68]

In the decade or so before World War I, France, the United States and Britain all provided models for the Australian infant welfare movement. French pediatricians, responding to the national concern about the falling birthrate, introduced two innovations: the *consultation de nourrisson* (infant health consultation), which was the forerunner of the baby health center, and the *goutte de lait,* or clean milk station. Pierre Budin, head of the obstetrical service at the Charité Hôpital in Paris, noticed that babies of poor families often left the hospital well, only to die at home. With the consent of the director of public assistance, Budin opened an outpatient clinic where babies could be assessed. His main aim was to promote breastfeeding, although sterilized milk was made available where the mother lacked adequate breast milk. Over the next two decades consultations (and milk stations) sprang up in many French cities and towns under the auspices of both public and charitable agencies. Not all municipalities were diligent. A 1910 survey of 150 of the largest cities found that only eight supervised the health of infants well. A milk station was opened in his Paris dispensary in 1892 by Gaston Variot, but the term *"goutte de lait"* was introduced by Leon Dufour, who opened a milk station at Fécamp in 1894. While advocates of consultations and milk stations defended the merits of each institution, both usually offered sterilized or pasteurized milk as well as advice to breastfeed wherever possible. French doctors were well aware that poverty was a serious bar to adequate mothering, and cash or payments in kind as well as instruction were often provided in infant health centers; short-term financial aid also became available under a 1904 law. The Strauss Law of 1913 offered maternity benefits to women who could show they provided proper care for their babies.[69]

In the United States, as in France and other Western countries, diarrheal disease—often brought into the home by flies from horse manure heaps and piles of garbage in urban areas—was the great threat to infant life that the reformers who established consultations and milk stations sought to combat. Progressives bent on integrating southern and Eastern European immigrants into society, and social workers seeking to turn tenement dwellers into responsible citizens, joined pediatricians and obstetricians, not unconcerned with advancing their professional interests, in promoting education of mothers as the solution to the problem of infant wastage. Despite the obvious connection between poverty and high infant mortality, reformers did not set out to banish or alleviate want. The American infant welfare movement drew on French experience, and the milk station was central to urban work in the United States. While a physician, Henry Koplik, established the first station in the country in 1889 to ensure that sick children on New York's Lower East Side obtained uncontaminated milk, it was a New York philanthropist, Nathan Straus, who established a network of stations in the 1890s; by 1896 his stations were providing six hundred thousand bottles of pasteurized milk a year to poor infants. He gave pasteurization plants to Philadelphia and Chicago. In 1908, the New York Milk Committee (of the Association for Improving the Condition of the Poor) established seven stations in addition to the six run by Straus and one by the Good Samaritan Dispensary. The new stations focused first of all on education of mothers in feeding and hygiene, encouraging breastfeeding; they also, however, offered modified and sterilized milk. The committee's approach became the model for stations established elsewhere in the country over the following decade. The City Council of New York financed an additional fifteen milk depots in 1910, so that by 1912, fifty-five stations functioned in the city.

In other cities, charitable and civic organizations set up milk and baby hygiene associations that established stations that employed visiting nurses and volunteer doctors. Chicago's system was typical of larger cities. Some charities offered clean milk for feeding babies of poor families. The Visiting Nurse Association and the Department of Health organized domiciliary visits by nurses. The Pediatric Society provided physician services. From 1911, the Infant Welfare Society acted as coordinator of milk stations, each station offering twice-weekly consultations and cheap, certified milk. In the smaller cities, infant welfare developed in a similar piecemeal fashion. Where the French emphasis was on consultations with doctors, the domiciliary visits of public health nurses were central in the United States. In fourteen cities, nurses made home visits to all babies born in poor areas and to all those delivered by midwives or in the charitable wards of hospitals. The public health nurse's contact with the mother opened the way for the mother's coming for a consultation. But it was also intended to improve the physical environment of the tenement along middle-class lines, as Progressivism dictated.[70]

The French model centered on the physician; the English model, like the American, gave much weight to the lady health visitor or nurse who visited the home. In the 1890s English health societies established training schools for lady health missioners, while nurses took up professional domiciliary work. The Board of Education provided grants for schools for mothers, of which St. Pancras School for Mothers (1907) was the best known, and the 1907 Notification of Births Act allowed local authorities quickly to obtain information about newborn children so that visiting could be arranged. In the 1900s milk centers and then clinics were created, usually by local authorities but sometimes by voluntary agencies. Home visitors aimed not only to encourage breastfeeding and infant care but also to improve domestic hygiene standards generally.

A major landmark in the development of maternity and child welfare services was the first National Conference on Infantile Mortality. This took place in London in 1906 under the presidency of John Burns, president of the Local Government Board, whose speech did much to mobilize public opinion behind the growing national effort to preserve infant lives. The loss of young men in World War I heightened concern about infant life wastage in Britain, as it did in Australia. A temporary decline in the birthrate in Britain in 1918–20 reinforced this concern. The Maternity and Child Welfare Act of 1918 confirmed the legality of local government expenditure on child and maternal health services, and a maternity and child welfare section was created within the new Ministry of Health. Nine organizations joined forces in 1917 to form the National League for Health, Maternity and Child Welfare. The Midwives Act of 1918 empowered local authorities to fund training of midwives and to pay doctors brought in on cases under the regulations of the Central Midwives Board.[71]

W.G. Armstrong began organized infant health work in Australia in late 1903, while the Royal Commission on the Decline of the Birth-rate was in progress. In the 1890s, he had seen the work of Budin and Dufour in France and was working in England when health visitors were beginning to be employed by the local authorities. Impressed by Newsholme's idea that the home was the focus of diarrheal infection, he concentrated on provision of advice in the home rather than creation of milk deposits or *consultations de nourrissons*. The core message for the mother, apart from domestic hygiene, was to breastfeed, but where this was impossible, advice was given on hygienic preparation of modified cow's milk. For the first ten to fifteen years the campaign was aimed at the working-class areas of the inner city, where the child was more at risk and the mother was less likely to consult a doctor.[72] Initially, Armstrong simply sent pamphlets (on precautions against diarrhea, along the lines standard in England) to homes in the inner city where births had been registered in the previous six months. From May 1904, he used the services of Margaret Ferguson, the City Council's lady sanitary inspector, who, besides reporting on the sanitary condition of houses, advised mothers to breastfeed and to take pains with domestic hygiene. By the end of that year, she had carried out 1,414 visits to 911 houses.

As in Britain, voluntary and charitable bodies developed services alongside those provided by local authorities, although the state took firmer control of infant welfare in NSW after World War I. The Benevolent Society set up in 1906 a consultation on the French model at the new Royal Hospital for Women (successor to the Benevolent Asylum's lying-in section) in the inner suburb of Paddington. Two years later it established an outpatient department at its Hospital for Infants, at which babies were examined. They were later checked at home by a visiting nurse. The society's outdoor aid department offered milk to mothers and babies in need. Unable to fund a milk depot of the French or American type offering pasteurized milk, it used donations of tinned condensed milk for this purpose. With the support of the National Council of Women, the Alice Rawson School for Mothers was established in 1908. It opened rooms in the inner suburbs of Darlinghurst, Newtown and Alexandria. In its third year of existence, its workers saw more than 750 babies in the rooms and carried out over two thousand home visits. Its visiting staff often assisted Armstrong's staff in domiciliary work.[73]

J.S.C. Elkington, newly appointed head of Tasmania's Department of Public Health, was the author of a Tasmanian pamphlet carrying advice similar to Armstrong's. His department distributed the pamphlet in 1906. Thomas Borthwick, the Adelaide City Council's medical officer, impressed by Armstrong's report on his work to the 1905 Australasian Medical Congress, had a pamphlet distributed from 1907. A nurse visited babies in inner-city locations, until her services were terminated in 1912. Dr. Helen Mayo, the first woman to obtain the Adelaide M.D. and in the 1920s South Australia's equivalent of director of infant welfare in other states, created, with Miss Harriet Stirling, a friend who was a visitor to boarded-out state children, the Adelaide School for Mothers in 1909. Mayo had been impressed by the work of the London St. Pancras School for Mothers. She had also observed the work of Budin in France and that done at Huddersfield in England. The Adelaide School educated mothers and regularly monitored the growth of babies.

Doctors Isabel Younger Ross and Constance Ellis, encouraged by work being done in London and Chicago, led the movement to create infant health clinics in working-class areas of Melbourne from 1917. At the earliest stage, milk depots were the preferred vehicles of assistance. The Lady Talbot Milk Institute—named for the wife of the governor of Victoria—was established in 1908. While the aim of the institute from 1909 was to offer pure bottled milk according to capacity to pay—the milk came with an ice chest, because of the hot Australian summers—encouragement of breastfeeding and domiciliary visiting were just as much a part of its remit. Doctors disagreed about the cost benefit of pasteurized milk for babies. Eminent physicians A. Jeffreys Wood and J.W. Barrett caused an uproar among milk reformers when they replaced pasteurized milk with raw milk from tuberculin-tested cows. In Queensland, the preferred approach was distribution of milk from a milk depot. In 1908, the Lady Chelmsford Milk Institute (here too named for the governor's wife) was established with the advice of Alfred Jefferis Turner, a pioneer Brisbane pediatrician. Turner, unlike his Melbourne confreres, insisted on pasteurized, cooled milk, because the greater heat of the Brisbane summer made other options too dangerous. In Western Australia, women's associations in Perth established a Children's Protection Society in 1906; it had the same objectives, fighting baby farming and other abuses, as were pursued by similar organizations in the eastern colonies in the 1880s and 1990s. Women's organizations like the local branch of the National Council of Women pressed from 1909 for improvement in midwifery standards, and their concerns included encouragement of breastfeeding. While the western state lacked a school for mothers or an infant health center until 1920, it experienced the decline in infant mortality that the rest of the country enjoyed in the early twentieth century.[74]

As we have seen, the great turning point in infant mortality in Australia in the 1900s, after which the infant death rate fell progressively, occurred just when the earliest piecemeal efforts to promote mothercraft took place. These pioneering efforts cannot account for the decline, although the institutional and educational developments of the interwar period reinforced the downward trend. The infant health movement nationwide did not gather real momentum until the loss of sixty thousand young men in the Great War pushed health authorities into establishing larger-scale facilities. Moreover, with 36 percent of military volunteers classified as unfit for overseas service, health authorities had become concerned about "race degeneration." Even then, as we shall see, they were careful to restrict the reach of the services so that they did not intrude on the preserves of private medical practitioners.

Among social reforms the NSW Labor government was required by party policy to pursue when it assumed office in 1910 was the state provision of a range of health services. Although committed to government control of public hospitals and other state initiatives, the reforming Labor government was constrained by the weakness of its parliamentary situation, by financial stringency (soon heightened by the demands of World War I) and the influence of a strong and organized medical profession, the nonprofit, self-help, mutual aid societies that funded much medical care in the private market, and of individuals running the public hospitals who wished to preserve their institutions' charitable orientation. In 1914, following consultation with Armstrong, the Labor minister for public health, the Hon. Fred Flowers decided to put infant health facilities under direct state control. Even so, he included voluntary and charitable bodies in the scheme, establishing the Baby Clinics, Pre-Maternity and Home Nursing Board to advise him on the development of his infant health clinics. Charles (later Sir Charles) Clubbe, a leading pediatrician, was chairman of the board; Neville Mayman, president of the Benevolent Society, was vice chairman; R.T. Paton, director general of public health, and Miss Alice Friend, secretary of the Rawson School, were members. This advisory board proposed to reduce the time taken to reach the mothers of newborn children by means of an early-notification-of-births program like that in England. In early 1915 the Notification of Births Act began to operate in the poorer areas of Sydney and Newcastle. That concern about infant health was commonly linked with population growth and protection of a "white Australia" can be seen in the parliamentary debate of this measure. J.J. Morrish, Labor member for the electorate of King (later a Nationalist), strongly supported government actions to save infants at a time when so many potential fathers were being killed in the war. Native-born citizens were to be preferred to immigrants, he proclaimed.[75]

Flowers opened the Lady Edeline Hospital for Babies in 1913 to accommodate diarrheal disease cases. Infants were not usually admitted to general hospitals, including children's hospitals, at this time because of the dangers of cross-infection and the potential high mortality. The infant welfare clinics referred infant patients to the new hospital. Flowers's wife, active in infant welfare, became president of the Hospital Board, and Ada Holman, wife of the premier, W.A. Holman (the only Labor member of the Royal Commission on the Birth-rate of 1903–1904) vice president, while the matron was a former public health nurse, Miss C.M. Burne. The Labor government also opened a convalescent home at Rose Bay in 1915 to assist debilitated working-class mothers to recuperate and maintain capacity to breastfeed.

By the end of 1915 there were nine baby-health clinics in NSW, mainly in areas of high infant mortality in Sydney and in the port city of Newcastle. By the close of 1919 there were fifteen clinics, and plans were being made for one in the inland mining town of Broken Hill. In Victoria there was rivalry between pioneering groups in the infant welfare movement. Dr. Isabel Younger Ross, who had been a leading student of pediatrician Dr. Eric Pritchard, Frederick Truby King's English rival, returned from London to Melbourne in 1917. She joined with women (including Nurse Peck, who had been a nurse visitor for the Talbot Milk Institute) associated with Boroondara Free Kindergarten in working-class Richmond to establish the first infant health center at the kindergarten. However, women from the Melbourne District Nursing Society, who carried out district nursing among the sick poor, and associates in the Victorian Ladies' Benevolent Society and Association of Crèches expected to run the infant health clinics in Melbourne. At the same time, Sister Maude Primrose of the Visiting Trained Nurses' Association of Victoria (founded in 1909), who had trained at Truby King's Karitane Hospital in New Zealand, was eager for a mothercraft body like King's Plunket Society to be established. Although the state's Liberal government publicly supported the idea of coordination of effort in a single organization, Dr. Younger Ross and her associates jumped the gun, establishing in 1917 three centers at kindergartens in the city and in the inner suburbs of Richmond and Carlton. From these developed the Infant Welfare Society, which emerged as the Victorian Baby Health Centres Association in mid-1918. Supported by the charity lobby and with the eminent pediatrician A. Jeffreys Wood at its head, the association by the end of 1919 had centers in the inner Melbourne suburbs of Richmond, South Richmond, Carlton, North Melbourne, Collingwood, Fitzroy, Port Melbourne, South Melbourne and Brunswick, and one in the port city of Geelong.

In Queensland, the Ryan Labor government established four clinics in Brisbane in 1918. There was no voluntary involvement in this state. In South Australia, the School for Mothers received its first funding from the Adelaide City Council in 1918. Tasmania and Western Australia were slower to develop facilities. The Child Welfare Association of Tasmania opened a clinic in Hobart in 1917 and another in Launceston, and government subsidies were made available from 1918. Nurses at the three Hobart clinics were being paid by the state government by the mid-1920s. By the latter date, the Mothers' School in Adelaide ran thirty-one part-time centers plus a small training school along Tresillian lines (about which more below). It offered a different service from that in other states in that more home visiting than clinic attendances took place—in 1924, almost sixty-five thousand home visits but only just under twenty-eight thousand clinic attendances. In Queensland by that date, four Brisbane and nine country clinics were in being, and a state-organized training school was in existence. Attendance rates were greater than in other, smaller states—almost fifty-three thousand clinic consultations and almost fourteen thousand home visits. In Western Australia an Infant Health Association was not established until 1922, but by the mid-1920s both the state and local authorities provided funds on a pound-for-pound basis for the operation of five clinics run by voluntary bodies. By 1925, all of the large cities in Australia (or at least the more densely populated sections and some suburbs) had clinics, even if country towns, particularly in the smaller states, were not well served. Although infant welfare services had been initially aimed at mothers and babies of the poorer classes, by this time mothers of all classes were eligible to use the facilities.[76]

The same coalition of interests tended to gather behind infant health initiatives throughout Australia (except in Queensland, where the state took the initiative): women doctors, wives of politicians and doctors, other women of the social elite who ran charitable bodies, the district nursing associations, the National Council of Women, the Women's Christian Temperance Union, and children's physicians, with the Australian branches of the British Medical Association offering qualified support.

The Great War saw attempts in the two largest states, where infant health developments had gone furthest, to rationalize organization. In 1918, the Royal Society for the Welfare of Mothers and Babies was created in Sydney. A grouping of doctors, interested politicians, public servants and private citizens, it was supposed to put a more human face on activities by reducing state involvement. In fact, it gave the private medical profession a dominating influence. Businessman and prominent Nationalist Party member S.R. Innes-Noad was asked to be president, in the belief he might be able to raise funds from the private sector. The vice presidents included J.D. Fitzgerald, the minister of public health; Fred Flowers, the ex-minister; W.A. Holman, the Nationalist premier and former Labor leader; and leading physicians Sir Charles Mackellar and Charles Clubbe. Those with the real influence on the day-to-day running of the clinics were the doctors—Clubbe, W.F. Litchfield and their protégée, Margaret Harper. In 1919 the society took over responsibility for administration of the baby health clinics. The Royal Society's aims were similar to those of the British Local Government Board's model scheme of 1917–18 in their emphasis on the health of both infant and mother. The NSW government had sent in 1918 Neville Mayman as a commissioner to investigate infant welfare work in New Zealand, which enjoyed a much lower infant mortality rate than NSW—in 1901–1905, seventy-four per thousand compared with ninety-seven. Dr. Frederick Truby King was absent in England, and Mayman was told by New Zealand's chief health officer, T.H.A Valintine, that his country's low infant death rate was due more to the work of the Health Department and climatic and social advantages over Australia than to King's Plunket Society. Even so, Mayman reported favorably on the society.

Margaret Harper went to New Zealand in 1920 to report to the society on King's system, even though some medical members pointed out that his strict ideas on infant feeding were not accepted by the profession in Australia. She recommended a training school like King's Karitane Hospital. The society opened the Tresillian Mothercraft Training Home at Petersham in Sydney in 1921, with Margaret Harper as first medical director. Nurses from all over the country came for postgraduate training in mothercraft, while mothers and babies were helped with feeding problems at Tresillian. The NSW government soon made Tresillian training plus Australian Trained Nurses Association certificates in general and obstetric nursing prerequisites for appointment as a clinic nurse. Tresillian North was established at Willoughby in 1927, and Tresillian Vaucluse was opened at the former Lady Edeline Hospital for Babies after the hospital closed in 1935; it was no longer needed, as infant diarrheal mortality had declined markedly. After an initial period of cooperation, the Royal Society's relations with King deteriorated. The Plunket-trained matron of Tresillian, Miss E. Martin, left her post in 1923 after disputes over departures from the Plunket approach and over use of King's New Zealand emulsion. She joined Karitane-Sydney, where King's system of infant care was followed strictly. The Australian Mothercraft Society, which adhered to the Plunket-King system and was formed in 1923, remained small. It never challenged the hegemony of the Royal Society.

In Victoria in 1917, the minister for health had convened meetings of organizations concerned with infant welfare work to try to rationalize efforts. A division developed between the Society for the Health of Women and Children, which followed the Plunket system, and the Baby Health Centres Association, the outlook of which was closer to the New South Wales Royal Society's approach. The association, with its nineteen-member council—twelve philanthropic women, three women doctors, two city councillors, a representative of the Salvation Army and a prominent Melbourne doctor, W.G. (later Sir George) Cuscaden—received from 1918 a government subsidy, on a pound-for-pound basis against funds supplied by local authorities. Municipal support gave the Victorian baby health centers some independence of state governments and a buffer against changes in state policy.

In 1925–26, the Royal Society for the Welfare of Mothers and Babies came under attack for an alleged failure to reduce infant mortality. J.S. Purdy, medical officer of health for Sydney, and others were publicly critical, while Truby King weighed in from New Zealand with criticism of the society's departure from his strict feeding regimen. The society defended itself by pointing out that apart from its inflexibility there was nothing special about King's approach, and that the much larger Australian cities and climatic differences made reduction of infant mortality more difficult in Australia than in New Zealand. The government responded by placing clinics under the control of the Health Department, creating a Division of Maternal and Baby Welfare within the department. The society's battle with King continued but had lost some of its vigor by the 1930s. When King died in 1938, Margaret Harper said that while he had been dictatorial in approach and that the Royal Society had developed its own style, drawing on its own experience and the results of work from all over the world, he had helped the society much in its early days.

Although it lost control of the clinics in 1926, the Royal Society continued to enjoy considerable influence on infant health services and infant care. It continued to run the Tresillian Homes, which were centers both of treatment and of the training of mothers and nurses. The dominance of the society and the common training it offered for clinic nurses ensured uniformity of instruction. The clinics and Tresillian Homes communicated the society's views on mothercraft directly to many urban mothers, but the publications and other publicity efforts of the society and the Health Department spread the net even more widely, reaching mothers not in personal contact with the society or the clinics.[77]

School Health Services

As early as the close of the eighteenth century in France, medical inspection of schoolchildren was being discussed. Indeed, the principle was endorsed by the Convention in 1793. However, only in the last three to four decades of the next century did European countries and the United States put into practice this idea. In 1874, regular inspection of students was initiated in Brussels. It was initiated in Paris in five years, and in Lyons six years later. It was implemented in Sweden in 1878.

In Germany and England, investigations into the eyesight of schoolchildren and efforts to prevent spread of communicable disease were the forerunners of state concern with the general health of students. In 1866, Dr. Hermann Cohn tested the eyesight of 7,568 schoolchildren in Breslau; his findings resulted in changes to classroom furniture and lighting. Thirty years later, the first school doctors were appointed—in Wiesbaden and soon in a number of other German towns as well. In 1880, Dr. Priestley Smith made public his findings concerning the eyesight of two thousand Birmingham children and adolescents, while in 1882 Dr. Clement Dukes, Rugby School's doctor, published *Health at School;* a decade later Dr. Francis Warner reported the results of his inspection of fifty thousand children in a variety of schools. In 1890, the London School Board appointed Professor W.R. Smith as the first full-time medical officer of a British education authority, although the board's intention, because of the size of its school population, at first was to use him to do medical examinations of candidates for board posts and for general advice. In 1901, when the board would not give him a salary increase unless he gave up his other public and private work, he resigned, to be succeeded by James Kerr. Kerr had since 1893 been a full-time medical officer with the smaller Bradford School Board, which, on dubious legal grounds, had employed its power to appoint "necessary officers" under the Elementary Education Act on 1870 to obtain his services. Kerr expanded the staff and activities of his medical department, appointing school nurses to inspect for ringworm and pediculosis. The eyesight testing service developed into more regular inspection of the general health of children.

By 1907, the London County Council had set up a general system of medical inspection that was largely due to Kerr's efforts. It influenced developments in the systems of other education authorities. Kerr saw his work as a specialized area of public medicine, not to be carried out by ordinary public health doctors. He refused to allow London public health officials to act as part-time school medical officers. Kerr's approach was not endorsed by Sir Robert Morant, permanent secretary to the Board of Education, who, like his friends the Fabian reformers Sidney and Beatrice Webb, saw school medical inspection as properly a part of a national public health service under a public health ministry. Since Beatrice Webb was working to influence the Royal Commission on the Poor Laws, 1905–1909, to this end, Morant delayed establishment of a medical department in the Board of Education, being pushed into action only by the failure of the Local Government Board (which had responsibility for public health) to act. Even so, both Morant and the Webbs wanted the officer appointed to build the medical service to do so in close cooperation with local health authorities. They chose George Newman, at the time medical officer of health for Finsbury. Kerr was much disappointed, not only because he saw himself as the most experienced person but because Newman's commitment to develop the school medical service in conjunction with the public health service was strongly at odds with Kerr's conception of the school service.

Both the report of the Royal Commission on Physical Training (Scotland), 1903, and the report of the Interdepartmental Committee on Physical Deterioration, 1904, had strongly recommended systematic medical inspection of schoolchildren. The second report also recommended a height and weight survey. The Education (Administrative Provisions) Act of 1907 created the Medical Department at the Board of Education under Sir George Newman (assisted by Doctors Alfred Eichholz, Janet Campbell and Ralph Crowley). The department's designated role was to encourage local education authorities to proceed with medical inspection of schoolchildren, who were supposed to be examined at least three times during their school lives. The parents had primary responsibility for actual treatment of defects, but as they were often unable to afford private practitioners and were unwilling to obtain medical assistance under the Poor Law, children not infrequently remained untreated or received treatment at voluntary hospitals, which were not happy about such an arrangement. In 1908, the London County Council (LCC) decided to continue to use voluntary hospitals under a reimbursement scheme rather than create school treatment clinics, as Kerr and other professionals advised. The BMA was hostile to the decision, and the LCC found itself in the "Gilbertian situation of its medical officer directing medical inspection in schools while the education officer directed medical treatment in hospitals."[78] In 1912, the Board of Education provided grants for treatment. Local authorities entered into arrangements with hospitals for treatment of minor conditions. A school clinic providing treatment was first set up in Bradford in 1908, and by 1912 a hundred clinics had been established through the country. The number had risen to two thousand by 1937. General practitioners at first opposed the clinics as threats to private practice, but as they came to see most of the clinics' work was preventive and eased their workload, they accepted them.[79]

In the United States in the 1870s and 1880s, doctors and concerned laymen wrote about school health, and the New York Board of Education briefly (1871–73) employed a physician to vaccinate schoolchildren and monitor the sanitary condition of schools. But the first organized service only came into being in 1894, in Boston, when Dr. S.H. Durgin, chairman of the Board of Health, facing a diphtheria epidemic, appointed fifty doctors to examine children and institute action to contain the disease. Philadelphia and Chicago introduced inspection systems in 1895, and two years later New York appointed 150 physicians as part-time inspectors to examine children for communicable disease. In 1902, Dr. Hermann Biggs broadened the scope of the service by requiring school doctors to carry out routine examinations for communicable diseases and minor eye and skin infections. With the cooperation of Lillian Wald of the Henry Street Settlement, he appointed school nurses. Three years later, routine inspection became the responsibility of nurses, freeing doctors to examine children for noncontagious defects. In 1903 Vermont required all schoolchildren to have annual eye examinations, and in 1906 Massachusetts required all to have annual physical examinations. The latter state, facing a situation where many local health departments were not well staffed, placed medical inspection under the aegis of the Education

Department, not the Health Department. Some communities in the United States followed this precedent, while others followed the New York model.

Continuing to lead the way, the New York City Health Department established a Division of Child Hygiene, under Dr. Josephine Baker. The school staff soon grew to 142 medical inspectors and 137 school nurses. Nurses did follow-up visits in homes and encouraged parents to have their children treated, but poverty was a major barrier. The department provided free treatment in its clinics from 1912, only to be criticized by local medical societies. In 1914, the New York Academy of Medicine proposed the closure of the five nose and throat clinics because surgery required hospital facilities; it went on to say that "the functions of the Department of Health should be restricted to the prevention of disease and that no therapeutic activities should be undertaken."[80] The department did close the nose and throat clinics but continued to operate other free treatment facilities for schoolchildren. Even so, there were never enough clinics. With Josephine Baker's resignation in 1920, school services tended to stagnate. A 1929 study revealed as few as 25 percent of defects identified by school doctors were being treated.

Like New York, Detroit early developed an inspection system. By 1915, it had dental and eye clinics and a corps of nurse visitors. But most cities and towns had at best limited programs. Thus, Seattle had only six nurses to inspect thirty-eight thousand children in 1915, and although medical inspectors were later appointed, a 1921 court decision saw medical inspectors reduced from twenty-six to twelve and its clinic taken over by the Red Cross. Baltimore had by 1920 eighteen school nurses. Yet inspection was so poorly organized that even reliable figures on the number of children with infectious disease were unavailable.[81]

Anthropometry—the measurement of physical and psychological characteristics of humans—was caught up in the beginnings of medical inspection of schoolchildren in Australia. Both were related to ideological concerns about "race deterioration" or "degeneration" and the future of the Anglo-Celtic "race" as it adapted to the Australian environment. The school medical services would monitor the trend of the national physique by periodic anthropometric surveys of children. The first systematic medical examination of children occurred as part of an anthropometric survey of Sydney schoolchildren in 1901. The survey had two primary aims: to record physical data so that the "development of the Anglo-Celtic race mixture" might be studied; and to reveal the extent of physical defects.[82] Concern about the fate of the "race" in Australia remained a primary aim of anthropometric studies for four decades, beginning in the 1890s, when the earliest proposals were made. As Dr. James Graham wrote to the Hon. F.B. Suttor, NSW minister for public instruction, in justification of a proposal for an anthropometric survey of the colony's children in the early 1890s, "The subject . . . would do much to answer the question whether the Australian born race is physically superior or inferior to the English speaking people in other parts of the world, and what causes are at work in producing such changes, if such are found to exist."[83]

In 1907, the commonwealth requested the states to carry out uniform physical examinations of all children. A conference of state representatives considered a motion put by the Hon. J.W. Evans of Tasmania for a uniform system of medical inspection so that the commonwealth statistician could compile statistically comparable results. Victoria and Queensland were not happy with the proposal, and it was withdrawn. But Tasmania listed both local and national advantages from such a scheme, including overcoming physical obstacles to efficient education, providing for the lower educational capacity of "defective" children, extending knowledge of the distribution of disease in children and of the influence of environment on "child life," and revealing defects liable to affect future military capacity and to influence the birthrate and health of future generations. At the 1908 premiers' conference, the states rejected the request but agreed to temporary cooperation with the commonwealth statistician. In 1906, the director of the NSW Department of Public Instruction, Peter Board, justifying regular medical inspection to the minister, cited in addition to anthropometric information the educational benefit of knowledge about eyesight, hearing and other physical defects, infectious disease, school hygiene, and mentally defective children. In 1909, the prime minister, Andrew Fisher, urging uniformity in inspection systems on the states, noted that they did not agree on the respective emphasis to be given to fitness and to anthropometric considerations. In the face of state rejection of uniform standards, nothing was done to create uniformity of examinations until 1916, when a school medical officers' conference agreed on standards for recording vision and hearing defects, deciding as well to notify parents about dental, nasal, throat, chest and skin disorders, and general health defects.[84]

In the course of an inquiry into administration of the Tasmanian Education Department in 1904, medical inspection of schools was mooted. The chief health officer, J.S.C. Elkington, reported on the hygienic condition of state schools and established a course on school hygiene at the Teachers' Training College. In 1906 he proposed to the government a systematic examination of schoolchildren in Hobart; a report on the examination of 1,200 children was presented to Parliament. The report recommended a medical inspection system. In 1907 a medical branch was formed in the Education Department under Elkington's direction. A full-time medical inspector, Gertrude Halley, and two part-time medical inspectors—one in Hobart, A.H. Clarke, and the other in Launceston, G.H. Hogg—were appointed. In 1911, two nurses were appointed, and in 1914 a second full-time inspector was appointed.

Interest was also rising in other parts of the country. In 1905, 384 Melbourne children in suburban schools were examined, and the Victorian government was pressed to appoint a schools medical officer. The medical officer of health of the Eaglehawk district in Victoria at the same time proposed a scheme for periodic medical inspection in his area. In NSW, a Royal Commission on Education recommended, inter alia, appointment of school physicians. The 1905 Intercolonial Medical Congress, a periodic national gathering of the medical profession since the 1880s, resolved that "in view of the profound influence of school life . . . upon the future of the race," hygiene should be taught in schools and in teacher training institutions; a full-time medical officer responsible for all matters of hygiene in schools should be appointed to each state education department; and a system of medical inspection should be introduced, especially in larger cities. In both Victoria and Queensland in 1906, deputations asked the minister for education to establish a medical inspection system. In the same year, medical inspections of 1,036 children in Perth and 490 in Kalgoorlie were carried out. In 1908 a school medical officer was appointed to the Western Australia Health Department. Under the 1911 Health Act in that state, all local medical officers of health became school doctors, carrying out examinations in their own districts under contract, while the Health Department's full-time officer focused on Perth. The 1911 act required all children to be examined at least twice during their school lives and defective children to be examined again within three months. The coming of war in 1914 saw curtailment of the service. It did not function on a permanent basis until 1918.

In 1907, following School Inspector Fox's reporting of the eye disease, trachoma ("blight"), as a terrible scourge among schoolchildren in Western Queensland, an ophthalmologist, William Taylor, examined almost two thousand people (mostly children) and reported that 90 percent suffered eye disease. Schools west of the trachoma line were fly-screened, and in 1909 doctors were engaged to treat children in nineteen hospitals. The campaign against trachoma was to continue for another fifty years. In 1910, Elkington became commissioner of public health in Queensland, and he persuaded the government to create a school medical branch in the Department of Public Instruction. Eleanor Bourne was appointed first medical inspector in 1911, and appointment of a school nurse and dental inspector soon followed. In 1912, a full-time ophthalmologist, Douglas Rodger, took up duty. In 1913 a second medical inspector, Elizabeth Sweet, was appointed. The Great War disrupted services, as Rodger was killed in France in 1916, and the two women doctors, having themselves joined the armed forces, did not return to the school medical service after the war. Part-time medical officers carried out examinations in some urban centers, while three school nurses and six dentists continued to examine children during the war. No full-time medical inspectors were appointed until the late 1920s, when the new chief medical officer, L.S. Welch, devised a new scheme that for reasons of cost relied heavily on the use of school nursing sisters. Queensland was divided into districts, each having a nurse to carry out screening examinations. A school medical officer would supervise the activities of a number of nurses.[85]

As early as 1904, the chief health inspector reported to the Central Board of Health in South Australia on the sanitary state of Adelaide and suburban state schools. In 1908, the South Australian government provided for examination of the eyesight and hearing of a thousand children selected from urban and rural schools. Regular medical inspection was introduced in 1913, and almost 4,500 children were examined in the first year of operation, of whom about 20 percent were found to have defects interfering with capacity to learn. The service began with a full-time medical inspector and a school nurse; later, school dentists were taken onto the staff. In 1925 the staff grew with the appointment of five additional medical inspectors, two dentists, three nurses and a psychologist. A metropolitan dental clinic was set up, and a traveling clinic treated country children. "Opportunity classes" for mentally slow children were established in five metropolitan schools; by 1926, nine classes were functioning. Victoria established a medical inspection branch in the Education Department in 1909, with three full-time doctors, who were assisted by an advisory committee of public health, medical, dental and education experts. On the recommendation of the medical staff, a school for "feeble-minded" children was opened in 1913, and a second school was opened the next year. In 1914 also, two nurses were appointed to work in Melbourne, and a fourth medical inspector was engaged. The medical staff proposed establishment of a dental clinic; a school dental center was operating from 1921. Four years later, four further medical officers were appointed to the service.

In NSW in 1907, medical inspection of Sydney and Newcastle schoolchildren was carried out by two part-time medical officers. In 1909, a third (but full-time) officer was engaged. In 1912, five nurses were taken on—four to follow up medical inspection by home visiting, and one to teach senior girls in metropolitan schools about infant care, personal and domestic hygiene, and nursing of the sick. The following year, a staff of nine full-time medical officers and a principal medical officer, C.S. Willis, was brought into being to fulfil a new commitment to carry out medical inspection of all state schoolchildren at regular intervals. Provision of services to private schools and treatment of children with defects demanded more staff, so in 1914 four additional medical officers and two nurses were recruited. By 1919, the staff consisted of eleven medical officers, twelve dental officers, six dental assistants and seven nurses.[86]

The medical inspection schemes unearthed a great deal of chronic, if usually minor, disease and ill health. In 1913 in Western Australia, 62 percent of children examined were defective, while in 1913–16 just over 59 percent of examinees had physical defects. The most typical conditions were dental caries, enlarged tonsils and adenoids, and defective eyesight. However, as the overall problem was less acute than in Britain, governments did not introduce a comprehensive service covering all children, as was done in the mother country. The services were restricted by poor funding and a focus on diagnosis. Treatment was normally expected to be provided by a child's own doctor.

In the years 1913 to 1926 the percentage of NSW children having defects and receiving treatment ranged from a low of 32.4 in 1913 to a high of 55.4 in 1924. The failure to provide state treatment services extensively resulted from two ideological positions. The first was that parents had to have the freedom (and responsibility) to decide about their children's welfare. This failed to protect children where irresponsible parents refused to ensure treatment was provided; more importantly, it left out of account those who wished to obtain treatment but could not afford to do so. The second obstacle was that the interests of private practitioners had to be respected. Everitt Atkinson, Western Australia commissioner of public health, clearly revealed both positions in a 1915 discussion of the issue of treatment: "Examination without treatment would certainly appear futile; but should the state be called upon to put into practice the suggestions of the school examiner? If this is done, will not many parents be rendered more helpless and heartless? . . . Will not medical practitioners be deprived of a large portion of their living? . . . Whilst to make indiscriminate use of hospitals . . . is incompatible with expediency in the public interest, or justice, either to the hospital concerned or to the gratuitous services of the honorary staff. Where such ability to pay does not exist, and the State must undertake the work, then would not this be best met by adequate remuneration to local medical practitioners?"[87]

The organized medical profession carefully guarded the preserves of private medicine against any intrusions by state treatment services. The BMA in Australia opposed efforts to extend services beyond the advisory sphere. In 1914, the NSW Education Department created a traveling hospital of two medical officers, a dentist and nurse to provide for children with defects in outback areas of the state where there was no resident doctor or dentist. The profession initially accepted the hospital. However, in 1916 two special branch meetings decided to oppose medical appointments to the hospital unless the government ensured that "the rights of private practitioners will be preserved."[88] Treatment of schoolchildren was to be abandoned. In 1917, a clinic was opened in Sydney to treat schoolchildren unable to afford private care for eye, ear, throat, nose, skin and other medical conditions. Although very popular with patients, the BMA local branch considered the clinic's activities harmful to the interests of members. Following conferences, the clinic's work was suspended on the understanding that certain metropolitan hospitals would treat the children. Education departments were, however, able to continue to provide treatment for dental cases.[89]

The private profession's concern for its own economic interests was also manifest in its attitude to infant health clinics. On the proviso that clinics would not be managed by nurses, the profession gave guarded support initially to their development. In NSW, each clinic had an honorary medical officer and two nurses, but the profession soon came out more strongly in defense of its interests. An extraordinary general meeting of the NSW branch of the BMA resolved in January 1916 that it would oppose the work of the clinics unless the government guaranteed that they would be used only by those unable to pay private fees. A medical member of the clinic's board, Dr. E. Ludowici, told the meeting that clinic nurses had been instructed not to attend babies whose parents could afford private care. He assured the meeting that the new health minister, unlike Fred Flowers, was not "an aggressive type." A conference of the BMA branch council, the medical members of the clinic's board and clinic doctors endorsed the following: clinics would deal only with babies under one year; only "hospital class" patients (those unable to afford private fees) would be received; treatment of sick babies would not be provided—the clinics' main function would be to advise mothers from poor families on infant care; and clinic nurses would work under medical supervision. The full board accepted the views of the conference.[90] But the clinics soon came to be used by mothers of all classes, although they were never allowed to offer treatment. In 1919, the Clinics Committee reaffirmed that medical officers should not provide treatment. In 1924, the committee accepted a BMA proposal that clinics should always be under medical control. In 1930, the annual meeting of local medical associations affiliated with the BMA protested the giving of medical advice by clinic nurses. Representatives of the profession and the health authorities agreed that the state should not become involved in treatment. In 1931, E.S. Morris, director of maternal and baby welfare, assured the profession that he would investigate any cases of trespass of these limits by the clinics.[91]

The clinics' work was similarly constrained in other states. In some remote districts, open hostility existed between the clinic and the local general practitioner. Tasmania alone provided treatment for minor problems of babies of indigent families. The BMA in Victoria would not permit honorary medical officers to be appointed; one full-time medical officer, Vera Scantlebury, had to serve all clinics. A set of operating rules intended to forestall criticism by the profession was in place by the mid-1920s. In South Australia, continuing friction resulted in the preparation of clear-cut guidelines and the creation of a medical board to resolve conflict. Even in 1933, it could still be asserted that "spoon-feeding the general public by the use of baby clinics free to all is totally unnecessary." The Adelaide clinic's Dr. Helen Mayo called for a more reasonable approach by the profession: "It must be difficult indeed for a nurse who had become expert, to stand by and watch a medical practitioner slowly starving a baby . . . or failing to diagnose a pyloric stenosis; yet these things have occurred, the nurse being powerless to intervene."[92]

In the United States too, when public health and medicine began to converge round the turn of the century, as public health's focus shifted from environmental to individual concerns, it came up against powerful barriers maintained by private practitioners. The first couple of decades of this century saw progress in medical science raise the standing of the medical profession. At the same time as public health began to concern itself with infant and child health, and with disorders like tuberculosis and venereal disease, awareness of the role of adverse social conditions in disease promotion increased. Awareness of the inability of the poor to pay for private care also increased. State and charitable agencies were seen by private practitioners, on the other hand, as taking patients away from them. Mass immunization carried out by public health agencies deprived private medicine of another source of income; individual immunizations by physicians were lucrative procedures.

Hermann Biggs of the New York City Health Department told the New York Academy of Medicine in 1897 that conflict between health departments and private practitioners might be expected from time to time, because the former represented the interests of the community, where the latter represented their own and those of their individual patients. Josephine Baker of the Federal Children's Bureau was to remember in her retirement how following the opening of baby health stations in New York, more than thirty Brooklyn doctors signed a petition saying the Bureau of Child Hygiene was destroying private practice. The New York Academy of Medicine condemned the Health Department's intention to set up a clinic to treat venereal disease cases, even though it endorsed the department's offering free diagnosis to poorer patients. The Academy's Public Health Committee in 1915 applauded the Bureau of Child Hygiene's closure of five nose and throat clinics for schoolchildren and stated that no therapeutic work should be done by a health department, the correct function of which was disease prevention.

In the years just before World War I, health insurance became a significant issue. Initially, the American Medical Association supported some form of insurance. The social insurance committee, reporting on the British national health insurance system, argued that a compulsory system was to be preferred to a voluntary one. In 1916, a *Journal of the American Medical Association* editorial endorsed insurance. But the organized profession soon turned against it. The war saw a marked increase in medical incomes, and the need for insurance to underwrite payment of fees disappeared. The defeat of health insurance is also partly to be explained by changes within medicine. A decline in the influence of socially conscious physicians like Hermann Biggs and Sigismund Goldwater (who had championed public health) came as a reorganized AMA was increasingly influenced by general practitioners and as the better-educated young graduates went into medical specialties and academic medicine. Moreover, the professionalization and institutional growth of public health distanced its practitioners from private medicine. The AMA acted more or less as a union defending its members' economic concerns.

By the beginning of the interwar period, the profession was becoming much less supportive of public health as it grew restive about health regulations. As we saw earlier, the AMA opposed the Sheppard-Towner Act, 1921, which provided federal grants for maternal and child health. It finally prevented its continuation in 1929. The AMA henceforward strongly opposed state schemes involving any care. Facing the fact that much public health now blurred the distinction between preventive and curative medicine, the organized profession responded by taking a narrow view of public health, seeing it as regulation of food and drugs, provision of pure water, and health education and research. Since public health is dependent on public funding, public and political opinion heavily influenced the direction of public health development. Since significant interest groups influence both, public health policy makers showed themselves very ready to defer to the interests of private medicine. Clinics opened to treat diseases and defects revealed by school medical inspections were closed in the face of opposition from local medical societies. Proposals for urban and rural health centers foundered in the face of the profession's hostility, and the 1940s saw marked decline in the health center and health district movement. The economic depression of the 1930s restricted the prospects of private practice. Public health became a more popular career option for young doctors, and some became the shapers of public health development over the next three decades or so. However, with economic recovery in train, the organized profession returned to a policy of employing its political influence to defend the preserves of private medicine.[93]

By the early part of the twentieth century, the medical profession in Australia was well on the way to achieving state-recognized autonomy as well as substantial social and economic status. It had achieved internal organizational unity, expressed in the dominance of the BMA (Australian branches) throughout the country. Externally it had largely won the nineteenth-century struggle with druggists and "quacks" for control of health care as well as the struggle with lay-controlled friendly societies and lodges for determination of conditions of work, including contract remuneration. Private practice attracted most local graduates and most medical immigrants. Few entered public service. Moreover, state health authorities wished to keep expenditure down and employed a bare minimum of full-time doctors in public health activities. Campaigns against major diseases like tuberculosis and venereal disease were rendered inefficient because they relied on the voluntary services of private doctors or on a few overworked public medical officers. Programs like school medical inspections were also inefficient, because so few doctors were involved; in 1924–40, full-time school medical officers carrying out examinations in Australia rose from twenty-five to thirty-nine. Yet in 1943 it was suggested that examining all public schoolchildren once a year would require 150 medical officers in service. "Ethical" considerations stopped public health doctors from carrying out treatment that would take patients away from private practitioner colleagues. Greater public provision of services was seen not only as harmful to private medicine but as the slippery slope leading to nationalization of medicine.[94]

In Australia the path of development of public health toward provision of personal services was more like that in the United States than that in Britain, because of the comparatively greater influence enjoyed by private medicine in Australia and the United States and the marginal position of public health doctors within the medical profession. Britain, having encountered the health consequences of urbanization and industrialization well before the United States, had initiated public health activities at an earlier time—when many in the medical profession, facing an uncertain market for their services, welcomed state salaries. By the 1900s, British medical officers of health were a mature subsection of the medical profession, with well-established control over preventive medicine. Indeed, nationalization of health care was discussed often at this time in their journal, *Public Health,* in terms of its organization around established public health services. On this view, medical officers of health would be central to a national system of preventative health care and be employed not by local but by central government. In contrast, in the United States by the second decade of this century the economic and professional power of the medical profession was in the ascendant, so the prospect of salaried posts was much less attractive. Only a few medical graduates wanted public health careers. The American Medical Association, the voice of the organized profession, was suspicious of state-derived or any other sources of income that had the potential to reduce professional autonomy. The British profession solved the problem of the competitive market pressures on income by accepting state subsidies through national health insurance, from 1911. The American profession, buoyed by good population growth and an expanding middle-class market for medical services, felt more secure about income from fee-for-service and private insurance.[95] It wanted neither national health insurance nor large employment opportunities in public health services.

NOTES

1. R. Taylor, M. Lewis and J. Powles, "The Australian Mortality Decline: Cause-Specific Mortality 1907–1990," *Australian and New Zealand Journal of Public Health* 22(1) (1998), 40–43.
2. H.J. Exley, "Infantile Mortality in Australia, 1906–1930," *Journal of Royal Statistical Society* 95 (4) (1932), 688; J.H.L. Cumpston, *Health and Disease in Australia: A History,* ed. M.J. Lewis (Canberra: Australian Government Printing Service [hereafter AGPS], 1989), 305, 316.
3. Cumpston, *Health and Disease in Australia,* 321–23.
4. Ibid., 270; Exley, "Infantile Mortality in Australia, 1906–1930," 692.

5. Cumpston, *Health and Disease in Australia,* 277, 284. See M.J. Lewis, "'Populate or Perish': Aspects of Infant Maternal Health in Sydney, 1870–1939" (Ph.D. dissertation, Australian National University, Canberra, 1976), 2, 66–67.

6. R.I. Woods, P.A. Watterson and J.H. Woodward, "The Causes of Rapid Infant Mortality Decline in England and Wales, 1861–1921. Part I," *Population Studies* 42(3) (1988), 348–49, 360–62.

7. R.I. Woods, P.A. Watterson and J.H. Woodward, "The Causes of Rapid Infant Mortality Decline in England and Wales, 1861–1921. Part II," *Population Studies* 43(1) (1989), 130.

8. Cumpston, *Health and Disease in Australia,* 112.

9. E.H. Ackerknecht, *History and Geography of the Most Important Diseases* (New York: Hofner, 1965), 7–22; A.B. Appleby, "The Disappearance of Plague: A Continuing Puzzle," *Economic History Review* 33(2) (1980), 161.

10. Cumpston, *Health and Disease in Australia,* 192–95.

11. D. Coward, *Out of Sight: Sydney's Environmental History 1851–1981* (Canberra: Department of Economic History, Research School of Social Sciences, Australian National University, 1988), 209–17.

12. See Lewis, "'Populate or Perish,'" 36–37.

13. Quoted in Coward, *Out of Sight,* 188.

14. Ibid.; *Sydney's Environmental History 1851–1981* (Canberra: Department of Economic History, Research School of Social Sciences, Australian National University, 1988), 188–91.

15. Quoted in R. Patrick, *A History of Health and Medicine in Queensland* (St. Lucia: University of Queensland Press, 1987), 227.

16. Ibid., 144, 211–12, 227–31; *Queensland Parliamentary Debates* 108 (15 August 1911), 512–19.

17. S. Petrow, *Sanatorium of the South? Public Health and Politics in Hobart and Launceston 1875–1914* (Hobart: Tasmanian Historical Research Association, 1995), 157–58.

18. E.H.G. Mathews, "A Review of the Administration of the Health Services in Tasmania" (Diploma of Public Administration dissertation, University of Tasmania, Hobart, 1959), 1–12.

19. Quoted in *Report of Commissioner of Public Health, Western Australia, 1979* (Perth: Government Printer, 1981), 3.

20. D. Snow, *The Progress of Public Health in Western Australia 1829–1977* (Perth: University of Western Australia Press, 1981), 18–20, 54–55; *Western Australia Parliamentary Debates* 39 (1 December 1910), 1963–68.

21. "Health Administration in Victoria 1834–1934," *Health Bulletin* 42 (1935), 1192; Cumpston, *Health and Disease in Australia,* 387.

22. A.J. Woodgyer and J.R.L. Forsyth, *Microbiological Diagnostic Unit 1897–1997: 100 Years of Service in Public Health Microbiology: A History* (Parkville, Victoria: Microbiological Diagnostic Unit, Department of Microbiology and Immunology, University of Melbourne, 1997), iii, 3; C.J. Cummins, *A History of Medical Administration in New South Wales, 1788–1973* (Sydney: Government Printer, 1979), 189; "Health Administration in Victoria 1834–1934," 1190.

23. "Health Administration in Victoria 1834–1934," 1190–91; "Public Health in Victoria," *Health Bulletin* 112 (1954), 19.

24. S. Holton, "Social Medicine in Nineteenth Century South Australia," *Community Health Studies* 7(2) (1983), 131–32.

25. W. Ramsay Smith, *The Control of Communicable Diseases in South Australia* (Adelaide: Government Printer, 1910), 22.

26. Cumpston, *Health and Disease in Australia,* 400; W.W. Holland and S. Stewart, *Public Health: The Vision and the Challenge* (London: Nuffield Trust, 1998), 19.

27. W.M. Frazer, *A History of English Public Health, 1834–1939* (London: Ballière, Tindall and Cox, 1950), 226; R. Walker and D. Roberts, *From Scarcity to Surfeit: A History of Food and Nutrition in New South Wales* (Kensington: New South Wales University Press, 1988), 58.

28. Walker and Roberts, *From Scarcity to Surfeit,* 52–54. See Lewis, "'Populate or Perish,'" 51–53.

29. E.H. Whetham, "The London Milk Trade, 1860–1900," *Economic History Review* 17 (1964), 379.

30. See Lewis, "'Populate or Perish,'" 55.

31. See ibid., 45–68.

32. Walker and Roberts, *From Scarcity to Surfeit,* 58–60; Cumpston, *Health and Disease in Australia,* 383; *Votes and Proceedings of Legislative Assembly of New South Wales* 11 (1883–84), 977; *New South Wales Parliamentary Debates* 85 (6 October 1896), 3757; *Report of Medical Officer of Health to Metropolitan Combined Sanitary Districts, 1901* (Sydney: Government Printer, 1901), 12.

33. Cumpston, *Health and Disease in Australia,* 400–403. See Lewis, "'Populate or Perish,'" 61.

34. Cumpston, *Health and Disease in Australia,* 403–404.

35. H. Collins, "Political Ideology in Australia: The Distinctiveness of a Benthamite Society," in *Australia: The Daedalus Symposium,* ed. S.R. Graubard (North Ryde: Angus and Robertson, 1985), 151.

36. B.K. De Garis, "1890–1900" in *A New History of Australia,* ed. F.K. Crowley (Melbourne: William Heinemann, 1974), 241–44.

37. Quoted in Collins, "Political Ideology in Australia," in *Australia: The Daedalus Symposium,* ed. Graubard, 151.

38. F.K. Crowley, "1901–14," in *A New History of Australia,* ed. F.K. Crowley (Melbourne: William Heinemann, 1974), 274–307.

39. M. Roe, *Nine Australian Progressives: Vitalism in Bourgeois Social Thought 1890–1960* (St. Lucia: University of Queensland Press, 1984), 7; A.M. McBriar, *Fabian Socialism and English Politics 1884–1918* (Cambridge: Cambridge University Press, 1966), 74–75; R. Porter and D. Porter, "AIDS: Law, Liberty and Public Health," in *Health, Rights and Resources: King's College Studies 1987–8,* ed. P. Byrne (London: Oxford University Press, 1988), 82.

40. C.D.W. Goodwin, *Economic Enquiry in Australia* (Durham, N.C.: Duke University Press, 1966), 370–71.

41. Roe, *Nine Australian Progressives,* 117–18. See Lewis, "'Populate or Perish,'" 307.

42. Roe, *Nine Australian Progressives,* 8–14.

43. See M.J. Lewis, "Editor's Introduction," in *Health and Disease in Australia,* ed. Lewis, 4, 24–25; Roe, *Nine Australian Progressives,* 66–68, 70, 157–58, 164–69, 176–77.

44. G. Rosen, *Preventive Medicine in the United States 1900–1975: Trends and Interpretations* (New York: Prodist, 1977), 15.

45. Goodwin, *Economic Enquiry in Australia,* 335–38, 344–49; G.R. Searle, *The Quest for National Efficiency: A Study in British Politics and Political Thought, 1899–1914* (Oxford: Blackwell, 1971), 95–96.

46. B. Semmel, *Imperialism and Social Reform: English Social-Imperial Thought, 1895–1914* (London: Allen and Unwin, 1960), 23.

47. B.B. Gilbert, *The Evolution of National Insurance in Great Britain: The Origins of the Welfare State* (London: Joseph, 1966), 59–61, 85, 90–91; Semmel, *Imperialism and Social Reform,* 24–25.

48. Quoted in S.R.S. Szreter, "The Genesis of the Registrar-General's Social Classification of Occupations," *British Journal of Sociology* 35(4) (1984), 529.

49. Gilbert, *The Evolution of National Insurance in Great Britain,* 92–101; Szreter, "The Genesis of the Registrar-General's Social Classification of Occupations," 543.

50. C. Thame, "Health and the State: The Development of Collective Responsibility for Health Care in Australia in the First Half of the Twentieth Century"(Ph.D. dissertation, Australian National University, Canberra, 1974), 156–58.

51. See Lewis, "'Populate or Perish,'" 124–25.

52. N.L. Stepan, *The Hour of Eugenics: Race, Gender, and Nation in Latin America* (Ithaca, N.Y.: Cornell University Press, 1991), 23–28; G.R. Searle, *Eugenics and Politics in Britain, 1900–1914* (Leyden: Noordhoff International, 1976), 74–105; K.M. Ludmerer, *Genetics and American Society: A Historical Approach* (Baltimore: Johns Hopkins University Press, 1972), 7–8.

53. Stepan, *The Hour of Eugenics,* 28–32; P. Weindling, "Public Health in Germany," in *The History of Public Health and the Modern State,* ed. D. Porter (Amsterdam, Atlanta: Editions Rodopi B.V., 1994), 124–26.

54. See M.J. Lewis, *Managing Madness: Psychiatry and Society in Australia, 1788–1980* (Canberra: AGPS, 1988), 130–31.

55. See ibid., 129–34.

56. G. Jones, *Social Hygiene in Twentieth Century Britain* (London: Croom Helm, 1986), 7.

57. A.S. Wohl, *Endangered Lives: Public Health in Victorian Britain* (London: Dent, 1983), 329.

58. Quoted in J. Lewis, *The Politics of Motherhood: Child and Maternal Welfare in England, 1900–1939* (London: Croom Helm, 1980), 28.

59. J. Walker-Smith, "Sir George Newman, Infant Diarrheal Mortality and the Paradox of Urbanism," *Medical History* 42 (1998), 349.

60. Quoted in P. Mein Smith, "Reformers, Mothers and Babies: Aspects of Infant Survival, Australia, 1890–1945" (Ph.D. dissertation, Australian National University, Canberra, 1990), 13–14.

61. J. Raftery, "'Mainly a Question of Motherhood': Professional Advice-Giving and Infant Welfare," *Journal of Australian Studies* 45 (1995), 67–71.

62. See Lewis, *Managing Madness,* 305; Frazer, *A History of English Public Health, 1834–1939,* 253.

63. See Lewis, *Managing Madness,* 302–306.

64. Report of Royal Commission on Decline of Birth-Rate and on Mortality of

Infants in New South Wales 1 1904, *New South Wales Parliamentary Papers* 4 (2nd session) (1904), 53.

65. Public Health Report of Commissioner, Mr. Neville Mayman, on Inquiry into Welfare of Mothers and Children in New Zealand, 1918, *New South Wales Parliamentary Papers* 5 (1918), 11.

66. *The Romance of St. Margaret's Hospital: Behind the Little Green Gate* (Sydney: St. Margaret's Hospital, 1925), n.p.

67. See Lewis, *Managing Madness,* 303.

68. M. Ladd-Taylor, "'Why Does Congress Wish Women and Children to Die?': The Rise and Fall of Public Maternal and Infant Health Care in the United States, 1921–1929," in *Women and Children First: International Maternal and Infant Welfare, 1870–1945,* ed. V. Fildes, L. Marks and H. Marland (London: Routledge, 1992), 121–25.

69. A. Klaus, *Every Child a Lion: The Origins of Maternal and Infant Health Policy in the United States and France, 1890–1920* (Ithaca, N.Y.: Cornell University Press, 1993), 62–67.

70. Ibid., 68–76.

71. See Lewis, *Managing Madness,* 309; Mein Smith, "Reformers, Mothers and Babies," 111; Frazer, *A History of English Public Health, 1834–1939,* 330–33, 412.

72. W.G. Armstrong, "Some Lessons from the Statistics of Infantile Mortality in Sydney," *Transactions of Australasian Medical Congress* (1905), 393–94, and "The Infant Welfare Movement in Australia," *Medical Journal of Australia* 2 (1939), 642.

73. Mein Smith, "Reformers, Mothers and Babies," 13–17. See Lewis, "'Populate or Perish,'" 33–35.

74. Mein Smith, "Reformers, Mothers and Babies," 117–21; Raftery, "'Mainly a Question of Motherhood,'" 71–72.

75. B. Dickey, "The Labor Government and Medical Services in NSW, 1910–1914," *Historical Studies* 12 (1967), 541–55; "Minutes of Baby Clinics, Pre-Maternity and Home Nursing Board" (7 August 1914), n.p., and (17 June 1915), n.p.; *New South Wales Parliamentary Debates* 57 (10 February 1915), 2386–87.

76. Mein Smith, "Reformers, Mothers and Babies," 142–46; Thame, "Health and the State," 215–16.

77. See Lewis, "'Populate or Perish,'" 153–59; Mein Smith, "Reformers, Mothers and Babies," 146–49.

78. Quoted in J.D. Hirst, "A Failure 'without Parallel': The School Medical Service and the London County Council 1907–12," *Medical History* 25 (1981), 291.

79. Hirst, "A Failure 'without Parallel,'" 281–91; B. Benjamin, "The Urban Background to Public Health Changes in England and Wales, 1900–50," *Population Studies* 17 (1964), 241; Frazer, *A History of English Public Health, 1834–1939,* 255–56, 323–27.

80. Quoted in J. Duffy, *The Sanitarians: A History of American Public Health* (Urbana: University of Illinois Press, 1990), 212.

81. G. Rosen, *A History of Public Health* (Baltimore: Johns Hopkins University Press, 1993), 342–44; N. Sutherland, "'To Create a Strong and Healthy Race': School Children in the Public Health Movement, 1880–1914," in *Medicine in Canadian Society: Historical Perspectives,* ed. S.E.D. Short (Montreal: McGill–Queen's University Press, 1981), 373–74; Duffy, *The Sanitarians,* 210–13.

82. M. Booth, "The Scope and Organisation of a School Medical Service," *Transactions of Australasian Medical Congress* 1 (1911), 651.

83. Quoted in A.M. Turtle, "Education, Social Science and the 'Common Weal,'" in *Commonwealth of Science: ANZAAS and the Scientific Enterprise in Australasia 1888–1988,* ed. R. MacLeod (Melbourne: Oxford University Press, 1988), 229.

84. *Commonwealth Parliamentary Papers* 3 (1907–1908), 316–19; 2 (1908), 109–12; Turtle, "Education, Social Science and the 'Common Weal,'" 231; Thame, "Health and the State," 232.

85. G. Halley, "Aims, Methods and Some Results of the Medical Examination of State School Children in Tasmania," *Transactions of Australasian Medical Congress* 2 (1908), 104; Thame, "Health and the State," 231; Cumpston, *Health and Disease in Australia,* 120–23; Patrick, *A History of Health and Medicine in Queensland,* 150–55.

86. "Public Health in Victoria," 20; Cumpston, *Health and Disease in Australia,* 122–25.

87. Quoted in Cumpston, *Health and Disease in Australia,* 124.

88. Quoted in Thame, "Health and the State," 233.

89. Ibid., 233; Cumpston, *Health and Disease in Australia,* 125.

90. "Baby Clinics," *Medical Journal of Australia* 1 (1916), 83–84; "Baby Clinics in Sydney," *Medical Journal of Australia* 2 (1916), 462–63; "Report of Preliminary Meeting Appended to Royal Society for Welfare of Mothers and Babies: Minutes of General and Executive Councils, 1918–23," n.p.; "Minutes of Baby Clinics, Pre-Maternity and Home Nursing Board" (10 July 1916), n.p.

91. "Minutes of Baby Clinics Committee" (5 August 1920), n.p., and (16 May 1924), n.p.; "Baby Clinics," *Medical Journal of Australia* 2 (1930), 741; "Baby Clinics," *Medical Journal of Australia* 2 (1931), 792.

92. Quoted in Thame, "Health and the State," 212.

93. J. Duffy, "The American Medical Profession and Public Health: From Support to Ambivalence," *Bulletin of History of Medicine* 53(1) (1979), 15–22; Duffy, *The Sanitarians,* 215–16, 247.

94. Thame, "Health and the State," 238; M. Lewis and R. MacLeod, "Medical Politics and the Professionalisation of Medicine in New South Wales, 1850–1901," *Journal of Australian Studies* 22 (1988), 81–82.

95. E. Fee and D. Porter, "Public Health, Preventive Medicine, and Professionalization: Britain and the United States in the Nineteenth Century," in *A History of Education in Public Health,* ed. E. Fee and R.M. Acheson (Oxford: Oxford University Press, 1991), 39–40; N. Bosanquet, "Health Economics: Finance, Budgeting, and Insurance," in *Companion Encyclopedia of the History of Medicine,* ed. W.F. Bynum and R. Porter (London: Routledge, 1993), vol. 2, 1378.

Chapter 5

The Health System in the Interwar Years

THE COMMONWEALTH AND HEALTH

As shown in the previous chapter, a significant force shaping public health development was the concern of an increasingly influential medical profession to keep treatment in the hands of private practitioners and so to limit the advance of public health into the area of personal health services. Another significant force in Australia, as in the United States, was the federal division of powers between the center and the states. Federation of the six colonies was an essentially conservative movement. Henry Parkes, the "father of federation," prefaced his list of resolutions for the National Australasian Convention of 1891 with the statement that "the powers and privileges . . . of the several existing colonies shall remain intact, except in respect to such surrenders as may be agreed upon as necessary . . . to the power and authority of the federal parliament."[1] The constitution protected the powers of the states while allowing achievement of the main aims of federation—establishment of a national market, creation of a national defense system and introduction of a national restrictive immigration policy ("white Australia"). Special interests could take advantage of the division of power in federations between center and constituent parts. The organized medical profession in the 1940s was to use to great advantage this division in the struggles over a national health service.

In a society that still looked to individual responsibility in health and welfare, supplemented by charity for the indigent, the new commonwealth enjoyed quite limited powers in health and welfare matters. Experience of a major economic depression in the early 1890s led a 1897–98 convention to support provision of a pensions power. However, the commonwealth's powers in health were limited to quarantine, and even here there were for some years disputes with the states. The commonwealth had the indirect means by which to fund health initiatives via conditional grants, but it had to curb its ambitions in this direction to have any chance of winning state agreement. In any case, the international economic depression in the 1930s drastically reduced expenditure on health, as on other areas of public administration. Until a referendum in 1946 gave the commonwealth new powers over medical and dental services (and social welfare benefits), it was forced to pursue an indirect approach to health policy—to pursue "cooperative federalism," as the first commonwealth director general of health, J.H.L. Cumpston, put it.

As early as 1884, an intercolonial conference had unsuccessfully asked colonial parliaments to agree on national quarantine legislation to establish uniformity of administration across the continent. Quarantine was not contested as a commonwealth responsibility at the federal conventions of 1891 and 1897–98. But R.E. O'Connor of New South Wales presciently questioned the extent of the commonwealth's power. He suggested restriction to maritime quarantine, because exercise of power over internal quarantine might clash with the states' prerogatives in public health matters.[2]

At a conference of experts in 1904, representatives of the states agreed to prompt transfer of quarantine administration, but New South Wales and Western Australia rejected the commonwealth's right to impose quarantine as an interference in their public health affairs. The states were unsuccessful in an attempt to have the scope of the Deakin government's 1907 bill confined to maritime quarantine, and the 1908 Federal Quarantine Act conferred on the commonwealth power over internal quarantine. However, the commonwealth assured the states in 1909 that it would not exercise this power. Four years later, the understanding was negated when the new director of quarantine, Cumpston, facing a smallpox outbreak in Sydney, quarantined an area within a radius of fifteen miles of the city center. The strongly states-rights Labor premier of NSW, W.A. Holman, suggesting that the disease was unlikely to spread to other states and that the quarantine was harming business, urged that the order be lifted. New South Wales agreed to controls laid down by the commonwealth, and the quarantine order was rescinded. Cumpston noted that the quarantining episode almost wrecked his career and in any case "started a long period of hostility between State Departments and myself."[3]

The influenza pandemic of 1918–19 was the worst on record; 15 to 50 percent of the populations of countries in Europe, the Americas, India, Africa, East Asia and the Pacific were affected, and twenty-one to thirty million people, depending on estimates, died worldwide. Just under twelve thousand of those who died because of the pandemic were European Australians; no reliable figures exist for Aboriginal deaths. The pandemic also brought new conflicts between the commonwealth and the states. Australia maintained strict maritime quarantine, particularly against ships from South Africa and New Zealand. New Zealand instituted no maritime quarantine, and its European population suffered more than double the death rate of Australia's. Cumpston's quarantine measures probably kept at bay for a while the more virulent strain from the Northern Hemisphere, perhaps mitigating the virulence and so producing the lower mortality rate in comparison to New Zealand. Commonwealth control of interstate quarantine had been accepted in November 1918, but the states broke ranks when outbreaks began in Melbourne and Sydney in January. NSW interdicted sea and land traffic with Victoria, where the first cases had appeared. Queensland indicated an intention to close its border with NSW, which suffered about half the country's deaths. Western Australia seized the commonwealth transcontinental train, suspending traffic on that line. The governmental crisis continued until June 1919, when it was clear that the states' unilateral actions had not protected them and the commonwealth took over quarantine again. The Federal Quarantine Act was amended in 1920 to incorporate a provision that in emergencies the commonwealth could override any state measure.[4]

The growth in commonwealth activities resulting from World War I, as well as the commonwealth's constitutional responsibility for invalid pensions and quarantine, increased its involvement in health matters. Sophisticated preventive techniques had been applied by Australian army doctors during the war. They returned to civil life enthusiastic about preventive work. Cumpston said in 1941 that "after the last war, my medical colleagues returned to Australia filled with a desire to apply to the civil community the great lessons of . . . prevention of disease which had been applied in the army." He also remembered "the progressive sense of depression and disillusion" as they came to realize the political and administrative obstacles to their application in peacetime.[5] Hygienic and preventive control measures had reduced troop morbidity due to communicable disease from 30.2 percent of total sick wastage in the Gallipoli campaign in 1915 to only 1.18 percent on the Western Front later in the war.

The war pushed the commonwealth into ongoing health responsibilities—rehabilitation of wounded servicemen, care for invalids and treatment of diseases like tuberculosis and venereal disease—VD among troops was of great public concern—acquired on active service. It also had international responsibilities under the League of Nations charter—for health services in the mandated territory of New Guinea and the provision of information on communicable diseases to the International Public Health Office. In addition, it had in 1916, as a result of a crisis in drug supplies brought on by the war, established the Commonwealth Serum Laboratories. Concern about loss of life during the war and the continuing obligation to pay invalid pensions led the commonwealth to establish in 1915 a Departmental Committee on the Causes of Death and Invalidity in the Commonwealth, of which Cumpston was a significant member. It produced a series of reports on a variety of public health problems: the health risks of middle age, tuberculosis, typhoid, venereal disease, infant mortality, maternal mortality, and diphtheria. Cumpston himself had examined twenty-three thousand of the 27,500 invalid pensioner medical certificates issued since 1910. He had decided that over 32 percent of cases of invalidity were the results of preventable causes. Yet, the commonwealth could do nothing to prevent such causes. The committee urged the commonwealth to fund the appointment of district medical inspectors throughout the country and to call an annual meeting between the states' chief health officers and the commonwealth director of quarantine. The committee was well on the way to calling for a federal health department.[6]

Cumpston had been arguing for creation of a national policy for some time. As early as 1915, in a lecture at the University of Melbourne on the implications of the war, he had claimed that the war would have produced a considerable amount of material good to Australia "if a coordinated national policy of public health" had emerged as a result.[7] In 1919, he discussed before another university audience the nationalization of medicine, observing that British social reformers like Bernard Shaw and Beatrice and Sidney Webb were advocating it. Dismissing nationalization of curative medicine as both impracticable and of negligible value to the community, he focused on national control of preventive work, which would advance beyond control of communicable disease to concern itself with all aspects of the health of the person.

In Cumpston's conception of nationalization, which he shared with the other "national hygienists" of this era, like J.S.C. Elkington, Harvey Sutton and Raphael Cilento, private practice would not be abolished. Rather, it would be subordinated to the objectives of a national public health policy directed from the center. The new partnership between the state and preventive medicine would, by reaching the basic causes of a great deal of illness, simply cut back demand for curative work. Moreover, as the sphere of preventive medicine grew, an increasing proportion of doctors' incomes would come from the state. Cumpston stated that his ambition was "to see every medical practitioner saddled with a definite responsibility for many functions in public health, and an orderly scheme of devolutionized local administration with paternal central supervision."[8] The acting prime minister, W.A. Watt, told a premiers' conference in January 1919 that Cumpston had proposed that the commonwealth take complete control of public health by a transfer of powers from the states, or, as in the United States, through creation of a federal health department. A federal health department would concern itself with investigation of causes of death and disease, methods of prevention, collection of data, and education of the public, but it would leave executive action to the states.

The states were slow in responding, so a resolution of the Executive Council to create a department was shelved. The states, when they did respond, declared that a department was desirable but made no mention of transfer of powers. Pressure for creation of a federal agency continued. A deputation from the Federal Committee of the British Medical Association (BMA) in mid-1919 pressed the federal government to increase its concern with health. In 1918 the *Medical Journal of Australia* had urged establishment of a comprehensive public health scheme under central direction. In early 1920 the Federal Committee of the BMA adopted a policy on preventive medicine calling for a federal department to coordinate the activities of the states, advance research, and establish diagnostic laboratories throughout the country. The commonwealth would not be involved in private practice, and "curative medicine and preventive medicine . . . should be kept distinct in any scheme which may be devised to meet present-day needs." Thus, preventive medicine would become "an organic part of the practice of medicine generally, without affecting the independence of the practitioner."[9] Cumpston told the Australasian Medical Congress of 1920 that if preventive medicine was to overcome its "infantile impotence," the current system of public health administration would have to be replaced by central and district staffs with laboratories and adequate funds; these staffs would supervise general practitioners and local authorities. He urged the congress to request that the commonwealth immediately appoint a royal commission to decide upon the best way to implement the new preventive medicine. The congress called for a federal health ministry as a matter of immediate national importance.[10]

Establishment of a federal department was finally secured by the visit to Australia of V.G. Heiser, representative in the Far East of the Rockefeller Foundation's International Health Board, whom Cumpston had met while visiting the Philippines in 1905. Heiser had been in Australia in 1916 as part of the foundation's campaign to promote health in the Asian and Pacific territories of the British Empire. Australians had been suspicious of Heiser, because of the then neutrality of the United States and because he was perceived in Labor circles as the agent of the arch-capitalist, Rockefeller. Heiser obtained the Queensland government's agreement to a campaign against hookworm, which the International Health Board sponsored, and he discussed creation of a federal health ministry with J.S.C. Elkington, then chief quarantine officer of Queensland and the Northern Territory.

When Heiser returned to Australia in January 1921, he offered to extend the hookworm program to NSW, and more importantly, he and Cumpston agreed that he would talk to the Nationalist prime minister, W.M. Hughes, about a federal health department. On behalf of the Rockefeller Foundation, Heiser offered Hughes, whose lack of enthusiasm for a department had delayed the project, the temporary services of American experts in industrial hygiene, public health engineering and public health administration; further, he offered to finance training of Australians to replace them, if Hughes would create a health ministry. Hughes, who had created the Institute of Science and Industry (a forerunner of the very successful Commonwealth Scientific and Industrial Research Organization) and whose highly developed sense of Australia's destiny in the Pacific—he had fought tenaciously for an Australian mandate over New Guinea at the Versailles peace conference—could be made to include health concerns, agreed. Cumpston became foundation director general of health as well as director of quarantine.

The new department's official functions were remarkably like those presented to Watt in 1918–19: administration of the Quarantine Act; investigation of the causes of disease and death, and establishment of laboratories to that end; control of the Commonwealth Serum Laboratories; collection of sanitary data, and investigation of health in industry; education of the public in public health; control of the Australian Institute of Tropical Medicine; and control of infectious disease among former members of the Australian Imperial Forces. The department was prevented from offering direct services, except in quarantine, associated laboratory work, and in the Federal Territories. But it sponsored research and, by provision of information and argument, it encouraged the states to initiate and coordinate activities. A Division of Marine Hygiene, under C.L. Park, pursued quarantine activities and also carried out medical inspection of seamen. A Division of Laboratories, under W.J. Penfold, formerly of the Lister Institute in London, ran the Commonwealth Serum Laboratories in Melbourne, as well as eight diagnostic laboratories located at strategic points around Australia. A Division of Tropical Hygiene, under J.S.C. Elkington, was responsible for the hookworm campaign and the Australian Institute of Tropical Medicine. A Division of Industrial Hygiene, under R.G. Robertson, collected data on occupational health, carried out inquiries, advised employer and employee groups and promoted cooperation between the states. Finally, a Division of Sanitary Engineering, under A.G. Gutteridge, carried out investigations—though it was constrained by the fact that state responsibility bulked so large in its area.

The Divisions of Marine Hygiene and of Sanitary Engineering essentially represented long-established public health concerns. But the other three divisions represented a larger vision of national public health policy—a vision that, harnessing centrally directed but locally implemented preventive medicine to health problems, would, the national hygienists believed, advance the national efficiency and vitality as well as the economic development of Australia.[11] For the hygienists, health was more fundamental to the welfare of the nation than were political and economic factors. The key issue of white settlement of tropical Australia would not be primarily resolved by economic factors to do with development of export industries and land settlement. The basic determinants of success were "(1) The successful institution of adequate measures of preventive medicine; (2) the exclusion of races with lower standards of life and higher rates of disease and reproduction; and (3) the continual increase in locally-born inhabitants."[12] European settlement of northern, tropical Australia was conceived of as primarily an issue of preventive medicine—an issue of control of prevalent diseases and establishment of an appropriate settler lifestyle, including suitable diet and hygiene.[13]

The idea that northern Australia was unhealthy for whites had been long established, and the experience of Europeans in other tropical areas of the world reinforced it. But by the end of the nineteenth century, the old geographic explanation of disease occurrence was giving way to the application of bacteriology and sanitation to tropical health problems. The British government, seeing commercial advantage and enhancement of imperial power in scientific investigation of tropical diseases, supported development of research facilities. Patrick Manson, adviser to the Colonial Office, was responsible for creation of the London School of Tropical Medicine (which focused on fundamental laboratory research into diseases), while Ronald Ross was responsible for the Liverpool School, which was more concerned with public health and preventive applications. Other European colonial powers created similar institutions. At the Intercolonial Medical Congress of Australian doctors in 1902, Dr. F. Goldsmith, a Northern Territory medical practitioner, pointing to these British developments, called for formation of a school of tropical medicine in Australia. The new commonwealth, responding to recommendations from the congress's Section of Medicine that a research school be established and that advice be sought from Manson, would only go so far as to allocate two hundred pounds a year for five years to support work in Britain.[14]

Meanwhile, George Frodsham, the Anglican bishop of North Queensland, was advocating creation of a local institute to investigate tropical diseases. Independently, the deans of the faculties of medicine at the Universities of Sydney, Melbourne and Adelaide were discussing establishment of a similar institute, probably to be located in Sydney. The 1908 Australasian (formerly Intercolonial) Medical Congress adopted a resolution supported by its Section of Public Health and State Medicine that the congress send a delegation to request that the prime minister appoint a royal commission on the colonization of tropical Australia by whites. Unable to see the prime minister, the delegation—which included J.W. Barrett of Melbourne, J.S.C. Elkington of Hobart and W. Ramsay Smith of Adelaide, as well as Richard Arthur of Sydney and doctors from other states—saw the federal minister for home affairs. The minister declared that the commonwealth was committed to funding the new Institute of Tropical Medicine in Townsville—Frodsham's proposal for an Australian Institute of Tropical Medicine in Townsville (AITM) had been approved in 1908. The deans of medicine hoped that an Australian might be appointed to head it. But Vienna-born Anton Brienl of the Liverpool School of Tropical Medicine, winner of the Mary Kingsley Medal for distinguished contributions to tropical medicine—he, with H.W. Thomas, had cured sleeping sickness with an organic arsenical, atoxyl—arrived in Townsville in 1910 to become director of the AITM.[15]

Because of the war, discussion of the "tropical question" at the 1914 Australasian Medical Congress was postponed to the 1920 congress. In 1920, a number of papers relating to the question were presented, and the congress discussed extensively a report from a subcommittee chaired by J.H.L. Cumpston's ally in the struggle for a federal department, J.S.C. Elkington. The report's central message was that no insuperable obstacles to settlement by "a healthy white race" existed. It was all a matter of applied public health, like the approach successfully taken to civil populations by American authorities in the Philippines before the Great War and in the military forces of the allies during that war. The congress also heard Anton Brienl's report on eleven years' work in Townsville, which showed from the viewpoint of physiology and vital statistics that the health status of North Queenslanders compared well with that of Europeans in temperate areas of Australia and that except for hookworm, tropical diseases were insignificant and easily brought under control. Cumpston put forward, and congress accepted, a range of recommendations concerning health improvements aimed at promoting white settlement of the North. A proposed tropical medical service would also halt the decline of Melanesian populations, thereby supporting Australia's economic development of Papua and New Guinea.[16]

The focus on the tropics, so significant in the infancy of the federal department, continued to be significant until the late 1920s, when Elkington resigned, although Cumpston foreshadowed reduction of support at the Federal Royal Commission on Health of 1925. When Elkington had joined the Federal Quarantine Service in 1913, he had become convinced the AITM would have to form part of a tropical medical service. By 1920 Director Brienl was in a difficult position. He had no security of tenure and was subject to departmental approval for the publication of scientific papers and the making of appointments. (P.A. Maplestone, briefly director after Brienl, would say later that the institute suffered from Cumpston's tight control as well as from its remote location.) In October 1921 Anton Brienl resigned. Elkington, who believed that unless northern Australia and New Guinea were developed, armed invasion from Asia or incursion of serious epidemic disease would occur, supported R.W. Cilento's idea of an Inland and Island Tropical Medical Service covering Queensland, the Northern Territory, Papua and New Guinea, the British Solomon Islands and the New Hebrides.

Cilento had been recruited in 1922 to reorganize the AITM. The service was to provide medical facilities for the Pacific islands but also to be a forward defense against importation of communicable disease into the heavily populated southeastern part of Australia. Cumpston was not keen on the proposal. Elkington had to work hard to get his support for a change of direction for the AITM: to carry out medical and sociological research to improve preventive work, provide diagnostic facilities, and offer a diploma in tropical medicine and hygiene. The last function never fully developed; from 1925 to 1930, when the AITM closed, only four diplomas were awarded, while another six people obtained certificates of completion of the course. Cilento left the AITM in 1923 to report on, and then reorganize, medical services in New Guinea. Remaining there until 1928, he established a health laboratory and a research station ready to serve the integrated island service wanted by Elkington and himself.

In the earlier 1920s, the future seemed bright for the tropical frontier strategy of departmental development. The Pan-Pacific Science Congress took place in Sydney in 1923, and a conference of colonial powers with western Pacific territories took place in Melbourne in 1926. The basis for greater medical cooperation seemed to be being laid. However, the grand plan never materialized. When Elkington resigned from the department in 1928, the tropical frontier closed. The focus of the commonwealth's interest shifted to the main centers of national population in the south and southeast of the country, very much because of Frank Hone's influence on Cumpston from 1924, according to Cilento. Hone was a major exponent of the importance of preventive medicine in the early interwar years. In his presidential address to the Section of Public Health and State Medicine at the 1920 Australasian Medical Congress, he strongly urged the teaching of preventive medicine to medical students, pointing out that no medical school taught it at the time. He wanted a preventive perspective to permeate all practical classes, not to be confined to particular parts of the curriculum. Hone was chief quarantine officer for South Australia, 1915–30, and lecturer in preventive medicine at Adelaide University from 1921. He became a member of the Council of the School of Public Health and Tropical Medicine at Sydney University after it opened in 1930.[17]

NATIONAL HEALTH INSURANCE

The national hygienists and their sympathizers in the medical profession sought to advance "national efficiency" and national health status by making public health and preventive medicine the focus of medical practice, which would remain largely in the hands of private practitioners. National health insurance as a cash-benefit scheme would do nothing to reduce the burden of disease and death by prevention, they believed; it would simply reinforce the existing curative orientation of medical services. But the system of medical care based on an ethic of individual responsibility, and inherited from the nineteenth century, was under stress. Access to good-quality care for low-income earners and their families was difficult. The traditional three-tiered system of charitable hospital care for the indigent, contract practice through friendly societies for the provident working and lower middle classes, and private, fee-for-service care for the well-to-do was coming to be seen as inadequate after World War I. The idea of a national health insurance scheme like Britain's began to seem a serious policy option.

INTERNATIONAL INTEREST IN NATIONAL HEALTH INSURANCE

State-mandated health care–funding systems appeared in Europe only a few decades after the emergence of centrally organized public health systems. Germany was the first country to introduce compulsory national sickness insurance. It was a political ploy by the conservative chancellor, Otto von Bismarck, to steal the thunder of the labor unions, which provided sickness benefits to members, and more generally, to win the loyalty of workers at a time of a rising tide of socialism. Introduced in 1883, it covered the services of general practitioners and specialists, and hospital care. It included dependants as well as wage earners, with payment both by fee-for-service and capitation. (So much per member for all visits for a range of services over an agreed period of time paid in lump sum by the scheme on behalf of members as opposed to so much per service per visit paid by private patient him/herself.) The British scheme, which was introduced in 1911, was more limited, covering only wage earners and giving access only to general practitioners willing to accept the capitation form of payment. In this period, national insurance was adopted across Europe to finance medical services. In France an insurance scheme similar to Germany's was in place from 1918, although later the patient was asked to pay a percentage of the doctor's fee. The German and French schemes encouraged use of specialists, whereas the British focused mainly on general practitioner care. In Britain the quality of care was widely questioned; the system was seen to promote superficial and speedy consultations. In 1910–20, there was a strong campaign to introduce health insurance in the United States. In the long run, it failed mainly because of the medical profession's opposition. The profession's opposition was strengthened by the fact that doctors' incomes improved significantly in the postwar years.[18]

When the Bruce-Page federal government proposed in 1923 introduction of a national health insurance scheme similar to that in Britain, both the BMA and the national hygienists opposed it. The Commonwealth Royal Commission of 1924–27 looked at contributory, superannuation, invalidity and sickness insurance. The commission, influenced by the profession's views, wanted health insurance kept separate from social welfare benefits, so that the profession's involvement would not be diluted and health insurance would not lose funds to pension and sickness payment obligations. Giving evidence, Cumpston emphasized the importance of including preventive health measures in a national insurance scheme, urging formation of health districts throughout the country. The commission did include in its recommendations a national public health scheme under the control of the federal department, but no action was taken on the recommendation.

THE ROYAL COMMISSION ON HEALTH

The national hygienists responded to the focus on cash benefits and curative services by working for another national inquiry into health. In any case, the obvious lack of an integrated policy on public health at the state level (a result of the piecemeal growth of services over a long period) made a national review of health policy desirable. Supported by Sir Neville Howse, the federal health minister and wartime director general of army medical services, and Dr. Earle Page, surgeon and the federal treasurer, a Royal Commission on Health was set up in 1925.

The commission was dominated by the medical profession. The chairman was Sir George Syme, chairman of the BMA Federal Committee and an eminent Melbourne surgeon; its members were Dr. R.H. Todd, federal secretary of the BMA; Dr. Frank Hone, who had been proposed by the Federal Health Department as well as the South Australian and Queensland branches of the BMA; and Dr. Jane Greig. The commission recognized that the constitutional division of powers in Australia made it impossible for the federal department to act like the Ministry of Health in Britain in relation to local authorities. It drew attention to the repeated failure of the states to cooperate with the commonwealth (or with each other) in health administration and to the lack of uniformity in health legislation. It was opposed to cash-benefit schemes not under medical control and wanted any growth in the state's role in health limited to the public health sphere. The commission's two most important recommendations were creation of a federal health council, to be composed of representatives of state health departments and the federal department, and a national public health scheme, to be directed by the commonwealth. Both had been put forward by Cumpston when he had appeared before the commission. He had wanted Australia divided into thirty-four health districts, each to have a health center supervised by a salaried doctor. Paramedical public health workers would be provided by local authorities; their salaries would be subsidized by the commonwealth. The salaried medical officer would coordinate preventive work relating to infectious disease control, tuberculosis and venereal disease clinics, maternal and infant health, school medical inspection and health education. He would also oversee private hospitals and bush nursing, if such functioned in his district. Local private practitioners, working on a fee-for-service basis, would do any clinical work required and would be expected to generate a wide range of clinical information. But this state health work was not intended to replace private practice as the main source of health care in the district.[19]

The grand plan for national public health coordination was not implemented. The great obstacle was that the degree of cooperation required of the states and of subordination to commonwealth direction went well beyond anything known at that time. Cost was almost certainly also a factor, as was the fact that there was no strong public demand for such a scheme. Further, the cooperation of doctors would have proven difficult to obtain. They were reluctant—as poor venereal disease notification records, for example, demonstrate—to furnish information to state authorities, being anxious about their professional independence and the confidentiality of the doctor-patient relationship. They were not keen either about direct remuneration on any scale by the state, fearing that this would reduce them to the status of public servants.

All that came out of the royal commission's wide-ranging plans for public health services development was the innocuous Federal Health Council, which held the first of its regular meetings in 1927. In retirement, Cumpston claimed a great deal for this body—that it reduced the distrust so common in commonwealth-state relations and that it markedly promoted cooperative activities. It achieved, in his phrase, "unity of purpose and harmony in action." But even he admitted that very often no action followed from the unity of purpose forged at meetings of the council. Certainly, the council discussed reports on a wide range of contemporary public health concerns: infectious disease control, tuberculosis, venereal disease, industrial hygiene, tropical medicine, maternal and child health, cancer, and immunization. The problem was that the states too often rejected commonwealth proposals for cooperative action, seeing them as erosion of their sovereignty. As James Stopford, Queensland's home secretary, put it, such projects were "nothing more than an attempt on the part of Dr. Cumpston to carry into effect what he had for a long while intended, namely, the control of the health services of Queensland."[20] The sometimes bitter politics of the federal compact always stood in the way of the national public health ambitions of the national hygienists, even in the relatively prosperous 1920s. Such ambitions withered altogether in the economically depressed early 1930s.[21]

THE PUBLIC HEALTH ACTIVITIES OF THE STATES

No general policy on public health prevailed at state level in the 1920s. New problems were dealt with on an ad hoc basis by state, municipal, or voluntary action. Ministries of health existed in all states but South Australia, where the Health Department was under the chief secretary. In most states the health minister held additional portfolio responsibilities. Delays in communication with the minister often arose because the medical head of the Health Department commonly contacted him via the department that represented his primary portfolio.

Another weakness was that authority remained divided in some states. The Board of Health in NSW, although part of the Health Department from 1913 and able to institute regulations, was without funds and lacked control of officers of the department. The director general of public health, while chairman of the board, had other responsibilities within the department and with other government bodies. In Victoria too there was a division of authority between the Health Commission and the chief health officer, whose functions were like those of the NSW director general. Public health activities came under different acts in different states. In NSW, supervision of dairies came under special legislation, but in Western Australia it was included in the Health Act. In Victoria, purity of milk was the responsibility of the Agriculture Department, and building regulations of the Public Works Department. In Queensland, the Health Act covered sewage and waste disposal, but in Victoria, while disposal of night soil was under the control of the Health Department, sewers and drainage were looked after by the Local Government Department. Other important activities were altogether outside the control of health departments. Education departments ran school medical inspections in all states other than Western Australia; infant health work was administered by the chief or home secretary in some jurisdictions, and in others no legislative control existed.

The geographical distribution of medical officers of health was uneven, although local, commonly part-time, officers were appointed in all states other than NSW. The senior state relied on municipal health inspectors at the local level. They were monitored by the department's traveling inspectors from time to time. Departmental medical officers would deal with difficult problems on a visiting basis. Few local general practitioners were well informed about preventive work. Many were only paid very small honoraria—ten to twenty pounds a year—for which little public work could be reasonably expected. Larger cities had medical officers, but often they were part-time. The cities of Melbourne (and the suburban Prahran municipality) and Sydney had full-time appointees, but Perth and Brisbane employed part-time officers. The more important provincial municipalities employed part-time medical officers in most states. In NSW, the Health Department employed full-time medical officers of health for the largest urban center, the Sydney metropolitan area, and for Newcastle and the Hunter River district. It later appointed a medical officer of health for the western mining town of Broken Hill. Victoria's Health Department went even farther, dividing the state into four rural and two metropolitan health districts and appointing a full-time medical officer to each district.[22]

By the Second World War, public health organization at state level had not significantly improved. Tasmania and Western Australia, with small populations, had always had simpler administrations. Although both had assembled most health responsibilities in a single jurisdiction, health was the second portfolio in the hands of the Western Australian minister for mines. Similarly, the South Australian chief secretary also held the health portfolio. Both the head of the South Australian Health Department and the chairman of the Central Board of Health were part-time. Voluntary bodies continued to run some health services in South Australia, as in Tasmania and Western Australia. The health department exercised little supervision. While health in NSW had its own minister, a number of health activities continued to be carried out in the Departments of Education, Local Government, and Labor and Industry. In Victoria, the Ministry of Health Act of 1943 brought all health services under the jurisdiction of the health minister; a nonmedical, permanent head ran the department. Under pressure from the BMA, departmental medical directors were given the right to communicate directly with the minister. Divisions of general health and mental hygiene were initially set up and, soon after, divisions of maternal and child hygiene and tuberculosis.

In the Australian colonies and states, for reasons discussed earlier, power was delegated by the center to local authorities, whereas in Britain it had been drawn in by the center. At the time of the Second World War, the position of local authorities was like that of local authorities in Britain before the Ministry of Health Act, 1919. This act had required local authorities to create specific services run by medical officers of health and health inspectors, while encouraging local initiatives in other areas. In Australia, state governments did neither, preferring to gain kudos with the electorate by establishing new services in the central health administration. On the other hand, fearing commonwealth encroachment, they opposed national coordination of services.

As state health ministers increasingly came to control policy, health boards were becoming simply advisory in function. As departments split into separate branches, capacity to develop a comprehensive policy was lost. A further, disabling split had developed between the local government level, which controlled traditional public health activities, especially environmental sanitation, and the state government level, where newer services involving some health care had been developing since the 1900s. Collective responsibility for health of a restrictive type had been successfully established in public health in sanitation and infectious disease control. It had been, in a more positive form, established up to a point in the services for particular social groups—mothers, babies and schoolchildren. But continuing widespread adherence to an ethic of individual responsibility for health, the influence of a powerful medical profession committed to private medicine, and the constraints on the power of the national government set by the federal system were to defeat attempts by the federal Labor governments of the 1940s to extend collective responsibility to medical and hospital services for all citizens. Had the federal Labor governments been successful in introducing a state-funded national health service integrating preventive and curative work, the extension of public health into personal services initiated in the early 1900s would have fully developed instead of being blocked by a medical profession wedded to private, fee-for-service practice.[23]

PUBLIC HEALTH AT THE FEDERAL LEVEL

The international economic depression had a severe impact on the Federal Health Department and the plans of the national hygienists. The Scullin Labor government initiated restrictions on spending in 1930, and the conservative Lyons United Australia Party government took them farther in 1932. Ceasing to subsidize activities in the states, the department retired altogether from industrial hygiene, maternal and infant welfare (it had only just formally entered this field, after a commissioned report calling for action had been prepared by Dame Janet Campbell of the British Ministry of Health), tuberculosis and venereal disease control, tropical hygiene and research. It withdrew almost completely from the hookworm campaign. Cumpston said that he had to fight "a hell of a fight" to prevent abolition of his department, sale of the Commonwealth Serum Laboratories, and transfer of health activities to the Department of the Interior. Cilento and the Queensland branch of the BMA fought to save tropical hygiene activities but were unsuccessful. With Elkington's encouragement, Cilento took up the Queensland Labor government's offer to make him head of the state's health services. This appointment provided opportunities to work in tropical health as well as to carry out public health reforms. As first director general of health and medical services, he made important changes, especially in state control of public hospitals and in movement toward provision of free hospital care. In the 1940s, Cilento was to join Cumpston and others in planning a national health service integrating curative and preventive work. He became a strong public advocate of full-time, salaried medicine, a position that deeply alienated the medical profession. As one senior public health figure has observed, "To say that the profession was alarmed and aghast at the Cilento plan was an understatement. Cilento became the socialistic ogre, the proponent of 'nationalisation' of medicine."[24]

A School of Public Health

One major plan that Cumpston managed to bring to fruition before contraction of federal health activities became unstoppable was establishment of a national school of public health. He had told the Royal Commission on Health that schools of public health should be established in the three medical schools—Sydney, Melbourne and Adelaide. However, he thought that for a start a school might be set up at the University of Sydney. A conference of commonwealth and state ministers in 1926 considered the recommendations of the royal commission, including one proposing a school where prospective medical officers of health might get postgraduate training in health administration and health inspectors and other public health personnel might also be trained. The commission also wanted a chair of preventive medicine created, with a chair of tropical medicine to follow. State governments approved the plan for a school, as did the university. In 1927 an agreement was signed between the commonwealth and the University of Sydney whereby the university was to provide the site and control academic functions while the commonwealth would fund the building, staff and equipment. The AITM was incorporated into the new school, which opened in May 1930.

The plans for the School of Public Health and Tropical Health were much influenced by the example of the London School of Hygiene and Tropical Medicine. In this sense it was indirectly the product of the Rockefeller Foundation's policy of promoting public health globally through its International Health Board. As we have seen, the International Board had already played a critical part in creation of Australia's Federal Health Department. Wycliffe Rose, director of the board, 1913–23, stated that the aim of the board was to create throughout the world agencies that would promote public health, and this required growing numbers of well-trained men. A major public health school or institute was to be established in each of the sectors into which the world had been divided. The first was the Johns Hopkins School of Hygiene and Public Health, opened in 1918, and the Harvard School came next, opening in 1921. The foundation had by 1950 established or provided funding for centers in Prague, Warsaw, London, Toronto, Copenhagen, Budapest, Oslo, Belgrade, Zagreb, Madrid, Cluj, Ankara, Sofia, Rome, Tokyo, Athens, Bucharest, Stockholm, Calcutta, Manila, Sao Paulo, and also at the University of Michigan. London was an early target because through London the policy would influence Britain's huge empire. In 1926, G.E. Vincent, president of the foundation, wrote:

> The progress of medical education and public health in the British Isles and in strategic parts of the commonwealth is of moment to vast areas of the world, to millions of human beings both within and without the borders of the commonwealth. The Rockefeller Foundation in carrying out a policy of international cooperation has found peculiarly valuable opportunities to aid British undertakings all the way from London to Edinburgh to Hong Kong and Sidney [*sic*].[25]

Both the foundation and the British government were motivated by humanitarianism, but they also saw scientific medicine and medical research as a form of "social capital." F.T. Gates, a trustee of the foundation and originator of its policy of support for medicine, saw disease as the primary source of virtually all other human ills, including poverty, crime, ignorance, vice, inefficiency and "hereditary taint." A healthier workforce meant greater labor efficiency, higher industrial output and a better return on capital investment. The London School was intended to be, and became, a model for Britain, the empire and the wider world. The Ministry of Health Committee on medical education stated in 1944 that the London School was the only public health school in the United Kingdom adequately equipped and staffed, and organized for research as well as postgraduate teaching. In the broad perspective, the foundation's support for public health (and medicine) not only promoted health, labor efficiency and the prospects of capital in Britain and the empire but prepared the way for a growing volume of American economic investment in economically underdeveloped countries.[26]

As early as 1913, after a visit to London to seek the Colonial Office's support for the hookworm campaign, Rose of the Rockefeller Foundation indicated to Professor R.T. Leiper, a specialist in helminthology (the study of parasitic worms) at the London School of Tropical Medicine, his interest in a future school of hygiene and public health based on the existing school and on the University College's Department of Hygiene. In 1921, as part of a growing movement to expand postgraduate education in medicine, a committee appointed by the health minister, Dr. Christopher Addison, recommended that a postgraduate medical school be attached to a London hospital and an Institute of State Medicine be located in London University. The institute would have students at postgraduate level in public health, industrial medicine, forensic medicine and medical economics.

Leiper let Sir James Michelli, secretary to the London School, know of the foundation's strong interest in establishing a new school. Michelli in turn worked to get Sir George Newman involved. Newman arranged for meetings between the Colonial Office and representatives of the foundation. Agreement was reached in principle on an international school. Rose promised that the foundation would provide fellowships to bring foreign public health personnel to the school. Details of the new establishment were worked out by the Mond Committee, including its location within the University of London, itself interested through its Board of Hygiene in centralizing teaching for the diploma of public health. In 1922 the foundation's Vincent and Rose, having returned to London, offered two million dollars to cover the capital cost of the school, on condition that staff and maintenance costs were met by another source. Mond, speaking for the British government, accepted their offer. The cabinet immediately agreed to furnish twenty-five thousand pounds per year, added to which would be assistance from the Ministry of Health and Medical Research Council grants, and tuition fees. In June 1923 in a formal contract involving the foundation, the Ministry of Health and London University, the parties agreed that the school would have "the purpose of promoting the study of public health and education in public health in Great Britain, the British Dominions, Colonies and Possessions and other countries."[27]

Dr. Andrew Balfour of the Wellcome Institute, who became the foundation director of the London School of Hygiene and Tropical Hygiene in late 1923, in January 1924 visited leading American medical and public heath schools to gain information to help him develop the new institution. Sir Patrick Manson endorsed incorporation of the School of Tropical Medicine, and apart from some opposition from the Royal Institute of Public Health, which felt it should have been the nucleus of any new public health education initiative, the progress of the new institution was smooth. Formally opened in 1929 by the Prince of Wales, the school's earliest teaching was in tropical medicine. In the same year, the professor of public health, W.W. Jameson, visited the United States at the expense of the foundation to see how public health was taught in American schools. By 1937, 422 students from twenty-seven countries were attending courses or doing research in the school, which consisted of the following divisions: public health, bacteriology and immunology, biochemistry, chemistry applied to hygiene, epidemiology and vital statistics, medical zoology and helminthology, entomology and protozoology. In addition, tropical hygiene and clinical tropical medicine were available at the Ross Institute, which had joined the school in 1934. True to its promise, the foundation established a fellowship scheme, which in 1922–39 brought fifty-nine public health fellows from sixteen countries to study at the school. Three fellows from Britain studied in the United States.[28]

The School of Public Health and Tropical Medicine at Sydney University was officially opened in March 1930 by the Scullin federal Labor government's health minister, Frank Anstey, who once said of the health portfolio that it needed "neither brains nor energy."[29] In his speech the commonwealth director general of health, J.H.L. Cumpston, showing a typically strong historical consciousness, paid tribute to the pioneering epidemiological inquiries of the earlier generation of public health doctors like Gresswell, Ashburton Thompson and Ham; to the pioneers of public health diplomas and proponents of tropical medicine at Sydney and Melbourne Medical Schools, Sir Harry Allen and Sir Thomas Anderson Stuart; and to the work of Anton Brienl at the AITM. He reminded his listeners that this was not to be a Sydney school but one designed to serve Australia and its Pacific dependencies, and also to cooperate with the British and French colonial medical services in the Pacific.

In the first year of its existence the school provided courses for the diploma of public health and the diploma of tropical medicine; in public health and preventive medicine, for senior medical students; in school hygiene, for diploma of education students; in architectural hygiene, for senior architecture students; in social aspects of public health, for the diploma of anthropology and the social service course; and also short courses in parasitology and tropical diseases. Except for short, specialized courses, the school never ventured into the projected area of training of health inspectors. The founding director of the school, who was also foundation professor of preventive medicine, Harvey Sutton—he remained in these posts from 1930 to 1947—had built a national reputation in school medical inspection and won the Order of the British Empire for disease prevention work with the Australian Light Horse Field Ambulance in the Middle East during World War I.

Sutton was a dedicated community health educator. He was very active in or on behalf of such voluntary health bodies as the Father and Son Welfare Movement (a pioneer of sex education), the annual Sydney Health Week, the Lifesaving Association of Australia (beachside patrols to rescue swimmers in difficulty), the eugenics-inspired Racial Hygiene Association (later the Family Planning Association, which was free of eugenic ideas and provided contraceptive advice) and the NSW branch of the Royal Society of Health. New courses were introduced to the school throughout the 1930s: in 1931 a lay course in tropical hygiene for anthropology students, cadet officers and medical assistants of territory administrations, and for Christian missionaries and the following year a mental hygiene course; in 1933–35 a training course for indigenous medical assistants from Papua, and in 1934 lectures on public health for hospital almoners (social workers) and on first aid and accident prevention for university staff and students. Special courses in bacteriology, entomology and parasitology were regularly taught for five decades, while extramural teaching in tropical medicine at Cairns and Townsville became an established part of the school's work.

From 1930, the school was part of the network of Commonwealth Health Laboratories. Eight years later, after the appointment of a consultant pathologist, a technical officer training program for staffing of the laboratories was instituted. Entomological and parasitological field surveys for diseases like malaria, filariasis, and amoebic dysentery in North Queensland, Papua, and New Guinea became established aspects of the school's research program. Health surveys of children in different parts of Australia were carried out. In the later 1930s the school became the headquarters for the work of the Commonwealth Advisory Council on Nutrition. Staff began to fill honorary posts—in 1930 the parasitologist being appointed honorary parasitologist to Sydney's Taronga Park Zoological Gardens, and in 1938 the lecturer in tropical medicine becoming an honorary consultant in tropical diseases to Royal Prince Alfred Hospital, one of the city's leading teaching hospitals.

During the Second World War, the school's staff provided invaluable assistance as teachers and researchers to the military forces. Their prewar disease surveys of areas in the Southwest Pacific that had now become campaign zones offered very important information for the Allied forces. Brigadier Sir Neil Hamilton Fairley, director general of medical services, Australian Military Forces—and chairman of the Combined Advisory Committee on Tropical Medicine and Hygiene, Headquarters, Southwest Pacific Area, an advisory committee to the Supreme Allied Commander, Southwest Pacific, Gen. Douglas MacArthur—noted that the specialist knowledge of the school's teachers was unique in the country at this time. Almost all military medical officers received brief training in tropical medicine, while longer-term instruction was provided for officers of the Army Hygiene Service. Personnel of the Army Pathological Services and the Malaria Control Service were also trained there. The research work of particular staff directly promoted the effectiveness of wartime medical organization; for example, the whole of the field malaria-control methods of the Allied Malaria Control Services in the southwest Pacific depended on G.A.M. Heydon's defining of anopheline vectors in Melanesia and Northern Australia. W.C. Sawers's extensive bacteriological and epidemiological knowledge of the southwest Pacific was frequently drawn upon by the Army Medical Directorate. Edward Ford's prewar medical surveys in the Trobriand and D'Entrecasteaux Islands, in Eastern Papua and in Northern Australia offered the only data available at the time allowing estimates of disease risks faced by troops. Ford (later Sir Edward Ford, director of the School of Public Health and Tropical Medicine, 1947–68) established and developed the Malaria Control Service, responsible for field control in all areas where Australian troops were located, and much praised in Australia and elsewhere for the high standard of its work. Colonel Ford later became army director of hygiene, pathology and entomology; as such, he was adviser on preventive medicine to the director general of medical services.[30]

The effectiveness of malaria prevention and treatment can be seen (table 5.1) in the low mortality relative to cases hospitalized in World War II—a conflict that saw Australian forces very much more exposed to malaria than in World War I.

The output of graduates from the school was not large, and, understandably, the number in public health fell notably during wartime. In 1930–45 thirty-three diplomas were conferred in public health, of which twenty-six were granted in 1930–39 (or an average of three per year). But the number of diplomates in tropical medicine during the war did not decline. In 1930–45 there were seventy-nine graduates in tropical medicine, of whom forty-six graduated in 1930–39 (for an annual average of five).[31] In these years, all graduates were medically qualified. Given the relatively slow growth of public health services in the 1930s—much affected by the impact of depression on the economy—the output of public health diploma graduates met the needs of health authorities in Australia.

Table 5.1
Malaria in the Australian Armed Forces, 1914–18 and 1939–45

Years	1914–18	1939–45
Armed forces personnel served overseas	330,000	360,000
Malaria cases in hospital	4,700	200,000
Deaths from malaria	139	76

Source: R.H. Black, *Malaria in Australia* (Canberra: Australian Government Publishing Service, 1972), 141.

Maternal Health

As the economy climbed out of depression and restrictions on bureaucratic expansion eased in the later 1930s, the Federal Health Department sought to advance its national public health policy again, this time with more emphasis on cooperation with the states and less on direct action by the commonwealth. For a number of these years, its minister was a former Labor leader who became a Nationalist and then a member of the United Australia Party government, the formidable W.M. Hughes—known for the slogan "Australia must populate or perish." Deeply concerned about defense, the declining birthrate and reduced migration, Hughes believed that maternal mortality, which, unlike infant mortality, had hardly declined, had to be brought down. Women's organizations had been pressing for improved obstetric facilities to reduce maternal deaths. A meeting of women's groups at the Feminist Club in Sydney in 1924 had called for a chair of obstetrics to be established immediately at the Sydney Medical School. In 1929, a motion calling for federal funding of chairs of obstetrics throughout Australia had been put to the Federal Council of the National Council of Women. In 1931, representatives of fifteen women's organizations discussed with the NSW health minister the unacceptable maternal death rate. In 1933, a conference of women's organizations passed resolutions demanding better obstetric education in medical training and better funding of the Obstetrics Department in the Sydney University Faculty of Medicine. In 1934 the prime minister, J.A. Lyons, promised in a policy speech to provide federal aid "to make motherhood safe." His health minister, Hughes, told the federal Parliament that a declining birthrate undermined the "white Australia" policy and so the very existence of the nation.

While the federal department lacked constitutional power and funds, it was active in the fields of infant, maternal and child health, encouraging the states to introduce measures or setting up model schemes, like the Lady Gowrie Centers for training in the care of preschool children. For the jubilee of the reign of King George V, the federal government created a fund to which the states and the public also contributed. In consultation with the states and women's organizations, a national scheme to advance maternal health was drawn up: advisory committees to coordinate activities in each state, a model maternity center in each capital, a consultant service; public antenatal clinics, rural maternity facilities, and a proper system for reporting of the vital statistics relating to maternal health. The commonwealth undertook to finance research in universities and have the Commonwealth Serum Laboratories undertake work on immunization against puerperal sepsis; finance obstetrics chairs and model maternity units; and convene annually a national conference on maternal health, as it already did for cancer. The reality was a far cry from this blueprint; the federal department's freedom of action was seriously limited by the national government's growing preoccupation with international affairs and war preparations; by the constitutional division of power in health matters; by the self-interest of private medicine, which supported state provision of antenatal care only for those unable to afford private supervision; and by widespread community acceptance of an ethic of individual responsibility for health care, despite some limited movement toward greater collective responsibility in the federal government's involvement in national health insurance.[32]

The intellectual and policy climate of the later 1930s was congenial to the renewed efforts of the national hygienists. Rationality in politics and a revivified state were seen by liberal and socialist planners alike as the key to reestablishing a national community of interest threatened by the mass poverty and unemployment of the depression years. Social and economic planning, intellectually underpinned by the arguments in J.M. Keynes's economics classic *The General Theory of Employment, Interest and Money,* was seen by an influential group of economists, public servants and political scientists who guided national policy in the 1930s and 1940s as the means by which to avoid a repetition of economic depression and later to construct a total war economy. Social welfare and health initiatives were implemented in the 1940s not only out of reformist idealism; they were seen as essential parts of the rational planning of national economic and fiscal policy.

SOCIAL FACTORS IN HEALTH

To a limited extent, the new ideas about social medicine, originating in Britain, the United States and the Soviet Union, influenced public health and thinking about disease in Australia. Social medicine was championed by politically progressive doctors and social reformers in Britain and the United States. Some were keen to follow the example of the socialized Soviet medical system, which pursued a social medicine that drew on social science and statistics and that promoted prevention. The health reformers Sidney and Beatrice Webb in Britain and the distinguished historian of medicine Henry Sigerist in the United States advocated the Soviet approach as a model. Sigerist, pointing in 1945 to the importance of the social sciences for medicine, saw social medicine less as a technique than as an approach to medicine that would eventually permeate the whole medical curriculum.

The figure who more than any other influenced thinking about social medicine in the British world was John Ryle, a distinguished clinician who had been the Regius Professor of Physic at Cambridge and became the first Professor of Social Medicine at Oxford in 1944, a chair specially established for him. F.A.E. Crew, a demographer and another influential figure, was appointed to a chair of social medicine at Edinburgh two years later. For Ryle, social medicine was inspired by his clinical experience; only late in his career did he see the significance of population-based research. Ryle viewed social medicine as the investigation of the influence of social, genetic, environmental and domestic factors on the incidence of disease and disability, and as the promotion of measures (other than therapy) for the protection of the individual and community from forces acting against the full development of mental and physical capacity.[33]

Social aspects of health and disease, and particularly the role of poverty, were explored by other British investigators in the 1930s: by G.C.M. McGonigle and J. Kirby, in *Poverty and Public Health* (1936); by J. Boyd Orr, in *Food, Health and Income: Report on a Survey of Adequacy of Diet in Relation to Income* (1937); and by R.M. Titmuss, in *Poverty and Population* (1938). In his reports for 1931–33, the chief medical officer, Sir George Newman, discussed the impact of economic depression on the health of the people of England and Wales. He reported that "the mortality of the country as a whole, with few exceptions, and even of many of the depressed areas themselves, has been uniformly decreasing." Neither, he added, was morbidity increasing.[34]

But one public health worker, G.C.M. McGonigle, medical officer of health for Stockton-on-Tees, showed the adverse effect of poor nutrition, arising from poverty, on health. He was the only medical officer of health of the time to pursue the matter at length. From a sample of local children attending child welfare centers in 1928, he did a comparison of the incidence of defective conditions in children having satisfactory and unsatisfactory diets. He found that poor diet correlated substantially with bone defects (rickety stigmata), pharyngeal conditions, dental decay, anaemia and squint. In another investigation he compared the death rates of former slum dwellers relocated in pleasant municipal housing and those who remained in slum areas. Surprisingly, the former showed a substantial increase in the standardized death rate, and the latter showed a reduction. He analysed weekly budgets from families in both areas, demonstrating that families who had stayed in the cheaper slum housing had much more money left for purchase of food. He concluded that the greater mortality was associated with the poorer diet of the better-housed community. Moreover, he showed that the diets of all families in both areas were seriously deficient in first-class protein and that those of the unemployed in both areas were badly deficient in all dietary constituents other than carbohydrates.[35]

As J.A. Gillespie has pointed out, ideas about social medicine in Australia were derived from overseas sources. Cumpston corresponded with John Ryle, but it was Cilento who publicly addressed issues raised by the social medicine perspective. Cilento used the Livingstone Lectures of 1936 to examine the role of nutrition in world history. The modern state, he argued, had to act to reestablish a balance between population and nutrition. He singled out the authoritarian regimes of Italy, Germany and Russia (representing 250 million white people) as the only governments taking effective action to combat a declining birthrate and to restore the balance between nutrition and numbers, offering hope to the young in an "ageing civilization."

Cilento's support for social medicine was informed by his belief that European superiority and dominance in world affairs would be soon challenged by non-European "races." As director general of health for Queensland, he was a key adviser to the Forgan Smith Labor government on the establishment of a faculty of medicine at the University of Queensland. In 1935, the advisory committee, much influenced by Cilento, strongly recommended that public health and tropical medicine be made routine parts of the proposed medical course. Offering a specific rationale for the medical school, the committee argued: "Queensland affords opportunities . . . greater than those of any other State at present in respect of anthropological studies with all that implies for the successful solution to the Aboriginal and coloured problem in the state, in tropical Australia elsewhere and in the tropical dependencies."[36] Cilento failed to have Aboriginal studies established as the basis for the teaching of anthropology within the medical course. But he became Honorary Professor of Tropical and Social Medicine in 1936 (the title of the chair was changed to Social and Preventive Medicine in 1956). Not only did Cilento introduce the teaching of social hygiene for the first time in an Australian university, but he may lay claim to having created the first chair in the English-speaking world that incorporated "Social Medicine" into its title. There are recurring discussions in his publications, travel diaries and professional reports on the relationship between social conditions and health in such areas as Aboriginal health; the poor diet, unsuitable housing and psychological problems of isolated Queensland populations; and the prevalence of parasitic infections in social conditions where poverty and ignorance held sway. As a medical educator, Cilento sought to produce a medical practitioner aware of his responsibilities to the community as well as to the individual patient.[37]

An overtly socialist perspective on the relationship between social conditions and ill health was held by E.P. Dark, a general practitioner from the provincial town of Katoomba, west of Sydney. The work of McGonigle and the other British writers concerned with the effect of poverty on health much influenced Dark, who produced a number of pieces in the *Medical Journal of Australia*.

Dark clearly related poverty to the inequities of the social order produced by capitalism. He was ready to go beyond mainstream prevention's preoccupation with immunization and disease surveillance to a fundamental redistribution of social and economic resources, in order to promote health. As one admirer wrote in the *Medical Journal of Australia*, "Dark's figures show quite clearly that healthier people come from those strata of society which have good food, good houses and good clothes. . . . [But] under the present organization of society very large groups of people are not able to get these things, and . . . until they can get them the nation cannot be healthy."[38] But Dark's socialist approach to health and medicine was very much a minority one. The mainstream conception of social medicine in

Australia was the much less radical view outlined by Cumpston at the first session of the new National Health and Medical Research Council in 1937—the NHMRC would give priority to prevention and develop a "widespread national campaign which will ensure complete and adequate supervision of an intelligent kind over the bodily health of infants, pre-school children and schoolchildren, over the physical culture of the school child and over the diet of the community."[39]

A NATIONAL HEALTH AND MEDICAL RESEARCH COUNCIL

The Royal Commission on Health of 1925 had called for a health or medical research council, as had medical researchers who appeared in 1928 before a Parliamentary Public Works Committee hearing on the proposed School of Public Health. In 1927–28 the various state branches of the BMA had asked the federal committee of the organization to press the federal government for a medical research council free of public service direction and with an endowment of thirty thousand pounds per year, as had been suggested by the royal commission. The National Health and Medical Research Council emerged as a compromise between the profession's demands and the revised preventive strategy of the national hygienists. Cumpston believed that research and its applications should be closely related. At the first session of the NHMRC he was critical of the British Medical Research Council for its aloofness from everyday medical practice. Thus public health practice and administration were made central to the work of the council. Its membership was dominated by the heads of state health departments, with the commonwealth director general of health as chairman. The two royal colleges (for surgeons and physicians), the BMA in Australia, and the university medical schools were also represented, together with two lay members. But even on the research subcommittee, academic researchers were in a minority. As scientific and medical research assumed unprecedented importance during the war of 1939–45, researchers pressed for an independent research council. The new director general of health, A.J. Metcalfe, created in 1946 a majority of researchers on the new research advisory committee, which advised about research grant allocations. The NHMRC annual endowment increased from thirty thousand pounds in 1937 to more than forty-six thousand pounds in 1947, and almost a million pounds a decade later.[40]

NATIONAL NUTRITION AND NATIONAL FITNESS

Investigation of nutritional problems became a major concern of Cumpston and the federal department in the later 1930s. This concern grew out of Australia's international trade interests as much as from health considerations. Facing considerable surpluses of agricultural products, Prime Minister Joseph Lyons visited Britain and Europe in 1935 with a view to promoting markets. Continuing the campaign, S.M. Bruce (later Lord Bruce), Australia's representative at the sixteenth session of the League of Nations in 1936, urged expansion in the international trade in foodstuffs to reduce malnutrition, calling for "the marriage of agriculture and medicine in the interests of the health of the peoples of the world."[41] Dr. Hazel Steibling, a leading nutritionist and member of the U.S. delegation to the League, proposed that member countries initiate studies of the nutritional status of their peoples. Having been prominent in the League debate, Australia was under some pressure to comply. Cumpston at the instruction of the government immediately established an Advisory Council on Nutrition, which took a similar British body as its model. The members were drawn from the federal department (Cumpston and Harvey Sutton), from the Council for Scientific and Industrial Research (Sir David Rivett and Sir George Julius), and from the universities (C.G. Lambie of Sydney, W.A. Osborne and S.M. Wadham from Melbourne, Sir Raphael Cilento and D.H.K. Lee of Queensland, Sir C. Stanton Hicks of Adelaide, and representing the BMA, Henry Priestley from the University of Sydney).

The council presented six pioneering reports in 1936–38, but immediate action on the recommendations was limited. The council then became the nutrition committee of the NHMRC. With the coming of war, it turned its attention to a national system of food rationing. The work of the Advisory Council fell into three areas: domestic food consumption patterns, the nutritional status of subgroups of the population, and the composition of Australian foods. The council's first report found no evidence of gross or general undernutrition and concluded that "the people of Australia are, by contrast with the older and more densely populated countries, well nourished and well-developed."[42] However, it did point to rickets in city slums, goiter in Tasmania, and the poor health of Aborigines after contact with Europeans, although the survey data did not themselves identify these problems. Moreover, there was serious bias in the collection of data, as the books recording domestic food budgets had been placed in households with young children and adolescents contacted through infant health clinics, kindergartens and schools, so that the very poor were greatly underrepresented. The director of the Queensland Bureau of Industry, Colin Clark, criticized the report for not employing the methodology of British surveys, which connected household income and nutrition. Trade unionists criticized it as an attempt to undermine the basic wage. From its surveys of the nutritional status of children living in inland communities, as well as in Sydney, the council argued that mothercraft was important to the nutritional welfare of children in both environments. No scurvy was identified, but mild rickets was present in a small percentage of infants.[43]

By the end of the 1930s, national fitness and physical education loomed larger than nutrition as a preventive issue. As the international political situation worsened, the NHMRC proposed in 1938 that a National Council of

Physical Fitness be created. The physical education program appealed to patriotism but also encouraged the Social Darwinist and national-efficiency perspectives of earlier decades. As E.S. Morris, NSW director general of public health, noted, the program would give rise to "a race of strong, virile, stalwart individuals who would provide an invincible bulwark for defence." Basically an individual responsibility, fitness was also "an essential quality of soundly efficient citizenship" and so was "obviously a matter of direct concern to the State."[44] To promote physical education in schools, universities and other institutions, a federal fund was established in 1941. The fund assisted programs run by state-based fitness councils. So prominent did national fitness become as a preventive issue that Frank Hone was moved to say in 1939 that the emphasis on physical fitness was obscuring other aspects of national prevention work.[45]

PUBLIC HEALTH AT THE FEDERAL LEVEL IN THE UNITED STATES

In 1912, the Marine Hospital Service had become the U.S. Public Health Service, an acknowledgement that the Hospital Service was in effect a federal public health body. As in Australia, preventive measures loomed large during World War I; the service was involved in environmental sanitation and disease control in military camps and war industries.

The service acquired a division of venereal disease. The American Expeditionary Force had experienced after arrival in France a sudden, substantial increase in incidence, from fifty-four per thousand a year in October to 201 in November 1917. The army director of urology, H.H. Young, impressed by the New Zealand army's policy of early treatment plus provision of chemical prophylaxis and condoms, combined this with the American practices of suppressing prostitution and providing "healthy" recreations and education. Prophylaxis stations proved particularly effective. In Paris they were set up in any building accommodating fifty or more troops. At home, two million dollars in federal funds were made available on a matching basis for prevention and treatment initiatives by the states. The service offered the states model laws for venereal disease control. Almost all introduced legislation aimed at containing the disease. California was particularly quick to respond, establishing in 1917 a bureau of venereal disease and isolating all persons testing positive until they were deemed noninfectious. The Board of Health in Illinois would place on the residence of any woman suspected of being infectious but refusing treatment a placard stating "suspected VD."[46]

We have earlier discussed the Sheppard-Towner Act of 1921 and the provision of federal funding to the states for the advancement of maternal and infant welfare. In 1929 the AMA and its allies succeeded in their campaign against the legislation. We have also traced the rise of schools of public health for the training of a range of public health professionals, demand for whom increased in the first three decades of this century as public health facilities at various levels of government developed. The economic depression of the early 1930s forced expenditure cuts on health departments as it did in Australia. For example, where health units in rural counties had grown from 467 in 1929 to 616 in 1932, they declined to 581 in 1933. Even before the New Deal, public health benefited from federal spending intended to stimulate economic activity. Under President Herbert Hoover, the Reconstruction Finance Corporation provided $1.5 billion in loans to state and local governments to construct public works including water and sewerage systems. Franklin D. Roosevelt's New Deal, 1933–35, developed public health infrastructure in various ways. Thus, in 1934 the Federal Emergency Relief Administration provided the Public Health Service with a million dollars to spend in rural locations. The Works Progress Administration and the Public Works Administration became involved in the construction of health centers, hospitals and laboratories as well as municipal water and sewerage systems.

In the second phase of the New Deal, the Social Security Act, 1935, channeled millions of dollars to public health work in the states. About eight million dollars were appropriated for grants to the states for maternal and child health, while an additional eight million was given to the Public Health Service for distribution to state and local governments. This money and funds used to construct public health facilities raised the standard of public health services across the United States. For example, in Wisconsin rural health work increased, children were tested for tuberculosis, maternal and child welfare activities expanded, and many communities were enabled to construct sewerage and water filtration facilities. Moreover, where in 1934 just 541 of 3,070 counties nationally enjoyed any public health facilities, by 1942, with a doubling of federal and state funding in the depression decade, 1,828 (about two-thirds) had full-time public health officers running health units. The growth of local facilities created greater demand for personnel. From 1935 federal funds were made available for training. In 1935–38, over four thousand people (including about a thousand medical practitioners) benefited from federal funding of training. Training facilities expanded to accommodate the new demand. By 1939, eighteen academic degrees in public health were being provided by various institutions.[47]

In the 1930s and '40s, Congress proved more ready to support programs focused on particular diseases or population subgroups than to provide general public health grants. Such vertical programs tended to fragment state public health services, and when applied to the structure of the National Institutes of Health they influenced the organization of biomedical research as well. Federal funds were made available for maternal and child health (and for crippled children) in 1935, as we have seen; for VD control in 1938; for tuberculosis in 1944; and for mental health, industrial hygiene, and dental health in 1947.

In the 1930s, as the traditional infectious diseases like smallpox and typhoid became better contained, public health workers focused on the more intractable mass infections like tuberculosis and venereal disease. Better living standards, specific educational efforts and isolation of sufferers in sanatoria were already working to contain tuberculosis. The federal Agriculture Department's efforts to remove tuberculosis from dairy herds and the spread of the practice of pasteurizing milk reinforced this trend. In the 1930s, efforts to rid herds of infected beasts increased. Health departments introduced X-ray screening to identify cases of human tuberculosis. The tuberculosis death rate in the United States fell from seventy-one per hundred thousand population in 1930 to forty-six per hundred thousand ten years later.[48]

The wartime political enthusiasm for venereal disease control soon fell away in peace. U.S. Public Health Service physicians curtailed their efforts in a moralistic climate stressing self-control in sexuality as the key to containment of VD. But the failure of moralism was clear in the rising incidence of syphilis and gonorrhea. An estimated one in ten Americans was infected with syphilis in the early 1930s. Surgeon General Thomas Parran led the way in opening up the subject to public discussion, advocating a medical, not a moral, solution. The print media began to discuss VD more often and more openly. To promote his national campaign, Parran called a national conference on VD control, and attracted almost a thousand health workers and other interested people. The Social Security Act of 1935 had already begun to provide grants to the states for this work. But Parran, now enjoying substantial public and professional attention, put pressure on Congress to pass the National Venereal Disease Control Act, 1938, which massively increased grants to the states, with just over three million dollars provided in 1939 and over $4.5 million the next year. The greater funding had a dramatic effect on public facilities. Where 1,746 clinics treated 197,000 new cases in 1938, 2,405 centers were treating 314,000 new cases in 1939. With about 50 percent of syphilis cases treated by private practitioners, the provision of free laboratory services, free drugs, a free mailing service for notifications, and hospital treatment of indigent patients represented further state intervention to contain venereal disease.[49]

PUBLIC HEALTH IN BRITAIN IN THE INTERWAR PERIOD

Because of Britain's unitary form of government, public health there did not have to cope with the division of powers that complicated development, especially at the national level, in Australia and in the United States. But it did have to cope with the problem, also encountered in the two other English-speaking nations, of the politics of private-practice medicine and the changing nature of public health itself within the preventive-curative relationship. The advent of bacteriology had drawn the focus of public health effort away from environmental sanitation and the quality of housing, with the potential for social reform which this environmental perspective possessed. If communication of germs was to be contained, personal hygiene, with its emphasis on individual behavioral change and health education as the mode of achieving that, became the core object of public health effort. We have seen how infant welfare work, one of the key frontiers of public health development in the early twentieth century in Britain (as in Australia and the United States), pursued health education as the key intervention, even as the epidemiological work of Newsholme and others showed that mortality from diarrheal disease and associated conditions was highest among the urban poor.

Public health eschewed advocacy of social and economic reform in favor of the education of mothers to produce behavioral change in the area of infant health, and in the case of school medical inspection, predominantly disease monitoring and education of children and parents. Social justice did not replace national efficiency as the superordinate goal of public health. In the 1930s, general practitioners were critical of what they saw as public health clinics' intrusion into the preserves of private practice. Private practitioners, who saw their professional independence (as in Australia) crucially connected with nongovernmental sources of payment, regarded the presence of salaried public health doctors as a threat. On the other side, the medical officers of health, now running municipal hospitals as well as other health services, saw themselves as well fitted to lead in the movement toward a national health service combining curative and preventive modalities. As it turned out, the National Health Service legislation of 1948 did not provide for local authority control. Moreover, it not only reduced the functions of public health departments but underwrote the future of general practitioners as independent contractors, and it took the voluntary hospital management structure as the model for the new hospital management committees. As Jane Lewis has observed, it "represented a victory for the mainstream of the medical profession."[50]

In the interwar period, state health services at the local level grew markedly, so that by 1939 a local authority might offer maternal and child health services; a school medical service (with treatment of minor problems); dentistry; school meals and milk; tuberculosis programs (including sanatoria, clinics and aftercare); infectious disease, ear, nose and throat, and venereal disease clinics; and health centers. The 1929 Local Government Act enabled local government to take control of Poor Law hospitals. A decade later acute-care beds available through this source were equivalent in number to those available through voluntary institutions. The 1939 Cancer Act enabled local authorities to develop regional cancer programs. When the National Health Service finally arrived in the 1940s, it entailed a much reduced public health sector. The sector lost domiciliary midwifery, health visiting and nursing services, immunization, ambulance services and environmental hygiene. But in retrospect, the difficulties of public health had begun in the interwar period, when public health departments, multiplying their responsibilities, failed to identify the distinctiveness of public health. When social medicine emerged in the 1940s as an attempt to provide a new approach to the determinants of health and disease, public health doctors soon dismissed it as neither offering anything new nor providing practical answers to health service issues.

Medical officers of health, caught up in responsibility for clinical services, failed to respond, in their traditional role as guardians of the public's health—with a very few exceptions, like G.C.M. McGonigle—to the new health challenges of the impact of unemployment on health or of the health consequences of malnutrition. Further, the services they controlled overlapped with those offered by the general practitioners and the voluntary hospitals, so they were often charged with trespassing on the preserves of private practice, which the BMA (the support of which was critical in their negotiations about salaries) would always support ahead of salaried service.[51]

The Consultative Council on Medical and Allied Services, set up by the new minister for health, Dr. Christopher Addison, and chaired by Lord Dawson, became concerned with the future provision of medical services in 1919. In 1920 the Dawson Report, in recommending integration of preventive and curative medicine, had proposed establishment of primary health centers to be run by general practitioners, and secondary health centers staffed by specialists and linked with teaching hospitals. Dawson was strongly supportive of private practice and proposed that the personal preventive services being developed by local authorities be taken over by general practitioners. The Ministry of Health quickly shelved the report because of severe financial restrictions, the failure of the report itself to deal with difficult questions of financing, and commitment to the educational work of salaried medical officers in the field of personal hygiene. Public health doctors themselves criticized the idea of general practitioners running preventive services on the simple ground that the latter lacked the capacity to do so. Although public health departments took care not to provide treatment except for minor conditions, the BMA on occasion became agitated about their alleged entry into the preserves of general practitioners. In 1928, the secretary, Dr. A. Cox, reported on the question of "encroachment." He found that in areas visited, public health departments tried hard to persuade patients to seek private care and then treated only minor problems. He also reminded the BMA that it had given its support to the 1907 Medical Inspection of School Children Act, which had given rise to public health services for infants and schoolchildren. The Committee on Encroachments on the Sphere of Private Practice by the Activities of Local Authorities (to which Cox had reported) was less conciliatory in its 1929 report. It argued that the general practitioner had greater clinical experience and knowledge of domestic conditions and that the public health doctor should carry out no clinical consultations that the general practitioner could perform.[52]

The 1930s saw the medical officer of health even more caught up in responsibilities for institutional treatment. He was now responsible for work in municipal hospitals, tuberculosis sanatoria, infectious disease isolation, and psychiatric hospitals. Administration and routine clinical work cut across involvement in epidemiological research. Responsibility for isolation hospitals even delayed implementation of new techniques in diphtheria immunization campaigns. Large trials of effective immunization agents were reported in the United States and Canada by the close of the 1920s; yet many British medical officers of health appear to have continued with older methods of control—identification of carriers by swabbing and their placement in isolation hospitals. Similarly, public health doctors working in tuberculosis control tended to remain stuck in older institutional approaches to treatment.

With the outstanding exception of Dr. McGonigle, it was not public health doctors who addressed issues to do with the health status of the population during the Depression; it was the Children's Minimum Council, the Committee against Malnutrition and the National Unemployed Workers Movement that demanded a larger unemployment benefit so that diets would reach the minimum nutritional level identified by the BMA. The Women's Health Inquiry investigated the health of 1,250 wives in working-class families and established that as few as 31 percent were in "good health." A social scientist, Richard Titmuss, found that while national aggregate infant mortality had fallen, the differences in infant mortality between social classes remained substantial. Obstetricians and gynecologists publicly raised the issue of the high level of maternal mortality and morbidity. Indeed, Sir James Young claimed that a large proportion of gynecological problems were the result of poor obstetrics. He said that the medical profession's "devotion to disease" had rendered it unable to see "the duties of health."[53] Sir George Newman said privately that the Health Ministry could not investigate the high maternal morbidity because it would reveal such an amount of illness associated with childbirth that the demand for state treatment facilities would be irresistible. The 1938 BMA scheme for a national medical service called for a focus on positive health and prevention as much as on treatment, but it saw the general practitioners at the center of such a service. Mass access would be enabled by extension of national health insurance. However, in the late 1930s, the Ministry of Health was not ready to support development of national health insurance—but then, neither was it ready to endorse the publicly funded service anticipated by the medical officers of health.

We have already discussed the advent of social medicine and John Ryle's desire to link social to clinical medicine. F.A.E. Crew claimed that what really distinguished it from preventive medicine and public health was the emphasis on social factors that promoted health. Neither Crew nor Major Greenwood, a distinguished medical statistician, nor George Rosen, a leading American public health professional and historian, believed that social medicine had developed beyond the concept of social hygiene formulated by Alfred Grotjahn, a German, in the early 1900s. As time passed, Ryle tended to stress its connection with clinical medicine and epidemiology rather than social science and health policy, and to focus on "social pathology" (the burden and causes of disease) rather than promotion of health. The movement away from social science and policy can be observed in the conflicts between Ryle and the Medical Research Council on one side, and the epidemiologist J.N. Morris and social scientist Richard Titmuss on the other. Ryle wanted social medicine to be seen as scientific, value free, and politically uninvolved. But Morris and Titmuss, who were strongly committed to the use of social science as well as epidemiology, wished to highlight social inequalities in their work. Ryle's response to their work on the epidemiology of rheumatic heart disease in 1943 was to say that "valuable though the enquiry has been it seems to protest the poverty factor too much and . . . it would be a pity to risk drawing adverse criticism in respect of a very important social disease."[54] In 1948 the Medical Research Council (MRC) established a social medicine unit at Central Middlesex Hospital. Morris and Titmuss proposed research be done on health services in the local borough of Willesden. But the MRC opposed the project, not seeing health services research as proper medical research.

Those supporting the new social medicine, believing public health was in an arrested state of development, distinguished between preventive medicine and public health on the one hand and the new field on the other. Ryle himself saw social medicine as studying the patient in his biological and sociological totality, whereas public health focused on environmental and personal health services. Further, social medicine pursued the epidemiology of all significant diseases, whereas public health focused on infectious diseases. Initially, public health doctors were sympathetic to the new discipline, but they soon became frustrated with the vagueness and academic remoteness of it. Social medicine ended up alienated from the practice of public health. By the later 1940s, public health doctors were finding it too clinical and too concerned with social pathology. Social medicine appears to have had a limited effect on medical education, even where new chairs were set up. Many medical schools just tinkered with existing departments of public health. With the coming of the National Health Service, district medical officers of health were stripped of a great many duties and much of their authority. The loss of hospitals and clinics, it was hoped, would be balanced soon by the acquisition of health centers; these, however, were not developed until the 1960s. Some saw the loss as a chance to return to traditional epidemiological work, a tradition that was more than ever needed, because the NHS was essentially a "sickness" service, devoting few resources to promotion of positive health. The split between academic exponents of social medicine and public health doctors was sustained over the next two decades. The Todd Commission on

Medical Education in 1968 was to propose introduction of a new specialty, community medicine, in the hope that it would heal the breach between the academics and the practitioners of public health.[55]

INFANT MORTALITY DECLINE IN AUSTRALIA, 1930–60

The neonatal death rate (deaths under one month of age) by the 1920s was greater than the postneonatal rate. It declined slowly from almost thirty-one per thousand births in 1906–10 to just over twenty-six per thousand in 1936–40. The turning point came in the 1940s, when it fell to just under twenty-four in 1941–45 and to just over nineteen in 1946–50. It fell again to 16.5 in 1951–55 and then went into a slower decline until 1970. While showing no improvement in the first four decades of the century, the early neonatal death rate (deaths under one week of age) followed a similar trend from about 1940. From almost twenty-one per thousand in 1906–10 and almost twenty-two in 1936–40, it fell to just above 16.5 in 1946–50 and just under twelve in 1966–70.

In 1950, the NSW director of maternal and baby welfare, Dr. Grace Cuthbert, said that if the infant mortality rate was to be reduced, deaths from malformations, prematurity and "other diseases peculiar to early infancy" had to come down. This required better antenatal care, better obstetrics, better maternal nutrition, and better neonatal care. Premature babies often died in Sydney because they arrived at mothercraft homes chilled or were carelessly handled. "Wrapping in cotton wool" had to be done in awareness that after chilling, exhaustion was the most common cause of death. Special nurseries for premature babies, for all infants exhausted from long labors or traumatic instrumental deliveries and for offspring of toxemic mothers had to be set up in large maternity hospitals.[56] Cuthbert's opposite number in Victoria, Dr. Barbara Meredith, made similar recommendations. A committee on medical aspects of the decline of the birthrate, reporting to the NHMRC, deplored the prevailing medical and official complacency about prematurity. In 1940, almost 46 percent of neonatal deaths in Australia were directly attributable to this cause. Meredith pointed out that premature babies were accommodated in overcrowded general nurseries and that nurses seldom took precautions against transfer of infection. Only a few hospitals had electrically heated cribs with automatic controls and employed specialist nursing staff. Only the Queen Victoria Hospital in Victoria had a humidicrib (an enclosed crib with carefully controlled temperature and humidity, in which premature babies are kept until able to survive outside). She proposed specific reforms: early notification, improved obstetrics training and practice, better equipped wards, infant welfare nurses in charge of all nurseries, and better transportation facilities to take babies to hospitals. Mothers, she recommended, should all receive regular antenatal care, and more municipal antenatal clinics should therefore be provided; mothers should also be educated about diet, hygiene and breastfeeding. They should receive more assistance in the form of mothercraft nurses, crèches, kindergartens and home delivery of food, as well as better-quality housing and general income security.[57]

Since the 1920s, reduction of neonatal mortality had been linked by experts to wider access to antenatal care and safer obstetrics. Marshall Allan, later professor of obstetrics at Melbourne University, had observed that birth injuries were higher in "residential areas" (where a general practitioner was most likely to be in attendance), whereas prematurity was higher in working-class areas of Melbourne. In New South Wales, illegitimate children had a higher neonatal death rate but a lower injury rate than legitimate babies—in 1924, 1.93 compared with 2.19 per thousand births. Younger mothers probably accounted for some of the difference, but the comparative absence of meddlesome midwifery (less instrumental intervention) because births took place in public maternity hospitals may well have contributed.[58]

A chorus of criticism of unnecessary and excessive interference in childbirth came from within the ranks of the medical profession in the interwar period.[59] E.S. Morris, senior medical officer of the NSW Department of Public Health, showed in a study of the causes of maternal mortality and morbidity in the 1920s that despite medical dominance of childbirth, mortality and morbidity associated with childbirth had not declined. The long-established belief in medical circles that the incompetent midwife was to blame for the high mortality would not hold up. Morris concluded that maternal mortality and morbidity varied in direct proportion to "the inefficiency or inadequacy of the professional care"; that the midwife's responsibility was not as great as customarily claimed; and that the medical profession, individually and collectively, carried a larger share of responsibility than had been thought the case.[60] Doctor attendances at births increased markedly (table 5.2) in the interwar years.

Where in 1919, 50 percent of births in Sydney occurred in hospitals—34 percent in small, private hospitals—by 1939, 91 percent of babies in New South Wales were delivered in hospitals. While there was a shift from home to hospital delivery in the interwar period, antenatal care for most mothers remained inadequate. There were some public antenatal clinics, mainly community centers for the poorer woman or outpatient clinics for patients admitted into public hospitals. The earliest clinics in Australia were among the first in the world. Inspired by the ideas of J.W. Ballantyne of Edinburgh, they opened at Royal Adelaide Hospital in 1910 and at the Royal Hospital for Women, Sydney, in 1912. But most women saw their general practitioners for antenatal supervision, if they saw anyone; 80 percent of pregnant women in NSW in the late 1920s failed to receive any supervision, partly because women themselves saw no need for it, and in part because general practitioners did not appreciate the importance of prevention in this area of practice. Only with the appointment of professors of obstetrics and the proper

Table 5.2
Percentage of Births Attended by Doctors, States and Australia, 1913–14 to 1934–35

Year	NSW	Victoria	Queensland	South Australia	West Australia	Tasmania	Australia
1913–14	58%	74%	48%	80%	64%	53%	63%
1922–23	73%	87%	67%	90%	71%	71%	77%
1928–29	85%	93%	—	—	—	—	87%
1934–35	81%	91%	—	—	—	—	83%

Source: P. Mein Smith, "Reformers, Mothers and Babies: Aspects of Infant Survival, Australia, 1890–1945" (Ph.D. dissertation, Australian National University, Canberra, 1990), 298.

organization of training for medical students did graduates emerge in the 1930s with an understanding of the need for adequate care and with the capacity to give it. Even so, as late as the 1940s many general practitioners still saw women only twice in their pregnancy, unless toxemia or other complications supervened.[61]

Infant welfare work in the community expanded considerably in the decade before World War II. Attendances at baby health centers (exclusive of home visits by nurses) increased nationally from 0.92 million in 1930 to 1.87 million in 1939, and centers grew in number from 301 to 664 (see table 5.3).[62] The infant welfare movement not only pioneered clinic work but promoted early neonatology in the hospitals through the teaching of mothercraft to nurses. Matrons and ward sisters at obstetric teaching hospitals were required to have infant welfare certificates. From the 1920s after the passage of nurses' registration legislation, mothercraft became part of the curriculum for student midwives and nurses. Mothercraft was especially important for the feeding and general care of premature babies. There is some evidence from the records of the Royal Hospital for Women in Sydney that mothercraft helped improve survival rates of premature infants, who from the mid-1920s were kept in the hospital until they gained sufficient weight and their mothers' milk was established. As seen in table 5.4, survival rates climbed from just over 50 percent immediately before creation of a mothercraft department to 70 to 80 percent afterward.

There is indirect evidence of the effect of better maternal nutrition on neonatal rates in particular areas of Australia, although a population-wide improvement probably did not take place until after the Second World War, as awareness of the importance of vitamins took hold. The gap between neonatal death rates in South Australia and Queensland widened from twenty-seven and twenty-eight per thousand, respectively, in 1926–30 to twenty-three and twenty-eight in 1931–35, and it narrowed to twenty-one and twenty-four in 1941–54. In South Australia the government supplied milk rations to the unemployed during the depression years of the early 1930s, whereas in Queensland a deficiency of milk was the most significant cause of malnutrition among women. Moreover, Victoria and New South Wales, which also supplied milk to the disadvantaged in these years, enjoyed lower neonatal mortality rates.[63]

As noted previously, the notable turning point in the trend of the neonatal death rate occurred in the 1940s. This was the result of a variety of factors, some longer term and some due to wartime conditions. The mothers of this generation were healthier than those of earlier generations, beneficiaries of the declining burden of infectious disease. Also, they were probably better nourished. Food was not in short supply in Australia during the 1939–45 war. Pregnant women and nursing mothers were supplied with fresh oranges by infant-clinic sisters. Further, Australians were generally influenced in their dietary habits by the expectations of American servicemen—a million

Table 5.3

Baby Health Centers and Bush Nursing Association Centers, 1930 and 1939

	NSW		VIC		QLD		SA		WA		TAS		ACT	
Year	**1930**	**1939**	**1930**	**1939**	**1930**	**1939**	**1930**	**1939**	**1930**	**1939**	**1930**	**1939**	**1930**	**1939**
Baby Health Centers:														
Metropolitan	39	57	74	72	5	21	39	43	10	13	4	2	1	—
Provincial Urban/Rural	45	154	55	135	10	101	6	24	8	11	5	22	—	9
Total	84	211	129	207	15	122	45	67	18	24	9	24	1	9
Attendances	431,445	852,422	244,800	520,819	116,304	241,911	70,706	116,397	47,531	95,406	24,692	39,241	2,415	3,574
Home Visits	100,103	72,597	55,749	73,490	14,224	13,601	38,471	23,210	10,111	17,970	12,358	15,315	971	1,676
Bush Nursing Association Centers:	38	46	69	70	11	12	30	32	5	6	16	18	—	—

Source: Commonwealth Yearbook, 24, 1931 (Canberra: Government Printer, 1931), 361; 33, 1940 (Canberra: Government Printer, 1940), 235.

Table 5.4
Survival Rates of Premature Babies at the Royal Hospital for Women, Sydney, before and after the Establishment of the Mothercraft Department

Before Establishment of Mothercraft Department

Year	Weight (kg)	Survived	Died	Total
1924	0.45–0.90	0	4	0
	0.90–1.35	2	9	11
	1.35–1.80	7	13	20
	1.80–2.25	19	11	30
	2.25–2.70	24	5	29
		52	42	94
1925	0.45–0.90	0	0	0
	0.90–1.35	0	3	3
	1.35–1.80	11	7	18
	1.80–2.25	11	14	25
	2.25–2.70	23	7	30
		45	31	76

After Establishment of Mothercraft Department

Year	Weight (kg)	Survived	Died	Total
1927	0.45–0.90	0	2	2
	0.90–1.35	4	5	9
	1.35-1.80	19	5	24
	1.80–2.25	34	5	39
	2.25–2.70	29	2	31
		86	19	105
1928	0.45–0.90	0	1	1
	0.90–1.35	2	10	12
	1.35–1.80	11	13	24
	1.80–2.25	32	2	34
	2.25–2.70	37	5	42
		82	31	113

Source: P. Mein Smith, "Reformers, Mothers and Babies: Aspects of Infant Survival, Australia, 1890–1945" (Ph.D. dissertation, Australian National University, Canberra, 1990), 315.

passed through Australia during the Pacific War—of access to fresh fruit and vegetables in abundance. Smaller families and spaced births due to the spread of contraception reduced risks to mothers and children despite the dangers of the increasing proportion of first births. The gradual decline in neonatal mortality in the prewar years and the sharp decline during the war were, then, the result of a number of factors. The effect of these factors was reinforced by improvements in medical and nursing practice in relation to the premature baby.[64]

HEALTH OF MOTHERS

We have seen how the general death rate and the infant mortality rate were declining in the first three decades of this century in Australia, as in Britain, as part of the great demographic and epidemiologic transition common to the Western world. But in this period the maternal mortality rate showed no inclination to fall. Indeed, in England and Wales it was 44.4 per ten thousand births in 1867, 44.1 in 1898, and 44.2 in 1934. In Australia, it was 58.6 in 1880 (Sydney and suburbs), 50.6 in 1910, and 53 in 1935.[65] The modern point of transition came in the later 1930s, when the sulfonamides, highly effective against *streptococcus pyogenes* and so against postpartum sepsis, dramatically reduced deaths from this cause. Penicillin, from the mid-1940s, was even more effective against puerperal infections. Thereafter, there was a sustained decline in Western countries, with a convergence of rates in countries that prior to 1935 had had considerably different ones. Thus, in 1920, rates in the United States, England and Wales, and the Netherlands were respectively 68.9, 43.3 and 24 per ten thousand births. They were 37.6, 26.1 and 23.5 in 1940 and in 1960 were 3.7, 3.9 and 3.7.

The availability and quality of clinical care were more significant in determining the maternal death rate than were socioeconomic conditions—that is, more significant than level of income. Domiciliary obstetric services of lying-in hospitals could attain low rates through high-quality attendance for women in poor urban areas. The Women's Hospital in Sydney reported in 1911 that in seven years of district work with women of the poorest class there had been only six deaths, including one from sepsis, in 3,281 cases. This was a maternal mortality rate of only 11.8 per ten thousand births. The London Royal Maternity Charity reported (in the period before antisepsis was practiced) remarkably low rates achieved in district work done by well-educated midwives (who could call on obstetricians): in the eastern district of the charity, 1828–50, 40.5 deaths per ten thousand births; in the western district, 1842–62, twenty-two per ten thousand births. Where well-educated midwives rather than doctors (or untrained midwives) carried out a large percentage of deliveries, the mortality rate was usually low. The reasons were that the midwives were less likely to interfere in labor and less likely to carry the streptococcus (doctors commonly came into contact with wounds, while midwives did not do general nursing); that they were often more practiced and more skilled in normal deliveries than general practitioners; and that they were better educated in basic obstetric care. Table 5.5 highlights the differences in rates in the pre-antibiotic era between countries where deliveries by

Table 5.5
Deaths per 10,000 Births from Puerperal Sepsis, 1921–27

Countries in Which Midwife Deliveries Predominated		Countries in Which Doctor Deliveries Predominated	
Britain*	3.3	New Zealand	18.2
The Netherlands	7.7	England and Wales	14.6
Denmark	9.5	Scotland	18.2
Norway	7.1	Ireland	17.9
		Australia	17.0

*British midwives working for the Queen's Institute of District Midwives and carrying out 317,758 deliveries.

Source: I. Loudon, "Some International Features of Maternal Mortality, 1880–1950," in *Women and Children First: International Maternal and Infant Welfare, 1870–1945*, eds. V. Fildes, L. Marks and H. Marland (London: Routledge, 1992), 17.

midwives were predominant and those where deliveries by doctors predominated.[66]

By the 1940s, a range of factors were working to bring down maternal mortality in Western countries. Wartime conditions caused the British, American and Australian governments to fund programs that helped lower-class mothers to be better nourished and receive better care. For example, the Emergency Care Program in the United States had offered care to 250,000 mothers by 1948, when it ceased to function. The contrast between occupied and unoccupied Europe is marked, with maternal mortality plateauing or increasing in the former but declining in the latter. In Britain, deaths from haemorrhage in childbirth much decreased because of the availability of blood transfusion and obstetric flying squads, and the coming of ergometrine (1942). Obstetric education and practice slowly improved, and more dramatically, penicillin after 1944 gave the clinician great control over infection. The international decline in maternal mortality continued in postwar decades. In Sydney and other Australian cities, the same technical factors significantly affected the quality of clinical care and therapy in the 1940s—the introduction of penicillin, the provision of blood transfusion services, and schemes to provide specialist care for patients otherwise unable to afford such care.[67]

Public provision of maternity services in Australia was very limited, and the organization of services in the predominant private sector itself probably delayed any improvement in maternal mortality. As early as 1874, a Sydney doctor called for proper training of midwives and for legislation to stop the unqualified from practicing. But while many doctors were keen to see such reforms, in the interests of their patients, fears of competition from a licensed body of competent midwives made them, at the same time, wary of legislation. A number of attempts to introduce registration failed for want of medical support before the Nurses Registration Bill (which provided for registration of general and psychiatric as well as obstetric nurses) was enacted in NSW.

By the late nineteenth century many members of the respectable working and the lower middle classes in Australia had joined contributory medical schemes run by friendly societies or lodges (self-help, non-profit, mutual-aid organizations)—about 25 percent of Sydney citizens by the early 1870s, and by 1913, 42 percent of people in New South Wales. The private fee-for-service system worked reasonably well in rural areas and in more prosperous urban areas, because a differential fee system meant that the well-to-do in effect subsidized visits by poor patients. But in inner-city and industrial localities, where a balance of classes did not exist, very few could afford private fees, and many could not afford to join mutual aid societies. Just as importantly, as a result of increasing medical specialization and hospital-based technological advances, contract or lodge practice (which was only a general practitioner service) failed too often to provide good-quality health care. Further, the large number of contract cases (in addition to private patients) typically seen reduced the standard of service women received. Lodge midwifery cases were attended for a reduced fee. Around the turn of the century, a general practitioner might have 150 to 180 midwifery cases a year under contract practice besides private cases. Forty years later an expert national committee could say of contract practice (still a significant provider of medical care in capital cities and industrial areas) that it often involved "fatigue and hurried work . . . to the detriment of the public welfare" and that to produce reasonable incomes, practitioners had to work "at the expense of their professional efficiency."[68] In 1929, Henry Jellett, an experienced obstetrician, told the Australasian Medical Congress that the primary preventable cause of maternal mortality was the fact that the average labor was conducted by a busy general practitioner, the demands on whose time led him to intervene to hasten delivery. Hubert Jacobs, obstetric surgeon to the Women's Hospital in Melbourne, also condemned the all too common practice of hastening a labor so that other commitments might be met. The resulting injuries could not be protected from infection even when asepsis was conscientiously pursued. On this and other evidence, excessive interference can be seen as in part the result of a bias in the maternity care system toward solo private practice.[69]

In New South Wales in the mid-1920s, when the total population was 2.1 million, only 419 public maternity beds were available, and only thirty-seven of these were in country centers. But there were 1,523 beds in private maternity hospitals, plus another 2,723 in those taking maternity and general cases. In Victoria, when the population was 1.5 million, only 109 public beds were available in Melbourne's two women's hospitals and about 1,600 private maternity beds at locations throughout the state. Until the late 1920s, public beds hardly existed in South Australia. Adelaide had a small lying-in home for indigent women; however, with the establishment of a new public obstetrics section at Adelaide Hospital, access to public facilities improved. Subsidized beds were available in the capitals of Tasmania and Western Australia, but in the two states country facilities were few and payment was required. Only Queensland provided small, government-built maternity units in country hospitals. Charges were levied, but people without means were not refused admission.

As the great women's hospitals in Sydney and Melbourne reported death rates much lower than state averages in the 1920s (even though they received emergencies from private hospitals) and as economic conditions improved in the later 1930s, demand for hospitalization increased. Many public hospitals now offered private and intermediate beds to paying patients. In 1934, 8,188 births took place in NSW public hospitals, and in 1942, 20,775. Domiciliary confinements fell from 39 to 9 percent in 1931–39. Small private hospitals, many of which were ill equipped, slowly disappeared, although wartime and immediate postwar constraints on resources for building plus a rising birthrate allowed many to survive. In 1943, of 1,403 Sydney maternity beds, 599 were located in private hospitals. Only Queensland moved decisively on the matter. In the late 1930s, 215 private hospitals were taken over, of which forty-one were closed straightaway and eighty-nine were required to carry out improvements. By 1938, 55 percent of Queensland births occurred in public institutions, where twelve years previously only 17 percent had.[70]

While hospitalization, especially in public facilities, increased in popularity, the growth of antenatal care was less impressive. From the late 1920s, more well-to-do women from urban and rural town backgrounds obtained antenatal care. Many women, however, did not. In 1929, 87 percent of mothers in receipt of the universal commonwealth maternity allowance had doctor-supervised deliveries, but most did not obtain supervision throughout their pregnancies. More starkly, half of forty-one women who died from eclampsia in 1930 in New South Wales had not consulted a doctor prior to the beginning of labor. The women's hospitals in the capitals required women booked to give birth in hospital to attend antenatal clinics, but since most were booked at a late stage in pregnancy, attendance was not good. In 1927, ten thousand women in NSW were estimated to have attended clinics on average on fewer than two occasions, and this when clinics were available in eight hospitals in Sydney and several larger hospitals in the country. By the mid-1930s, doctors were generally convinced of the importance of proper antenatal care; notable progress in convincing women was not achieved for almost another decade. Dr. Constance D'Arcy, a leading figure in obstetrics in Sydney, complained in 1935 that "amongst the educated class, especially amongst young women, there is no difficulty about inducing expectant mothers to present themselves for regular examination, particularly when a composite fee . . . is agreed upon. But in public maternity clinics and, . . . in lodge practice, it is still difficult to get women to attend regularly."[71]

Reference has already been made to the commonwealth's grant to the states of fifty thousand pounds in 1935 to celebrate King George V's jubilee by promoting measures to reduce the unacceptably high maternal mortality rate. State grants and public subscriptions raised the amount to 175,000 pounds by mid-1936. However, the jubilee initiative led to few new services; it was used largely to support established facilities. It did not lead to a comprehensive maternity service. The focus of state efforts was on regulating private hospitals and midwives, with the result that the established system in which the majority of women purchased services in the private sector was reinforced, as the NSW history shows.

The NSW Labor government set up two small hospitals for poorer mothers in western Sydney in 1920, one for maternity and the other for convalescent cases. A free service, they were much in demand, but they were closed in 1930 on the ground that the buildings were not functional. E.S. Morris, foundation director of maternal and infant welfare from 1925, publicized the need for antenatal supervision through the press, radio, leaflets and lectures to schoolgirls and Girl Guides. Greater resources from 1929 allowed him to open an antenatal clinic one evening each week at the inner working-class suburb of Newtown. Nine more were set up in 1930 in urban areas distant from public hospital clinics. Attendances stabilized at about 2,500 a year during the 1930s. They went into decline in the 1940s, as public hospital clinics expanded. Moreover, they never managed to attract local general practitioners into doing clinic work. All this hardly amounted to substantial state provision, and subsequent initiatives encouraged private-sector development of maternity services. From 1939, an effort was made to implement 1935 Federal Health Council recommendations on maternity: an expert committee to review all maternal deaths offered an obstetrical advisory service; a panel of private obstetricians, willing to attend poorer women for a lower fee, was set up (in a few instances the Health Department itself paid the fees); a mobile blood transfusion service was established in Sydney (the department paid for the cost of blood for those unable to afford the fee).

In the other states, there was very limited state provision. The thrust was largely support for private-sector services. The Queensland government after 1923 funded public maternity units in country hospitals and paid subsidies for the Lady Bowen Maternity Hospital in Brisbane as well. Some antenatal care was provided at infant health clinics, and after 1929 a departmental doctor conducted two evening clinics a week in Brisbane. Tasmania, South Australia and Western Australia simply gave the jubilee fund monies to voluntary and subsidized maternity hospitals, which expended them on buildings. In Victoria such monies were spent on laboratories at the Women's Hospital, Melbourne, a research scholarship, and grants to voluntary bodies working in child welfare. Several local authorities (including the Melbourne City Council) offered antenatal supervision, but only for women not receiving it from a public hospital or private practitioner, and in most instances no medical examination took place.

After establishment of a Maternal and Child Hygiene Section in the Victorian Health Department in 1944, six metropolitan councils joined a scheme whereby the department furnished a doctor and nurse one half-day a week (or paid a subsidy) for antenatal work in municipal clinics. The scheme's ambit was not large—in 1945–46, just under five hundred new cases involving 2,165 visits. In the same year in the state as a whole, fourteen thousand attendances took place at local authority clinics.

Thus, state provision of maternity services did not develop beyond a very limited area, although health authorities publicly encouraged women to seek antenatal supervision and skilled attendance at the birth to reduce the embarrassingly high maternal death rates. Cost considerations and opposition from a medical profession deeply committed to private practice were factors standing in the way of further development of public health services in the direction of health care for individuals. But an ethic of individual responsibility for health, which was widely accepted in the community (and by public health professionals), also acted as an obstacle to such development.[72]

CONTROL OF TUBERCULOSIS

Tuberculosis is an ancient disease of humankind. Evidence of the disease has been found in the bones of mummies from ancient Egypt. It became established as a major source of illness and death in Europe in the eighteenth and nineteenth centuries, as a result of rapid urbanization and industrialization.[73] The great migrations of people to European settlements in North America and the Antipodes made it a major cause of death and disability in the United States and Australia, though they helped constrain tuberculosis (TB) rates in the United Kingdom.

Although the precise relationship between poverty and the disease is unclear (overcrowding, inadequate housing and poor nutrition are considered to facilitate the spread of the disease), it is clear that improvement in living standards in Britain over the 120 years or so after 1840 coincided with a decline in the overall infectious-disease death rate from more than 11 to 2.5 per thousand population. Almost half the decline was due to a fall in TB mortality. William Farr computed the mortality rate in London in 1660–79 from consumption (pulmonary tuberculosis—also known as phthisis, graveyard cough or wasting disease) as thirteen per thousand population. It seems that tuberculosis emerged as the leading cause of death when plague and malaria declined in the second half of the seventeenth century. In 1680, John Bunyan had called tuberculosis "the captain of all these men of death."

Farr identified the beginning of a long-term downward trend as occurring in 1831–35, when the death rate declined for the first time to nine per thousand. Respiratory tuberculosis mortality in England and Wales fell from 2.77 per thousand in 1851 to 1.28 per thousand in 1901, and in Scotland from 2.6 in 1861 to 1.55 in 1901. But in Ireland it rose from 1.89 in 1871 to 2.16 in 1901. It declined substantially in the three countries in the twentieth century: in England, from 1.04 in 1911 to zero in 1981, although there was a regression from 0.74 in 1931 to 0.95 in 1941 and to 0.98 in 1951; in Scotland, from 1.15 in 1911 to 0.01 in 1981; and in Ireland from 1.73 in 1911 to 0.025 (all forms) in 1981.[74] The reasons for the great decline in TB have been much disputed. Better nutrition and other improvements in living standards have been significant long-term factors across the Western world. Increasing real wages paralleled declining TB mortality in Britain. Economic growth in the United States and Belgium was also accompanied by a decline in TB mortality. The isolation in workhouses of destitute sufferers, as well as of some patients in sanatoria, probably reduced the risk of spread to others in the community. But it was the antibiotic streptomycin and adjuvant drugs—the former was distributed in Britain from 1947—that gave the coup de grace to TB. Deaths fell by 51 percent in 1948–61—that is, 140,000 lives were saved.[75]

As mentioned above, the secular decline in TB commenced in England and Wales about 1840 and in Scotland about 1870, when it also began in the United States. It began in Australia and New Zealand about 1880, and in various European countries somewhat later: Bavaria and Switzerland, about 1890; Hungary, about 1901–1905; and Czechoslovakia, about 1905. It got under way in Japan about 1909. At this time clean, fresh air, bed rest and good diet were seen as curative; the first sanatorium was opened in Nordach, Germany, in the nineteenth century. But the comfortable rest homes for private patients were very different from the often spartan state establishments for working-class sufferers.

State-funded treatment was introduced in Britain, France and Germany. The British National Insurance scheme from 1911 provided a benefit for hospitalized patients. Indeed, those receiving Poor Law relief or state sickness benefits could be compulsorily hospitalized by the health authorities. Sanatorium and dispensary promoters in Britain, like Sir Robert Philip, could not produce rates of cure to match their high hopes for such institutions. There was an 85 percent level of mortality among former inmates five years after discharge. Sanatoria, with a total of four to five thousand beds (1910)—more cases were housed in Poor Law institutions, and they were the only places to take advanced cases—provided for but a small proportion of sufferers. Moreover, changes in personal hygienic habits—like the safe disposal of sputum—which sanatoria aimed to promote, do not appear to have had a large impact; spitting in public remained common in the 1930s. Similarly, the educational work of the National Association for Prevention of Tuberculosis was very limited in its impact.

Lack of success with therapies based on bed rest and graduated labor in sanatoria led to a search for other cures. Surgery to collapse the diseased lung in the hope that rest would lead to regeneration (pneumothorax) never achieved the level of success that enthusiasts envisaged, although the scientific nature of the approach gave hope to patients and increased the interest of medical staff. While X-ray procedures were employed in the 1930s to detect cases, many rural districts and boroughs lacked equipment; in any case, not only were treatment facilities insufficient to the demand but treatment itself was ineffective. Only in the 1940s and '50s, when effective chemotherapy became available, did mass radiography become significant.[76]

In the half century from 1861, ten million people—six million from England, a million from Scotland and three million from Ireland—emigrated from Great Britain. Many of them migrated to North America and Australasia. The Australian death rate from TB (all forms) declined notably from a peak in the 1880s. In Victoria, the worst affected of the colonies, it peaked at 1.83 per thousand population in 1886–90 and fell to 0.77 in 1911–15. Low death rates in the early nineteenth century produced an erroneous belief that Australians enjoyed immunity to the disease, although this was dispelled by the 1850s. This and the idea that warmer, drier climates were beneficial for consumptives had led doctors in Britain commonly to recommend emigration to Australia. A Melbourne doctor, S.D. Bird, a TB sufferer who had emigrated from London, published in 1863 *On Australasian Climates and their Influence in the Prevention and Arrest of Pulmonary Consumption*. Well received in medical circles in Britain, the book encouraged further migration of consumptives. In the 1870s William Thomson, another Melbourne doctor, carried out epidemiological investigations into TB deaths in Victoria. He showed that the rising mortality was not due to an influx of consumptive immigrants and that the native-born did not enjoy any natural immunity. In the age of bacteriology after Koch identified the TB bacillus in 1882, an increasing number of colonial doctors rejected Bird's claims about the curative capacity of Australia's climate. But British professionals and laymen alike continued to believe in the therapeutic benefits of emigration, partly because the arguments of critical colonial doctors were little heard "at Home."[77]

In the period up to about 1880, colonial governments did not concern themselves with TB control. Consumptives were cared for in benevolent asylums (and some voluntary hospitals) if indigent. They received friendly-society medical and sickness benefits if they were members of the provident working and lower middle classes; the well-to-do obtained private medical care. Of 343 deaths at the Melbourne Benevolent Asylum in 1855–60, just over 50 percent were from phthisis. Phthisis was reported as the cause of death in 23.5 percent of friendly-society-member deaths in Victoria in 1866–67, but because in Australia sickness benefits usually ceased after twelve months, deaths after that time would not be recorded. In Britain, consumptive members of the Hearts of Oak Friendly Society received sickness benefits on average for fifty-eight weeks. In the last years of the nineteenth century in the Australian colonies, as we have noted, limited efforts to control TB were initiated. The development of inspection of the meat and milk supplies in colonial cities very probably helped to reduce nonpulmonary TB deaths, most of which were due to the bovine bacillus.

The health authorities made some attempt to educate a more receptive people—universal primary education was now in place—about the need for hygiene and the infectious nature of the disease. D.A. Gresswell's *Tuberculosis and its Prevention* went through six editions in Victoria in 1893–1902. Sydney and Melbourne health officers disinfected rooms that had been occupied by consumptives, and sanitary inspectors inspected lodging houses. The latter were required to provide more ventilation and more space per bed. The NSW Board of Health in 1905 asked all local authorities to prohibit spitting in public places—7 percent of sputum collected from Birmingham streets had been found to contain bacilli. Five years later the Victorian Board of Health did the same.

J.H. Goodlet, a Sydney philanthropist, opened the first sanatorium in Australia, at Thirlmere, in 1877. A small sanatorium was established at Echuca, Victoria, in 1889, and Kalyra Sanatorium was opened in South Australia in 1895. The Queen Victoria Homes (which drew on the Queen's Jubilee Fund) assumed control of Thirlmere and established in 1903 a male sanatorium in the Blue Mountains, west of Sydney. Charitable effort established a small sanatorium in Hobart in 1906 and one at Hazelbrook in 1909; Mount Macedon in Victoria had opened in 1899 as summer accommodation for Echuca inmates. The Victorian government opened the first state institution, Greenvale, in 1905, and the NSW government opened one at Waterfall, south of Sydney, in 1909. By 1920, critics were questioning the effectiveness of sanatoria. Certainly sufferers in the early stage of the disease had a good chance of emerging with the disease arrested, but advanced cases had no hope. In 1909–12, of 1,146 people admitted to Waterfall in 1913, 18.6 percent were still resident, 26.9 had died, 9.9 percent were unimproved, 30.7 had improved, and 13.7 percent were in an "arrested" status. For those discharged, there was the serious problem of finding work. The stigma attaching to the disease, as well as the sufferer's sometimes precarious state of health, could make this a difficult task. In Scotland and England experiments with farm colonies were tried. The commonwealth's Committee on Causes of Death and Invalidity of 1914–17 recommended the same be created in Australia. Because of cost, both capital and recurrent, the recommendation was not implemented.

Inadequate economic support for working-class TB sufferers was the weakness of the schemes to control TB. It was not adequately addressed till after World War II. Until then, great poverty was the lot of TB sufferers, and the stigma of poverty reinforced that arising from popular (and professional) fears about the deadliness of tuberculosis. Poverty meant overcrowding and spread of infection to other members of families. Moreover, many sufferers after diagnosis tried to disguise their illness for as long as they could, because they feared loss of employment or eviction from rented accommodations. This put not only them at greater risk but also those with whom they came in contact. NSW had in 1907, in a world first, introduced a noncontributory invalid pension for the permanently incapacitated, but as with the commonwealth invalid pension that replaced it in 1910, the rate of ten shillings per week—twenty shillings to the Australian pound—was quite inadequate to provide decent food and accommodation. The pension remained below 25 percent of the basic wage, which the national arbitration system set as a minimum acceptable income for a working man. Thus, the basic wage was eighty-two shillings in 1925, when the invalid pension was seventeen shillings and sixpence. With extra family allowances, a TB sufferer with a wife and two children received thirty-seven shillings and sixpence. Dr. Richard Arthur reported in 1925 that in the Sydney working-class suburb of Surry Hills he knew of two families that lived in single rooms; one of the rooms was a cellar twelve feet below the level of the street.[78]

Institutional facilities were quite inadequate. Only 474 beds, fewer than 50 percent of annual deaths, were available in NSW, which also had the only dispensary system. In 1912, Fred Flowers, the Labor minister of public health, won the agreement of a small number of friendly societies to use their dispensaries for ambulant care. The plan did not proceed, because of opposition from private medical practitioners and pharmacists.[79] But Flowers's aim to extend outpatient dispensary facilities did not altogether fail. The state government subsidized dispensaries at Marrickville and in the Royal North Shore, Royal Prince Alfred and Newcastle Hospitals; it also funded the dispensary run in the city by the National Association for Prevention and Cure of Consumption.

Victoria differed from NSW in its control policy. NSW put advanced cases into sanatoria; the result was that if beds were increased in number, dispensary facilities dealing with early cases and contacts had to be increased. Victoria tried to get early cases into sanatoria on a short-stay (up to three months) basis to educate them in self-care. Some help was also provided by visiting nurses, and Austin Hospital took incurables. Altogether there were 372 beds in the state in 1915. The other states simply provided sanatoria beds: 157 in Queensland's state institutions and three hundred in Western Australia's state-run Wooroloo; fifty-two and 120 in subsidized sanatoria in

Tasmania and South Australia, respectively, plus homes for the terminally ill attached to the general hospitals in Hobart and Adelaide.[80]

The growing need for government funding of treatment and premises drew the Australian state into developing control policy. The commonwealth became involved because of responsibility for ex-servicemen with the disease. The repatriation pension paid to ambulant incapacitated veterans was more generous than support for civilian pensioners. For a couple with two children it was four pounds, four shillings. By 1924, 2,116 pensions were being paid, and 340 patients were in sanatoria. Five years later, as the need for commonwealth benefits declined, only 1,572 pensions were paid at the full rate and 2,902 at a partial rate. The Federal Health Department's director of tuberculosis, M.J. Holmes, in the late 1920s presented national reports on TB, but the commonwealth limited direct provision of services to repatriation cases. Moreover, bed capacity in the states expanded only slowly. In the decade and a half from 1915, nationally, beds increased by 656, but 420 of these were in NSW.

Nor did outpatient facilities expand very much. In South Australia, Tasmania and Queensland local authorities did not usually carry out at all well their responsibilities for domiciliary visits and disinfection. In Western Australia, where constitutional and economic development was retarded until late in the nineteenth century, the state rather than local government ran public health services, and a comprehensive TB control scheme was established. This involved strict notification procedures, a departmental diagnostic clinic, and supervision by nurse visitors of patients not under the care of a general practitioner. Yet, mortality there came down more slowly than in any other state, although it needs to be borne in mind that Western Australia (like Victoria) had a considerable underground mining industry, which had not yet achieved a dust-free working environment. The Victorian Public Health Commission after 1922 regularly proposed expansion of diagnostic capacity and maintenance allowances, but a policy of government financial constraint prevented implementation. After a director of tuberculosis was appointed in 1927, a plan for regional dispensaries under local authority control was drawn up. By 1930, a dispensary functioned in Melbourne. The organized medical profession ensured that no dispensary would do more than educate; treatment remained in the hands of private practitioners. NSW came nearest to constructing a coordinated system of care, although with only four dispensaries and nine nurse visitors in 1930, capacity was still inadequate. A director of tuberculosis appointed in 1926 took responsibility for contacts, sanatoria admissions and discharges, and most of the domiciliary visiting.

The Commonwealth Royal Commission on Health of 1925 had put forward a national plan involving local diagnostic clinics working with neighboring general practitioners, a state bureau to ensure that patients were channeled to appropriate institutions, commonwealth-funded pensions of a size adequate to support families, and educational efforts to encourage early diagnosis and treatment. Thus, education and personal financial support would be used to induce voluntary involvement, and the traditional necessity to compel compliance with infection containment would be avoided. In turn this would help reduce the serious problem of concealment of infection, which resulted from economic necessity and social stigma. Victoria, with its dispensaries promoting education, and NSW, with the Health Department and the National Association for Prevention of Tuberculosis distributing leaflets and mounting radio broadcasts, were already taking this path. However, the commission's national plan was not realized, although the Federal Health Council in 1929, following a report on established facilities by the federal director of tuberculosis, made similar recommendations.

As we have seen, the coming of the economic depression markedly reduced federal activity in health. The Health Council's proposals—and indeed, the Division of Tuberculosis and Venereal Disease in the federal department—were casualties of this restrictive policy. An expert national committee, reviewing the tuberculosis services in 1943, said that little had changed since the 1929 report of the federal director of tuberculosis; growth of facilities in Queensland, Tasmania and South Australia had been negligible. Western Australia had a coordinated administration in metropolitan and nearby areas, but remote areas were poorly served, because of inadequate funds. Better working conditions and mandatory medical examinations had reduced the proportion of miners suffering from silicosis and tuberculosis from 3.5 to 0.4 percent over the previous two decades. Services in NSW and Victoria had become more alike. NSW had focused less on dispensary development—only Newcastle outside the metropolitan area had a clinic. Victoria had increased outpatient facilities. NSW still lacked the central control of sanatoria and clinics that Victoria enjoyed. Victoria had opened branches of the Central TB Bureau of Melbourne at Prahran and regional centers at Ballarat, Bendigo and Geelong.

Public health officers and medical specialists had spearheaded the development of control facilities in the 1920s. They had failed to achieve much growth in the 1930s; however, educational efforts concerning the potential for control helped in the long term to change traditional fatalistic attitudes, at both the community and political levels. They facilitated the introduction of mass prevention schemes in the two decades after World War II. Other forces at work were medical interest in new treatments and methods of diagnosis, and with the coming of the Second World War, the successful mass X-raying of army recruits. New treatments, like artificial pneumothorax and other collapse therapies, and the question of treatment standardization were of growing concern in medical circles. Miniature radiography, the Mantoux skin test, and improved laboratory analysis made population screening realistic. The Australasian Medical Congress, which took place in Adelaide in

1937, expressed formal support for an NHMRC resolution that the "economic factor"—income support for poorer sufferers—was the key to success in control of TB.

Miniature radiography, developed in the late 1930s, was both inexpensive and speedy enough in application to permit screening of substantial numbers. In 1939, the Australian Army Medical Corps decided to use it with all recruits. Greater military efficiency was one objective, but the long-term cost of caring for tuberculous servicemen was also a consideration. Seven million pounds had been spent by 1940 on cases arising from World War I. The immediate effectiveness of X-raying was shown when tuberculosis was discovered in 0.5 percent of men who had already been passed as fit after a complete medical examination. In 1940, the NHMRC proposed that mass X-raying be made available to the civilian population on a voluntary basis. The development of TB control after the 1940s will be discussed in volume 2 of this history.[81]

CONTROL OF VENEREAL DISEASE

As a public health problem, venereal disease had a good deal in common with tuberculosis. Both carried a social stigma that made many sufferers avoid diagnosis and treatment. Both impacted heavily on people of lower socioeconomic status, who could not afford long-term, private medical care and so needed to use public services. These expanded in the interwar period but remained inadequate to needs. Both were very prevalent, especially among young adults and their children, to the extent that national economic efficiency and "racial" vigor were particularly at risk. Unlike tuberculosis, venereal disease did not kill—congenital and tertiary syphilis excepted—but it did give rise to conditions that were fatal or produced disability: a large percentage of abortions and of premature and still births, and a good proportion of infant mortality from malformations and debility; an estimated 25 percent of child blindness from maternal gonorrhea, plus 33 percent of gynecological problems in public hospital patients; perhaps 20 to 25 percent of psychiatric illness (neurosyphilis); 33 percent of intellectual disability, and a good deal of heart and vascular disease, as well as nephritis. VD was notoriously underreported, so official notification figures in themselves are not reliable indicators of incidence.

In 1921, 17 percent of just over three thousand hospital patients in Melbourne reacted positively to the Wassermann test for syphilis. In 1930, 10.5 percent of almost three thousand men and 13.6 percent of one thousand women in state hospitals in Sydney were carrying syphilis. While these groups are not fully representative of the general population, it would seem that around 10 percent of lower-class people had syphilis and that probably more had gonorrhea.[82]

Australian doctors had, like their colleagues overseas, been encouraged by the growth in knowledge of, and capacity to treat, syphilis in the decade before World War I. They had been pressing governments to act to reduce its prevalence by encouraging early treatment. In this they were supported by the labor movement and significant community organizations, like the patriotic Australian Natives' Association. However, it was the high levels of VD among Australian troops during World War I that led directly to the emergence of a national campaign.

In Britain, philanthropists and doctors since the late 1890s had been urging the government to take measures to contain the "Red plague." Governments were reluctant to take a first step and establish an official inquiry, for fear of reawakening the bitter controversies surrounding the Contagious Diseases Acts of the 1860s, when middle-class feminists, working-class men and concerned Christians all criticized the state for introducing compulsory examination of (working-class) women suspected of having a venereal disease. Nevertheless, various official bodies had over a number of years commented on the problem, including the Royal Commissions on Feeblemindedness, on Divorce, and on the Poor Law. Before the International Medical Congress held its meeting in London in 1913, Sir Malcolm Morris, an internationally known venereologist, and some colleagues set out to obtain public support for an inquiry. Morris publicly stressed the threat VD represented to national health and vigor at a time when German power loomed so menacingly. Strong support was forthcoming from the press and ultimately the congress itself. Prime Minister Asquith indicated that a royal commission would soon be set up.

The Royal Commission on Venereal Diseases, 1913–16, saw the existing prevalence of VD as a "terrible peril to our Imperial race" and the economic losses involved as "a powerful argument for the initiation of general measures of prevention and treatment at the earliest possible date."[83] The commission made thirty-five specific recommendations, most of which related to diagnosis and treatment. For example, larger local authorities were to establish diagnostic laboratories, with substantial subsidies from the central government. Free treatment should be offered at general hospitals to minimize stigma, and opening hours should be "convenient to the working classes." Poor Law patients and military and naval patients, the congress recommended, were to be detained until cured, and all prisons were to have treatment facilities. Notification of cases should be introduced only after the new national treatment system was in place. Using the Public Health (Venereal Diseases) Act of 1917 and regulations of the Local Government Board issued in mid-1916, the British government speedily implemented a number of the commission's key proposals. County councils and county borough councils were required to provide diagnostic facilities, free institutional treatment and free supplies of arseno-benzol for domiciliary care by private practitioners. A nationwide clinic system providing voluntary, confidential and free therapy was quickly established. Clinics increased from 113 in 1917 to 193 in 1925.[84]

The royal commission's report, the most authoritative of this period, became well known in Australia. More significant, however, in initiating official action was professional and political concern about high VD rates among Australian troops and the threat these rates represented to the civilian population. The prime minister, Andrew Fisher, wrote to the state premiers in 1915 encouraging them to introduce compulsory reporting of VD cases. Western Australia responded almost immediately, amending its Health Act in 1915. The new legislation established compulsory, anonymous notification. Treatment defaulters could be compelled to resume treatment. Free outpatient and inpatient care was provided for those not able to purchase private care, and free pathology services were introduced. Knowingly communicating VD and the carrying out of treatment by persons not medically qualified were made illegal. Anyone suspected of being infected could be detained for a medical examination. The commonwealth, influenced by the call of its Committee on the Causes of Death and Invalidity for legislation like Western Australia's to be passed in the other states, offered up to fifteen thousand pounds on a matching basis to the states to help establish a national control system. That it acted so promptly on this matter while ignoring other concerns of the committee shows the importance attached to VD control. This was the first financial support for national health services provided by the commonwealth. Victoria enacted legislation in 1916 and Tasmania and Queensland in 1917. New South Wales did not pass legislation until the end of 1918, largely because opposition in political circles to the use of compulsion in communicable disease control was strong. South Australia passed an act in 1920 but did not proclaim it. The chief health officer of South Australia argued in 1933 that compulsory notification was probably less important than adequate provision of treatment facilities and education of the community concerning the risks of infection.[85]

Unlike the Australian states, Britain did not employ compulsion in its approach to VD control, in part because of the history of bitter political conflict over compulsory medical examination of women under the Contagious Diseases Acts. In the late 1930s, a British expert group compared the effectiveness of control systems in Scandinavia, which employed notification and compulsion in treatment, and Holland which did neither. It concluded that "the degree of success in reducing the incidence of syphilis and of relative failure in gonorrhoea are broadly similar" in the two systems and that "compulsory treatment does not seem to us to be a major factor influencing the results of the antivenereal measures in the countries where it is employed."[86] Sir Arthur Newsholme in 1926 certainly thought that the post-1917 "remarkable reduction in the mortality from and incidence of venereal diseases" was significantly influenced by the clinic system's provision of "prophylaxis by treatment."[87] The combined mortality from syphilis, neurosyphilis and aneurism fell from 166 per million in 1901 to 118 per million in 1924. The age-standardized death rate from syphilis per million males declined from sixty-eight in 1911–20 to thirty-five in 1936. Infant mortality attributable to syphilis fell from 2.03 per thousand live births in 1917 to 0.2 in 1938. New syphilis cases fell progressively from forty thousand in 1919 to eighteen thousand in 1938. Since the majority of cases were seen in public clinics (to the annoyance of private venereologists who said the more well-to-do should not use public facilities), these figures are a not unreasonable indication of the national trend in incidence.

The mayor of New York City appointed in 1936 a commission to inquire into the control of VD in Britain and Scandinavia. The commission found that the disinclination of general practitioners to treat VD, together with people's inability to pay the fees of private specialists, resulted in the British clinics' becoming centers for the practice of venereology; that the decline in syphilis seemed to be due to medical measures and not moral restraint promoted by educational initiatives, since gonorrhea remained at a high level; that in Britain and Scandinavia the official prevention programs did not promote use of condoms or chemical prophylaxis; and that social and cultural factors contributed to reduction of syphilis—factors such as homogeneity of language, customs and moral standards, respect for authority, high standards of general education and of medicine, and minimization of quack and druggist treatment of VD. Of the various causes of the reduction, none was more significant than that "diagnosis and treatments are free, accessible, and generally good."[88]

In this era public health services in Britain, as in Australia, expanded into health care areas traditionally the preserves of private medicine—infant, child and maternal health, tuberculosis, and venereal diseases. The creation of a national system of VD treatment centers induced debate about the limits of state provision. But the 1914–1918 war normalized state intervention in many new areas of social life, and in any case, private practitioners who wished to do clinic work were rewarded for their services. Moreover, many practitioners had no desire to treat such stigmatized diseases and were happy to allow the clinics to do the work.[89]

Syphilis mortality in Australia declined in the interwar years, although it had already been in decline before World War I. In males, mortality fell from 121 per million (all forms except aortic aneurism) in 1908–10 to twenty-nine in 1946–50, and in females from forty-six to six per million. The decline was due in part to the availability of the arsenical drugs—Salvarsan and its successors—which provided the first effective treatment, and from the mid-1940s, penicillin. But the greater access to treatment, at least in large urban centers, that free public clinics provided must have contributed a good deal to this decline. Similarly, the considerable decline in mortality from general paralysis of the insane (GPI), a long-term consequence of untreated syphilis, must have owed something to the clinics, which in reducing the acute syphilis cases helped cut down mortality from GPI itself.[90]

Early provision of public facilities in Australia was inadequate. In the early 1920s in all states, only the capital cities had diagnostic facilities, although it should be remembered that a large proportion of the national population lived in these cities. Clinics were understaffed, poorly equipped, and often overcrowded. In early 1922, the commonwealth convened a conference of federal and state health administrators and BMA representatives "to ascertain whether the best results are being obtained for the expenditure of the money" on the control system.[91] The conference supported continuance of the system, believing a larger percentage of people were then receiving more effective treatment, even if private practitioners were too often failing to send in notifications. It was too early to decide whether the system was responsible for the decline in VD.

The Royal Commission on Health of 1925 criticized the quality of the public clinic system. All capital cities, it declared, required more clinic accommodation. Some clinics were so overcrowded that gonorrhea patients requiring long-term irrigation could not be properly treated. Equipment was inadequate. Laboratories in Sydney, Brisbane and Hobart were in various respects not able to perform their tasks efficiently. The Federal Health Department, the commission advised, should create a VD division to assist the states to improve the clinics. Enforcement of penalties against unqualified therapists and individuals knowingly spreading VD was almost impossible, because patients would not admit in court that they were infected. As noted earlier, M.J. Holmes was appointed director of a Division of Tuberculosis and VD within the commonwealth health department, and in 1928 he carried out a national review of the VD control system. Holmes noted that syphilis incidence had fallen considerably in all states but NSW since the inauguration of the system. This might have resulted from increasing failure to notify, but that failure should also have been reflected in gonorrhea incidence, and gonorrhea had not undergone a similar decline. He believed that as facilities improved and the community became educated, the need for compulsory treatment and notification would disappear. He proposed that doctors try persuasion before resorting to legal action to obtain patient compliance. He advocated full-time specialists within state health departments to run VD control, and subsidized hospital clinics directed by specialists to function as branches of the central departmental clinic. He praised Western Australia for its success in VD control but said that even there diagnostic and treatment facilities needed to be improved. With some frustration, Robert Dick, a senior public health doctor in Sydney, pointed out that in a small city like Perth it was reasonably easy to administer VD control legislation successfully. In much larger cities like Sydney and Melbourne, "compulsory notification was a hopeless procedure."[92]

In 1929 the Federal Health Council endorsed Holmes's recommendations for improving clinics and state organization of services as well as education of the community and the medical profession. As we have seen, the coming of the economic depression saw abolition of the Division of Tuberculosis and VD in the Federal Health Department in 1932. It also saw the end of commonwealth subsidization of state VD control. Despite the urging of the Royal Commission on Health, this had never been increased beyond the original total of fifteen thousand pounds per year. Political concern with VD had been evoked by the high levels of infection during World War I; in the longer term, as the sense of emergency diminished and syphilis incidence seemed to be falling, concern evaporated. There was some shift away from compulsion toward persuasion in the control system. But traditional moral condemnation of "illicit" sexuality and, by association, sexually transmitted diseases remained an obstacle. At the end of the 1930s, the chief health officer of Victoria, H.N. Featonby, observed that Australia's approach was located midway between the English approach (which abjured compulsion because it allegedly deterred people from obtaining treatment) and the Scandinavian (which allowed ample coercive powers). With syphilis in decline and the new treatment of gonorrhea with the sulfa drugs promising speedy and effective cures, Featonby said the way forward involved the provision of more and better clinics and large increases in hospital beds, although in the long term public education in its own right might be expected to have a marked preventive effect.[93]

The standards of comfort and privacy in public clinics left much to be desired. However, there was no groundswell of community opinion pushing for improvements, because all who could afford it sought private care, and this generally included the more articulate middle and upper classes. The situation contrasted with that of public tuberculosis treatment facilities. Because these offered sophisticated therapy, they attracted a growing number of more well-to-do patients. The "criminalizing" of VD treatment and control—legal sanctions could be and were applied to those failing to seek, or defaulting on, treatment—disempowered poorer patients who, having nowhere else to go, could not easily call for better facilities. Moreover, because of the general inhibition against public discussion of sexual matters, there was little public education, whether through leaflets, posters, radio or in schools. As with everything to do with sexuality, the quality of treatment facilities for sexually transmitted diseases was not a legitimate topic of public debate at this time.[94]

A more civilized control program involving more attractive public facilities would have elicited the ire of private practitioners objecting to the loss of paying patients to free public clinics. Public health authorities were always careful not to alienate private medicine, as we have observed. By the 1940s, antibiotics promised to solve the problem, both because they offered swift and sure cures (and so containment of infections) and because the ease with which they could be administered meant general practitioners in private practice could deal with VD cases. Special public facilities seemed redundant. The illusion of containment was, of course, to be shattered in the 1960s as VD became strongly resurgent just when the freedom of the "sexual revolution" was beginning to be enjoyed by increasing numbers of younger people.

THE INTRODUCTION OF MASS IMMUNIZATION

Corynebacterium diphtheriae, the pathogen causing diphtheria, appears as three types—*gravis, intermedius* and *mitis*—and each type differs in virulence. Case fatality rates vary according to the type involved. It is an old disease. The ancient world knew diphtheria; it was epidemic in Spain from the 1580s. From there it spread to other parts of Europe.

Diphtheria burst suddenly onto the English epidemiological scene in 1858. The English cases were part of an international upsurge of epidemic throat infection. It probably entered Australia some time between 1827, when Surgeon Peter Cunningham reported that it was not known here, and 1842, when three deaths in Hobart were attributed to "croup." Diphtheria certainly arrived in Victoria in 1858. Not only was it very prevalent in England then, but Victoria was experiencing the largest inflow of immigrants from the United Kingdom of any of the Australian colonies. It soon spread to the other colonies, although it was not reported in Western Australia until 1864. Antitoxin treatment was first employed by J.W. Springthorpe of Melbourne in 1895. The practice spread so quickly that by 1903 it was used in most cases. Case mortality fell greatly after the new treatment was introduced: around 1900, 10 to 20 percent; by 1920, 5 to 10 percent; 2 to 5 percent by 1930, where it plateaued until the 1940s.[95]

Diphtheria mortality in infants and very young children began to decline from about 1930. With the introduction of an effective toxoid in the 1920s, control became possible. At first only administered to case contacts, from the early 1930s on it was employed in school immunization programs. But real control only came with the widespread immunization of infants in the 1940s and '50s.[96] While immunization campaigns were a significant cause of decline, nonspecific factors like improved nutrition and the advent of small families contributed. At any time, the greatest mortality took place in the second year of life, with rates falling slowly up to five years of age, and then more quickly so that rates at five to nine years are much lower (table 5.6). Diphtheria still caused notable mortality among ten to fifteen year olds.[97]

Death rates in Australia for one to four year olds, in 1911–45, were very similar to those in England and Wales (see table 5.7). From the close of 1941, English medical officers of health pursued a vigorous diphtheria immunization campaign, although they had no legal capacity to immunize against any infection other than smallpox before the National Health Service Act of

Table 5.6

Deaths from Diphtheria per Million per Annum, Australia, 1908–10 to 1941–45

Period	Gender	0–4 yrs	5–9 yrs	10–14 yrs	Gender	0–4 yrs	5–9 yrs	10–14 yrs
1908–10	Male	584	318	68	Female	477	351	88
1911–20	Male	776	388	87	Female	706	470	103
1921–30	Male	527	165	27	Female	445	185	38
1931–40	Male	398	201	23	Female	370	201	27
1941–45	Male	233	127	26	Female	218	109	18

Source: H.O. Lancaster, "The Mortality in Australia from Measles, Scarlatina and Diphtheria," *Medical Journal of Australia* 2 (1952): 276.

Table 5.7
Deaths of Children Aged 1–4 Years from Diphtheria per Million per Annum, Australia and England/Wales, 1911–20 to 1941–45

Australia			England and Wales	
Period	Males	Females	Period	
1911–20	833	791	1911–20	830
1921–30	564	489	1921–30	531
1931–40	442	411	1931–39	511
1941–45	267	258	1940–45	272

Source: H.O. Lancaster, "The Mortality in Australia from Measles, Scarlatina and Diphtheria," *Medical Journal of Australia* 2 (1952): 275–76.

1946. After one year, deaths had declined by 33 percent. By 1946, mortality and incidence had fallen by 75 percent.[98]

Diphtheria was notifiable in Australia from the close of the nineteenth century. Cases were isolated in hospitals or at home. Household and often school contacts were swabbed to identify carriers. The *Medical Journal of Australia* argued from the 1920s for routine throat swabbing of all children, as proposed by the Commonwealth Committee on the Causes of Death and Invalidity in 1916. Campaigns to promote inoculation in NSW were not very successful. The Health Department used the Schick test in 1923–24 in some country towns and at the Cleveland Street Public School in inner Sydney to find out the proportion of susceptibles. The department found that 18 to 30 percent of children in mining towns and the city, and as many as 70 percent in isolated country locations, had neither natural nor acquired immunity. When the Health Department proposed to immunize them, the parental response was poor. It was clear that mass education was necessary. Preliminary testing continued, and susceptibles were advised to see private practitioners for immunization. The campaigns in Victoria were better run. In 1922 and again in 1923, the Health Commission and the municipal council of the provincial town of Bendigo (which had a high prevalence) tested 40 percent of schoolchildren, after which five to six hundred were immunized. Diphtheria cases declined from 374 in 1921 to ninety in 1923. The Melbourne City Council tested schoolchildren. Those without immunity were immunized, with minimal protest. As the *Medical Journal of Australia* commented, the problem, however, was that few children in total were being immunized; also, the important preschool population was being overlooked.[99]

In New York City, by 1928 half a million schoolchildren had been actively immunized under a program which had commenced in 1920. The preschool child now became the focus of efforts, and by 1940 an estimated 60 percent had been given immunity. From 785 per hundred thousand in 1894, diphtheria mortality declined to 1.1 per hundred thousand in 1940. The decline cannot be all attributed to immunization, as the death rate among children up to ten years old had fallen from 785 per hundred thousand in 1894 to below three hundred in 1900. It was below one hundred in 1920. The national mortality rate also declined, as the practice of immunization spread to other large cities. The incidence of diphtheria increased considerably in Germany and some occupied countries during the Second World War. After 1945, immunization was widely pursued in Europe, with a consequent fall in incidence.[100]

The attempt to promote immunization in Australia was set back by events in Bundaberg, a Queensland country town. In January 1928, twelve children died there after receiving toxin-antitoxin. Although a federal royal commission came to the conclusion that accidental contamination of the serum during preparation of the injections had been the cause of the deaths, heavy damage to public confidence had been done. Neither the pronouncements of national politicians—the prime minister, S.M. Bruce, claimed that the federal inquiry would soon restore people's confidence—nor the assertions of the *Medical Journal of Australia* that high overseas success rates with immunization, particularly in New York City, justified campaigns in Australia could quickly change the negative image of immunization. Since compulsory immunization was never a serious possibility, it was not a matter of individual freedom and rights, as it had been in relation to compulsory vaccination against smallpox in the nineteenth century. It was undoubtedly fear of harm to their children that made parents reject immunization for a time after the tragic events at Bundaberg.

In 1930, the Melbourne City Council began immunizing again, using anatoxin, a safer serum employed extensively overseas. As well as schoolchildren, some preschoolers were being immunized by the mid-1930s. The council reported a gradual change in parental behavior from reluctance to the active seeking of immunization. It could also report, and continue to report, a lower incidence for the city than for the Melbourne region as a whole. In the early 1930s some country local authorities in Queensland began to provide immunization services again. Where fewer than 1 percent of Brisbane children had protection, 25 percent of country children soon had it. Bundaberg began immunizing once more in 1934, and Brisbane followed the next year. By 1942, 80 percent of Queensland children had been immunized. Local authorities were responsible for promotion and facilities and for obtaining parental consent, while the Health Department provided the serum and paid local general practitioners five shillings for each child immunized. The service was provided gratis to children. The other states were slower to mount community campaigns. In 1934, a member of the Victorian parliament could deny flatly that immunization prevented diphtheria. Four years later the Western Australian Health Department bemoaned the fact that many people still preferred the views of unqualified opponents of immunization to the informed opinion of the department. Even in 1946, at a public meeting in a large country center in NSW, the argument could be advanced that immunization caused a number of serious illnesses, from tuberculosis to cancer.

In 1934, the BMA Federal Council had stated that mass immunization ought to be pursued. In 1936 the NSW branch agreed that its state health department should initiate a campaign. Yet the affiliated local associations, which represented both Sydney and country doctors, condemned the department's plan to supply gratis a medical officer to carry out immunizations and to allow local authorities to levy a fee of four shillings per child to cover their costs. The associations wanted local doctors (who would be given free serum) to do the work and to receive five shillings from parents plus another five shillings from the department for each child. Friendly societies would be charged one guinea for each child covered by family contract membership. The NSW department in May 1936 initiated a mass campaign, involving 311 local authorities. A major promotion effort sought to convince parents that the process was both safe and effective against diphtheria. The target of a hundred thousand inoculations in twelve months was not achieved, but forty-three thousand were carried out in the first seven months. By mid-1940, almost 216,000 children had been immunized.

Prior to the Second World War this was the only statewide campaign. However, a growing number of local authorities in other states became involved. In 1935–38, twenty thousand South Australian children were immunized, although fewer than 50 percent of children were immune by 1940. Western Australia achieved more, but Tasmania and some areas of Victoria were only beginning their campaigns. Mortality reports, as noted above, reflected the efficacy of immunization by the early 1940s. Moreover, by the end of the interwar period the obstacles to mass immunization were not so much negative community attitudes as lack of public funds. Most local authorities lacked adequate funding for health. The commitment to carrying out preventive measures depended very much on the attitude of the local medical officer of health. Central health authorities also lacked adequate funding; almost the whole of their budgets went for salaries and established activities. Little was available for new initiatives.[101]

In the following chapter, the rise and fall in the 1940s of the idea of a state-funded national health service will be discussed. This approach sought to solve the problem of inadequate public health funding by drawing on the extensive resources of the commonwealth, and the problem of the divorce between public health and clinical medicine by organizationally integrating preventive and curative work in a proposed national system of local health centers.

NOTES

1. Quoted in C. Thame, "Health and the State: The Development of Collective Responsibility for Health Care in Australia in the First Half of the Twentieth Century" (Ph.D. dissertation, Australian National University, Canberra, 1974), 13.

2. See M.J. Lewis, "Editor's Introduction," in J.H.L. Cumpston, *Health and Disease in Australia: A History,* ed. M.J. Lewis (Canberra: Australian Government Printing Service [hereafter AGPS], 1989), 7–8; Thame, "Health and the State," 13–14.

3. Quoted in Lewis, "Editor's Introduction," 26.

4. Ibid., 8–9; Cumpston, *Health and Disease in Australia,* 320; G.W. Rice, "Australia and New Zealand in the 1918–1919 Influenza Pandemic," in *New Perspectives on the History of Medicine,* ed. H. Attwood, R. Gillespie and M. Lewis (Parkville: Medical History Unit, University of Melbourne, 1990), 68–73.

5. Quoted in G. Rodwell, "Lessons from the First World War: Drs. Harvey Sutton and J.S. Purdy: Sydney's Health Week: 1921–1950," in *Individuals and Institutions in the History of Medicine Proceedings of 6th Biennial Conference of Australian Society of History of Medicine,* Occasional Papers in Medical History Australia 9, Organizing Committee of 6th Biennial Conference of Australian Society of History of Medicine, Sydney, 1999, n.p.

6. Thame, "Health and the State," 27. See Lewis, "Editor's Introduction," 26; M. James, "'A System of Industrial Hygiene': The Commonwealth Government and Occupational Health, 1921–1932" (M.A. dissertation, Australian National University, Canberra, 1990), 13.

7. Quoted in Lewis, "Editor's Introduction," 9–10.

8. Quoted in J.A. Gillespie, *The Price of Health: Australian Governments and Medical Politics 1910–1960* (Cambridge: Cambridge University Press, 1991), 40.

9. Quoted in ibid., 42.

10. See Lewis, "Editor's Introduction," 9–10; Gillespie, *The Price of Health,* 42; J.H.L. Cumpston, "The New Preventive Medicine," *Transactions of Australasian Medical Congress* (1920), 86.

11. See Lewis, "Editor's Introduction," 10–11.

12. Quoted in Gillespie, *The Price of Health,* 35.

13. Ibid., 34–35.

14. F. Goldsmith, "The Necessity for the Study of Tropical Medicine in Australia," *Transactions of Intercolonial Medical Congress* (1902), 178–79; "School of Tropical Medicine," *Transactions of Intercolonial Medical Congress* (1902), xxxviii; L. Harloe, "Anton Breinl and the Australian Institute of Tropical Medicine," in *Health and Healing in Tropical Australia and Papua New Guinea,* eds. R. MacLeod and D. Denoon (Townsville, Australia: James Cook University, 1991), 37–39.

15. Harloe, "Anton Breinl and the Australian Institute of Tropical Medicine," 39–40; "Tropical Australia," *Transactions of Australasian Medical Congress* 1 (1908), 100–103.

16. See Lewis, "Editor's Introduction," 10; Harloe, "Anton Breinl and the Australian Institute of Tropical Medicine," 44; Gillespie, *The Price of Health,* 41.

17. See Lewis, "Editor's Introduction," 11–12; F.S. Hone, "The Teaching of Preventive Medicine to Medical Students," *Transactions of Australasian Medical Congress* (1920), 273–75.

18. N. Bosanquet, "Health Economics: Finance, Budgeting, and Insurance," in *Companion Encyclopedia of the History of Medicine,* ed. W.F. Bynum and R. Porter (London: Routledge, 1993), vol. 2, 1379–81; *The World Health Report, 2000: Health Systems Improving Performance* (Geneva: World Health Organization, 2000), 12.

19. Gillespie, *The Price of Health,* 43–45; "The Report of the Health Commission," *Medical Journal of Australia* 1 (1926), 81. See Lewis, "Editor's Introduction," 12–13.

20. Quoted in Gillespie, *The Price of Health,* 45.

21. Ibid., 45. See Lewis, "Editor's Introduction," 13.

22. Thame, "Health and the State," 39–43.

23. Ibid., 44–50.

24. R. Doherty, "Elkington and After: Public Health, Queensland Style," *Australian Journal of Public Health* 19(1) (1995), 10.

25. Quoted in D. Fisher, "Rockefeller Philanthropy and the British Empire: The Creation of the London School of Hygiene and Tropical Medicine," *History of Education* 7(2) (1978), 130.

26. D.J. Lee, *The School of Public Health and Tropical Medicine, 1930–1980* (Sydney: School of Public Health and Tropical Medicine, 1980), 3–7; Fisher, "Rockefeller Philanthropy and the British Empire," 27.

27. Quoted in Fisher, "Rockefeller Philanthropy and the British Empire," 139.

28. Ibid., 129–43.

29. Quoted in L.F. Fitzhardinge, *The Little Digger 1914–1952: William Morris Hughes. A Political Biography* (Sydney: Angus and Robertson, 1979), vol. 2, 630.

30. Lee, *The School of Public Health and Tropical Medicine, 1930–1980,* 13–18.

31. Ibid., 54–60.

32. See Lewis, "Editor's Introduction," 14, 28.

33. P. Beilharz, M. Considine and R. Watts, *Arguing about the Welfare State: The Australian Experience* (North Sydney: Allen and Unwin, 1992), 83; G. Rosen, "What Is Social Medicine? A Genetic Analysis of the Concept," *Bulletin of History of Medicine* 21 (1947), 722–24; R. Acheson, "The British Diploma in Public Health: Heyday and Decline," in *A History of Education in Public Health,* ed. E. Fee and R.M. Acheson (Oxford: Oxford University Press, 1991), 299; R. Porter, *The Greatest Benefit to Mankind: A Medical History of Humanity from Antiquity to the Present* (London: HarperCollins, 1997), 643.

34. Quoted in W.W. Holland and S. Stewart, *Public Health: The Vision and the Challenge* (London: Nuffield Trust, 1998), 48.

35. Rosen, "What Is Social Medicine?" 722; Holland and Stewart, *Public Health,* 50–56.

36. Quoted in F.G. Fisher, "Raphael West Cilento, Medical Administrator, Legislator and Visionary, 1893–1945" (M.A. dissertation, University of Queensland, Brisbane, 1984), 179.

37. Gillespie, *The Price of Health,* 50–51; Fisher, "Raphael West Cilento, Medical Administrator, Legislator and Visionary, 1893–1945," 179–85.

38. P. Parkinson, "Correspondence: Property and Health," *Medical Journal of Australia* 1 (1939), 525.

39. Quoted in Gillespie, *The Price of Health,* 52.

40. "A Medical Research Council," *Medical Journal of Australia* 1 (1928), 529;

"A Medical Research Council for Australia," *Medical Journal of Australia* 1 (1935), 497; Gillespie, *The Price of Health,* 51. See Lewis, "Editor's Introduction," 15–16.

41. Quoted in F.W. Clements, *A History of Human Nutrition in Australia* (Melbourne: Longman Cheshire, 1987), 87.

42. Quoted in Gillespie, *The Price of Health,* 54.

43. Clements, *A History of Human Nutrition in Australia,* 87–112; Gillespie, *The Price of Health,* 54–55. See Lewis, "Editor's Introduction," 14–15.

44. Quoted in Gillespie, *The Price of Health,* 55.

45. Ibid., 55. See Lewis, "Editor's Introduction," 15.

46. M. Lewis, *Thorns on the Rose: The History of Sexually Transmitted Diseases in Australia in International Perspective* (Canberra: AGPS, 1998), 155–56; J. Duffy, *The Sanitarians: A History of American Public Health* (Urbana: University of Illinois Press, 1990), 240–43; E. Fee, "Public Health and the State: The United States," in *The History of Public Health and the Modern State,* ed. D. Porter (Amsterdam: Editions Rodopi B.V., 1994), 241.

47. Duffy, *The Sanitarians,* 256–60; E. Fee and B. Rosenkrantz, "Professional Education for Public Health in the United States," in *A History of Education in Public Health,* ed. E. Fee and R.M. Acheson (Oxford: Oxford University Press, 1991), 234–36.

48. Fee, "Public Health and the State," 247–48; Duffy, *The Sanitarians,* 263.

49. Lewis, *Thorns on the Rose,* 209–11; Duffy, *The Sanitarians,* 266.

50. J. Lewis, *What Price Community Medicine? The Philosophy, Practice and Politics of Public Health since 1919* (Brighton, England: Wheatsheaf Books, 1986), 5–10.

51. Ibid., 15–17.

52. Holland and Stewart, *Public Health,* 40–41; Lewis, *What Price Community Medicine?* 22–24.

53. Quoted in Lewis, *What Price Community Medicine?* 31.

54. Quoted in ibid., 40.

55. Ibid., 26–48.

56. G.J. Cuthbert, "Infant Mortality in New South Wales," *Medical Journal of Australia* 1 (1950), 75.

57. B. Meredith, "Statistical and Public Health Aspects of Prematurity," *Medical Journal of Australia* 1 (1950), 258–62.

58. P. Mein Smith, "Reformers, Mothers and Babies: Aspects of Infant Survival, Australia, 1890–1945" (Ph.D. dissertation, Australian National University, Canberra, 1990), 295.

59. See M.J. Lewis, "'Populate or Perish': Aspects of Infant and Maternal Health in Sydney, 1870–1939" (Ph.D. dissertation, Australian National University, Canberra, 1976), 213–19.

60. E.S. Morris, "An Essay on the Causes and Prevention of Maternal Morbidity and Mortality," *Medical Journal of Australia* 2 (1925), 338.

61. Mein Smith, "Reformers, Mothers and Babies," 302–307.

62. *Official Year Book of Commonwealth of Australia,* 24 (Canberra: Government Printer, 1931), 361; *Official Year Book of Commonwealth of Australia,* 33 (Canberra: Government Printer, 1940), 235.

63. Mein Smith, "Reformers, Mothers and Babies," 318–19.

64. Ibid., 322–23.

65. I. Loudon, "Some International Features of Maternal Mortality, 1880–1950," in *Women and Children First: International Maternal and Infant Welfare, 1870–1945,* ed. V. Fildes, L. Marks and H. Marland (London: Routledge, 1992), 5; J. Jamieson, "Contributions to the Vital Statistics of Australia: Puerperal Fever, Its Prevalence and Pathological Affinities," *Australasian Medical Gazette* 1 (1882), 130; Lewis, *What Price Community Medicine?* 109.

66. I. Loudon, "On Maternal and Infant Mortality 1900–1960," *Social History of Medicine* 4(1) (1991), 39; Loudon, "Some International Features of Maternal Mortality, 1880–1950," 15–17; E. Ludowici, "District Midwifery Practice," *Transactions of Australasian Medical Congress* 1 (1911), 391–95; J.M. Munro Kerr, R.W. Johnstone and M.H. Phillips, *Historical Review of British Obstetrics and Gynaecology, 1800–1950* (Edinburgh: Livingstone, 1954), 262–63.

67. Loudon, "Some International Features of Maternal Mortality, 1880–1950," 23–28; M. Lewis, "Maternity Care and the Threat of Puerperal Fever in Sydney, 1870–1939," in *Women and Children First: International Maternal and Infant Welfare, 1870–1945,* ed. V. Fildes, L. Marks, and H. Marland (London: Routledge, 1992), 42.

68. Quoted in Lewis, "Maternity Care and the Threat of Puerperal Fever in Sydney, 1870–1939," 39.

69. Ibid., 35–42.

70. Thame, "Health and the State," 175–78; J.C. Caldwell, "Population," in *Australians. Historical Statistics,* ed. W. Vamplew (Broadway: Fairfax, Syme and Weldon Associates, 1987), 36.

71. C.E. D'Arcy, "The Problem of Maternal Welfare," *Medical Journal of Australia* 1 (1935), 389.

72. Thame, "Health and the State," 179–98.

73. M. Humphreys, "Tuberculosis: The 'Consumption' and Civilization," in *Plague, Pox and Pestilence,* ed. K.F. Kiple (London: Weidenfeld and Nicolson, 1997), 136.

74. F.B. Smith, *The Retreat of Tuberculosis 1850–1950* (London: Croom Helm, 1988), 1–7.

75. Ibid., 243–47.

76. Ibid., 237–40; D. Porter, *Health, Civilization and the State: A History of Public Health from Ancient to Modern Times* (London: Routledge, 1999), 283–84.

77. Smith, *The Retreat of Tuberculosis 1850–1950,* 241; R. Walker, "The Struggle against Pulmonary Tuberculosis in Australia, 1788–1950," *Historical Studies* 20 (1983), 441; Cumpston, *Health and Disease in Australia,* 291.

78. Walker, "The Struggle against Pulmonary Tuberculosis in Australia, 1788–1950," 440–53.

79. Ibid., 447; Thame, "Health and the State," 23.

80. Thame, "Health and the State," 87–89.

81. Ibid., 91–109.

82. Ibid., 115–18.

83. Quoted in Lewis, *Thorns on the Rose,* 136.

84. Ibid., 135–52.

85. Ibid., 163–68, 211.

86. L.W. Harrison, D.C.L. Ward, T. Ferguson and M. Rorke, *Report on Anti-Venereal Measures in Certain Scandinavian Countries and Holland,* Reports on Public Health and Medical Subjects 83 (London: N.p., 1938), 3, 120.

87. Sir Arthur Newsholme, "The Decline in the Registered Mortality from Syphilis in England: To What Is It Due?" *Journal of Social Hygiene* 12(9) (1926), 519–20.

88. New York City Commission, "Control of Syphilis and Gonorrhoea in the Scandinavian Countries and Great Britain: A Report of New York City Commission to Investigate Prevention and Control of Syphilis and Gonorrhoea in Scandinavian Countries and Great Britain," *American Journal of Syphilis, Gonorrhoea and Venereal Diseases* 20(1) (1936), 56–61.

89. D. Evans, "Tackling the 'Hideous Scourge': The Creation of the Venereal Disease Treatment Centres in Early Twentieth-Century Britain," *Social History of Medicine* 5 (1992), 433.

90. Lewis, *Thorns on the Rose,* 232–33.

91. Quoted in ibid., 225.

92. Quoted in ibid., 229.

93. Ibid., 211–33; Thame, "Health and the State," 127–28.

94. Thame, "Health and the State," 142.

95. Cumpston, *Health and Disease in Australia,* 292–93; Thame, "Health and the State," 74.

96. B. Feery, "Impact of Immunization on Disease Patterns in Australia," *Medical Journal of Australia* 2 (1981), 174.

97. H.O. Lancaster, "The Mortality in Australia from Measles, Scarlatina and Diphtheria," *Medical Journal of Australia* 2 (1952), 276.

98. Holland and Stewart, *Public Health,* 68.

99. Thame, "Health and the State," 74–77.

100. G. Rosen, *A History of Public Health* (Baltimore: Johns Hopkins University Press, 1993), 313–14.

101. Thame, "Health and the State," 77–83.

Chapter 6

A National Health Service, 1939–49?

STATE-MANDATED HEALTH CARE FUNDING

State-mandated health care funding systems began to appear only a few decades after a centrally organized public health system emerged in the United Kingdom in the mid-nineteenth century. Arising in the industrializing nations of Europe as modern industrial capitalism transformed their economies and as the organized labor movement made demands on the state for welfare provision for workers, such systems spread to economically advanced countries in other parts of the world. Three models emerged: (1) mandated payments by employers and employees (and sometimes also contributions by the state); (2) centrally planned, tax-funded schemes, sometimes with public provision of services; and (3) more limited state funding of care for the disadvantaged or other special sections of the population, like war veterans or the aged, with the rest of the population making private arrangements.

As noted earlier, the first compulsory national insurance scheme originated in Bismarckian Germany in the 1880s. Belgium and Norway followed suit in 1894 and 1909, respectively, and Britain in 1911. The German model was adopted in Japan in 1922.[1] Australia seriously contemplated a compulsory national health insurance scheme in the 1930s. The conservative United Australia Party government introduced legislation. The Labor opposition rejected it, and in the end the scheme was not implemented. Labor had started on the path to the idea of access to publicly funded health care as a right of citizenship and a matter of social justice. As we shall see, the period 1941–49 was marked by fierce debate about the federal Labor government's ill-fated plan for a tax-funded national health service intended to deliver, in a socially just way, universal access to health care.

NATIONAL INSURANCE IN AUSTRALIA

It had become increasingly clear in the interwar period in Australia that the tripartite system of medical care inherited from the nineteenth century was not providing an adequate range of services for the population. Both income and geography were limiting access. Perhaps 50 percent of people obtained treatment from private practitioners on a fee-for-service basis, but many, being unable to afford fees except on a very occasional basis, sought care only when forced by an emergency to do so. About 20 to 25 percent were treated under friendly society–contract arrangements with private practitioners. These arrangements allowed a very limited range of primary-care services and normally did not provide for specialist consultations, at a time when specialization was becoming more common as medical care became more technologically complex. One doctor described contract medical practice in a mining town around World War I in this way: "The medical tactics . . . consisted in recognizing promptly the patient who was acutely ill and packing him off to hospital. As for the others, the doctors always adopted a stonewalling game. They kept their wicket up while Nature scored all the runs."[2] Those unable to pay private fees or friendly society membership dues were forced to use the charitable services of the public hospitals. In 1929, 25 percent of Melbourne people sought free outpatient treatment at public hospitals.[3]

The origins of interest in national insurance in Australia, however, go back beyond the interwar years. As early as 1876, a Victorian royal commission on friendly societies had looked at the possibility of introducing government sickness insurance. The commission had rejected the proposal, because it would inevitably have "something of the appearance of a relief system," and Australian working men, even more than their English cousins, were opposed to any scheme carrying the stigma of poor relief.[4]

The introduction of legislation in 1908 to provide a commonwealth revenue–funded aged pension had stimulated Liberal interest in the contributory method of paying for social benefits. In 1909, the Deakin government had arranged for inquiry into the matter of social insurance. Commonwealth statistician G. H. Knibbs in 1910 reported after a study tour concerning social insurance in various European countries that the "fundamental doctrine underlying the whole fabric of social insurance . . . is that a proper regard for the solidity of each community requires that all classes . . . should be protected by the strength of the community as a whole, against the incidents of misfortune on the class or on the individual."[5] Knibbs claimed that Germany had benefited morally and materially from national insurance. Insurance had strengthened in the working class the habits of thrift and of self-reliance.

Political interest in the contributory principle had increased because of Knibbs's report. It was also fostered by the British legislation on health and unemployment insurance of 1911, and by a 1911 report to the commonwealth by Sir John Cockburn, former premier of South Australia, on a conference on social insurance held at The Hague. The Labor Party showed some interest in the contributory principle. Three state branches favored contributory schemes in motions submitted to the 1912 commonwealth conference of the Australian Labor Party. But a conference motion calling for compulsory, contributory insurance against sickness, accidents, motherhood, and old age received very little support on the floor, mainly because most delegates believed that social benefits should be funded from general tax revenue. The labor movement was coming to believe that like education, social benefits should be universally available. In the light of this groundswell of opinion, the Fisher Labor government abandoned any thought of introducing contributory insurance schemes.

Fisher's introduction of a tax-funded, noncontributory, national maternity allowance scheme in 1912 pushed the federal Liberal Party farther toward endorsement of insurance-based funding of social services. At the federal election of June 1913, the Liberals proposed a contributory national insurance scheme offering sickness, accident, maternity, widowhood and unemployment benefits. There was doubt concerning the constitutional propriety of the scheme, but the main obstacle was the opposition of the friendly societies. Contributory state schemes appealed to modern Liberals not only as a self-help means of providing for individual security but as a way of mitigating class conflict (as industrial arbitration did) and promoting social cohesion. The employers' contributions even represented a small redistribution of wealth between capital and labor.

The short-lived Cook Liberal government had given way in late 1914 to a Labor administration. Soon after, Australia had followed the mother country into World War I. The conservative Bruce-Page government in 1923 established a royal commission to inquire into national insurance. The treasurer, Dr. (later Sir) Earle Page, expressed the conservative view of social welfare in his perception of the commonwealth tax-funded pension scheme as being as much a charity "as the poorhouse or the soup-kitchen."[6] Introducing the National Insurance Bill, Page called it "the most comprehensive and progressive measure of social reform . . . ever brought forward."[7] The compulsory, contributory scheme covered sickness, invalidity and old age, and it also provided for widows and orphans. But the government parties were not enthusiastic, and more importantly, the friendly societies, employers and insurance companies were hostile. The first declared that it would destroy the sturdy independence fostered by their mutual aid movement; they opposed the acceptance of other organizations, like commercial insurers, as approved societies. The second feared that employees would seek wage increases to cover their contributions, so making local products less competitive with imports. With doctors hostile to national health insurance, medical benefits had not been included. The royal commission recommended that they be investigated, together with public health services, by the Royal Commission on Health of 1925. However, in the course of discussion of national insurance, the medical profession publicly stated its position on payment for medical services, a position it was to adhere to strongly thereafter. It opposed the provision of services and opposed cash payments by any third party, whether the state or a friendly society. It argued that payment should be in the form of a reimbursement of the patient for settlement of the fee, not direct payment of the doctor. All this was justified by the claim that only in this manner could the integrity of the doctor-patient relationship be preserved. The Bruce-Page government won the election of November 1928, but the electorate had been cool toward its insurance plans, and nothing further was done.

The Scullin Labor government, which came to office in late 1929, was soon caught up in coping with the effects of worldwide economic depression and had no interest in the insurance idea. The Depression had an especially harsh financial effect on doctors in poorer areas, as many patients were forced to seek free outpatient hospital care and contract practice became more significant as a source of medical incomes. The profession became more interested in national health insurance. In 1933, F. Antill Pockley, a senior medical practitioner, had urged the profession to pursue voluntary insurance or see "nationalization" forced on it. In 1937, L.A. Dey, president of the NSW branch of the British Medical Association, predicted that the growing sophistication of hospital care would attract more and more people and that nationalization would ensue unless a way was found to provide for citizens who could not afford private fees. In August 1936, the BMA had put forward its own plan, in which general-practitioner services would be delivered to low-income earners on a capitation basis, while specialists would receive fees for services. Doctors would have majority status on the bodies administering the state scheme.[8]

The Lyons United Australia Party government became concerned about the increasing cost of invalid and aged pensions and decided to revisit the idea of a contributory scheme for pensions. Richard Casey, the federal treasurer, was a keen supporter of contributory insurance. Moreover, as the economy rose out of depression, attention to social services became more feasible. Sir Walter Kinnear, controller of the Insurance Department of the British Ministry of Health, at the invitation of the Lyons government presented a scheme of national insurance in 1937. This much resembled the scheme operating in the United Kingdom: compulsory contributions by employees, employers and the state and an income limit of 365 pounds per annum for membership. Under the Kinnear scheme, cash benefits for sickness, disability, old age and widowhood would be administered by a commonwealth insurance department. Medical benefits would be available to contributors for general practitioner services, for which private practitioners would be paid on a capitation basis. Considerable limitations applied, in that the self-employed, unemployed and dependents of contributors were excluded from medical benefits, and midwifery and specialist services were not included in the scheme.[9]

The Kinnear plan was primarily concerned with financial management, not health advancement. For the national hygienists like Cumpston, keen to promote preventive and social medicine, it simply provided more funds for curative medicine, doing nothing to advance the nation's health status. The Federal Health Department was excluded from the planning work, as Cumpston made clear: "The whole attitude of this type of approach was condensed in one remark made to me by Sir Walter Kinnear. . . . [W]hen I called on him to offer any assistance I could give, his reply to me was that the only concern a Health Insurance Scheme had with doctors was to police them. He declined my assistance and did not again discuss Health Insurance with me."[10] After some ambivalence, the federal Labor Party, concerned about the principle of a contributory pension and wanting a more socially equitable scheme funded from taxation revenue, opposed national insurance. Opposition also came from sections of the governing coalition concerned about the exclusion of farmers and other self-employed people, and from friendly societies, which did not relish the prospect of competition from life insurance companies as approved agents.

The Federal Council of the BMA, preferring national insurance to nationalization, agreed to the capitation fee of eleven shillings per patient per year offered by the federal government. However, after the rank and file rejected the fee as inadequate, the council sought to renegotiate its position. The government announced an inquiry into payments. Other concessions were made to various interests, including a voluntary contributory scheme for the self-employed and medical benefits for dependents of members of the compulsory scheme. In mid-1938 the National Health and Pensions Insurance Bill was enacted. The report of the inquiry into fees was delayed, and with the likelihood of war looming larger, defense preparations took precedence among federal policy preoccupations. An internal crisis gripped the government when the attorney general, R.G. (later Sir Robert) Menzies, resigned, ostensibly over the repeal of the pensions provisions. The BMA and friendly societies said that they would withdraw from negotiations. Then, Lyons died. Menzies became prime minister. But with the advent of war, the introduction of the scheme was indefinitely postponed. Of course, if the BMA had not withdrawn its initial support, the scheme might well have been implemented at the beginning of 1939 as originally planned. In its victory over the friendly societies in the 1920s and now its decisive role in the sinking of national insurance, the organized medical profession was emerging as a formidable player in national health policy.[11] It was to expand this role in the protracted struggle over the nature of the national health service in the 1940s.

PLANNING A NATIONAL HEALTH SERVICE

After the 1940 federal election, the political fortunes of the Menzies government were on the wane. It turned its attention to social welfare issues to bolster its position. The Australian government, like other Allied governments, sought to promote a national consensus to advance the war effort. The leaders of the liberal democracies talked not only about defeat of fascism but about the creation of a new, more just social order that would protect citizens against the economic insecurities of the interwar years. As Labor prime minister, John Curtin addressed the National Conference of the Labor Party in 1943. He promised that the four freedoms mentioned in the Atlantic Charter (freedom of speech and expression, freedom to worship, freedom from want, and freedom from fear) would become the basis of a new national and international order able to offer security from war, oppression and want for all people.[12] In 1941, the Menzies government had established the Ministry of Labor and National Service with a brief to look at postwar reconstruction issues and also an all-party Joint Parliamentary Committee on Social Security, with a brief to investigate social security issues on a wide front.

In the first phase of postwar reconstruction planning, 1940–43, the national hygienists' vision of a major reform—a national health service integrating preventive and curative medicine and drawing on the skills of a corps of salaried doctors without excluding private practice—dominated policy making. By 1944, however, the hope of such radical reform of health services had faded. The Labor government made the health program a subordinate part of its larger, cash benefits–based social welfare scheme. In pursuing this cash-benefits approach, the Labor government was reaffirming Labor's long-established goal of state provision of income support for socially disadvantaged citizens. The Labor government was not therefore primarily focused, as were the national hygienists, on advancement of the health status of the population through more efficient, more rationally integrated organization of preventive and curative health services.

In the policy gap left by the demise of national health insurance, the national hygienists worked to revive the ideas of the 1920s for a centrally directed reconciliation of public health and curative medicine. In late 1940, Cumpston urged the federal health minister, Sir Frederick Stewart, to allow the National Health and Medical Research Council to plan a health service. Cumpston was thus able to separate health policy from other social security concerns and so avoid its subordination, which had happened with national insurance. The NHMRC was well suited to his purposes, because public health doctor-bureaucrats were in control there, while it still provided channels to the wider medical world, including the BMA.

Members of the NHMRC were asked to offer individual critiques of the existing system, as well as proposals for change. Sir Raphael Cilento's contribution was both visionary and typically concerned with promoting the idea of state-directed prevention on a national scale. Salaried doctors practicing in group clinics would replace private general practitioners. The honorary system in hospitals would be replaced by salaried specialists, while hospitals would be under central control. Administration of services would remain with local and state health authorities, but general policy and finances would become the responsibility of the commonwealth. A subcommittee consisting of Cumpston, Cilento, John Newman Morris (of the BMA) and Professor Harold Dew (Royal Australasian College of Surgeons) produced a report, *Recommendations of the National Health and Medical Research Council on Reorganization,* to which the full NHMRC gave its approval in July 1941.

Recognizing that population health was determined by social and economic conditions, the report nevertheless was driven by notions less of social justice than of national efficiency. The primary goal was a fit population able to defend and develop Australia. It was an updated version of the 1920s plan to elevate preventive over curative services, with both functioning under the guidance of health departments. A national system of hospitals and district clinics would be staffed by a salaried service. Salaried doctors would be located, in the first place, in more remote parts of the country, where private practitioners were in short supply. Official supervision of the preventive efforts of private practitioners would be increased. General taxes, not individual contributions to a national insurance scheme, would fund the proposed program. The long-term role of private practice was left rather unclear. On the one hand, it was viewed as continuing alongside the salaried service. On the other, it was expected ultimately to be replaced by state-funded facilities, although the question of the means of compensation for the loss of a practice as a saleable asset—a major issue in the formation of the National Health Service in the United Kingdom—was not adequately addressed.

Cumpston played a dominant part in the formulation of this NHMRC plan, which envisaged the eventual demise of private medicine. He told a progressive industrialist who had praised the plan that he had personally written the report. Yet in retrospective accounts of the proposal written after his retirement in 1945, Cumpston tended to stress the tentativeness of the 1941 plan and to attack Labor's unrealistic, "socialist" objectives. Cumpston appears to have appreciated the strength of the contemporary shift toward collective responsibility for health and welfare; even the BMA and the Royal Australasian Colleges of Physicians and Surgeons at this time saw the advance of state intervention as inevitable. He wanted in 1941 to devise a national health scheme having the national hygienist imprint and forestalling the ill-informed contributions of "socialist" politicians and lay social reformers.[13]

The Joint Parliamentary Committee on Social Security (JPCSS) met first in July 1941, not long before the Curtin Labor government came to power.

It soon asked the NHMRC for another report on health services. This *Outline of a Possible Scheme for a Salaried Medical Service* costed the salaried scheme and proposed a set of planning regions and employment conditions for medical officers. The report also proposed that service be made available to all citizens irrespective of income. The press, comparing the NHMRC plan with Britain's Beveridge Report *(Report on Social Insurance and Allied Services)* in late 1943, asserted that the Australian noncontributory scheme was preferable to Beveridge's contributory health program. When the Labor cabinet began to consider postwar social security, the treasurer's input referred to the salaried service concept but also mentioned pharmaceutical and dental benefits as part of income support. The cash-benefit concept was at odds with the concept of state provision of medical services.

At the same time, the NHMRC plan was beginning to lose the profession's support. Dew argued that the profession had to be consulted fully over the salaried service. The BMA was angry about Cumpston's input to the JPCSS asking for immediate introduction of salaried services in large provincial towns like Cairns and Albury. The BMA saw this as a breach of the assurances by E.J. Holloway, the federal health minister, that nothing major would be done till the war was over. In mid-1943 the JPCSS released its sixth interim report. This report on health services set out to solve the basic problem of adequate provision for those in the middle rank, neither so poor as to be eligible for charitable aid nor well-to-do enough to meet medical costs out of their own resources. The answer was a salaried service under central direction and greater commonwealth control over public health and over medical education and registration. Aware of the BMA's commitment to fee-for-service, it envisaged gradual introduction of the salaried service. The JPCSS believed that the financial and technical attractions of salaried group-practice clinics would ultimately win over most practitioners, with the result that private practice would survive only in well-to-do areas. The great financial resources of the commonwealth would finally achieve national control over the curative and preventive health system. But the report, while indicating preference for the salaried concept, discussed the advantages of alternative means of financing services; accordingly, it constituted a confusing guide to reform of the medical services. Indeed, the committee's plan, like that of the NHMRC, remained rather abstract. Insofar as it looked to means by which the profession might be persuaded to support the scheme, it relied on large-scale funding of new facilities—regional group clinics and base hospitals—to persuade practitioners that the new system would overwhelmingly outperform private facilities. Moreover, strong insistence on commonwealth departmental control antagonized doctors and other politically significant interests. Even medical supporters of the salaried concept were attacked by national hygienists who, like Arthur Brown of Victoria, questioned the wisdom of public service control. Spokespersons for the Roman Catholic Church were concerned about the prospect of Catholic hospitals coming under the centralized control of state planners, who allegedly lacked respect for the religious principles to which the hospitals were devoted.[14]

With the war situation requiring less than its total attention as the outlook for the Allied cause improved, the Curtin government began in 1943 to address seriously postwar planning. In the process, the center of health planning moved from the NHMRC and the JPCSS to the Treasury, as the objective of policy shifted from "socialization" of medical practice to payment of cash benefits to citizens, who would purchase services from the established system of private practitioners. This also meant the end of the national hygienists' ambition to shift the balance of medical practice from the curative and remedial to the preventive side. At the beginning of 1943, the cabinet had accepted a Treasury-devised program of social welfare cash benefits; these included hospital, pharmaceutical and tuberculosis benefits. Having failed to persuade the states to refer voluntarily the necessary powers, the commonwealth government sought fourteen new powers by popular referendum, as it was allowed to do under the Australian constitution. The health power, like the other powers sought, was limited to a duration of five years after the end of the war, and in any case, the referendum did not pass. Health was becoming subsumed in a larger social welfare program based on income redistribution through cash benefits, and the Treasury was shaping national health policy. Macroeconomic concerns about inflation were influencing economic policy in such a way that the national hygienists' idea of huge infrastructure investment in new medical and health facilities was fast becoming unattractive.

In mid-1944, the states accepted the fundamentals of the hospital and tuberculosis benefit schemes. The federal government terminated negotiations between the BMA and the JPCSS—which, having offended the treasurer (J.B. Chifley), the health minister (J.M. Fraser), Cumpston, the Treasury and the BMA, was quickly losing influence. After two years there was still no agreement between the two sides. Cumpston, eager to place the Health Department closer to the center of health policy making, arranged a conference involving Fraser, Chifley, the NHMRC, the BMA Federal Council and the royal colleges. The meeting produced no clear outcome. Indeed, apart from insistence that a protective and corrective medical service be tax funded and universal, the government offered no coherent plan. However, the new developments showed that henceforth the government would take the initiative and not rely on proxies like the JPCSS to negotiate with the medical profession. Cumpston and J.H. Goodes of the Treasury now undertook talks with the BMA, talks that were really an effort to discover the organized profession's attitude to policy specifics. They also had the effect of unsettling the BMA about the government's intentions, raising suspicions that it was probing to discover the profession's internal divisions. The negotiations were to be halted by a constitutional challenge to the powers of the commonwealth.

In March 1944 the Pharmaceutical Benefits Act was passed. The medical profession (and the anti-Labor opposition) argued that it was a threat to professional independence. The profession added that it disadvantaged poorer patients because it was not free or universal. The government argued that a limited formulary of prescription medications was necessary to contain costs, although 80 to 90 percent of prescriptions would be included. Deciding not to cooperate, the BMA declined to put forward representatives for a formulary committee. In the second half of 1945, the Liberal attorney general of Victoria pursued an action in the High Court on behalf of a group of Victorian medical practitioners. He made two basic claims: that as the legislation was about medical and pharmaceutical services, it was beyond the powers of the commonwealth, a claim the court accepted; and that the commonwealth's expenditure power concerned only matters falling within its legislative, executive and judicial capacity. The act having been invalidated on the first ground, the second was not conclusively decided. However, observations by various justices pointed to a restrictive view of the spending power, a view that raised concern about the validity of spending on social services other than pensions, and on research. In the referendum of 1946, the government felt obliged to seek from the electorate constitutional power over specific social and health services.

Success in the referendum conferred on the commonwealth power to provide maternity allowances and widows' pensions; child endowment, unemployment, pharmaceutical, sickness and hospital benefits; medical and dental services (but not so as to authorize any form of civil conscription); and student benefits and family allowances. The restriction on its power over medical services was accepted by the Chifley Labor government, because it wanted to demonstrate that it would not exercise compulsion against doctors. The restriction was exploited by the profession to prevent implementation of the second Pharmaceutical Benefits Act, passed in 1947. The successful challenge to commonwealth constitutional powers in 1945 considerably delayed the movement toward a national health scheme. It meant that the fundamentals of such a scheme were not introduced along with the other social welfare measures like hospital and tuberculosis benefits. In the immediate postwar years, the ideological and political environment was to prove much less favorable than it had been to the idea of a state-funded health scheme.[15]

The profession in the interwar period had been split between doctors supporting insurance and conservatives unwilling to go beyond the existing tripartite system of medical practice. By 1940, the idea of a salaried service had gained support, albeit minority support. A.E. Brown, a member of the BMA's Victorian Council, was identified with this third way. He advocated doctor control of any national service through a statutory body, and he stressed the advantages to the individual practitioner in terms of time for preventive work. Supporters of the salaried service were mainly younger practitioners working in the armed forces. The majority of the profession, while accepting that change had to come, was keen to preserve both professional independence and social status, and it was wary of a state-funded, salaried service. At the end of 1941, as we have seen, the NHMRC brought out its report, *Outline of a Possible Scheme for a Salaried Medical Service.* A little earlier the BMA had officially endorsed the Bell-Simmons Report, which relied on the insurance principle, while a plan emanating from a subcommittee of the Victorian branch chaired by Brown advocated the salaried principle. The official BMA report was published under the title *A General Medical Service in Australia.* The three drew on a scheme, first endorsed by the Royal Commission on Health of 1925, to create across the country regional clinics providing the complete range of preventive services. But they differed over means of funding and administration. The official BMA plan had at the apex a statutory authority composed of representatives of the profession and other relevant parties. A compulsory insurance scheme would cover all with incomes below 416 pounds per year, and private practitioners would provide services on a capitation basis. The Brown committee's plan envisaged a universal salaried service funded from tax revenue and replacing private practice. A board of doctors would control the scheme.

The NHMRC plan was similar to the Brown committee scheme, except that private practice would be allowed to continue. The scheme would be run by regional medical officers reporting to the commonwealth Health Department. Criticism from within the profession of the BMA's own plan led to the Federal Council's asking the state branches to consider the three plans. Early in 1943 the New South Wales branch convened a meeting of members, the conclusions of which were to be binding on the branch membership. After considering the three reports, the meeting resolved that each person had a moral responsibility for his or her health and that of dependents; that the salaried concept was thus unacceptable; and that government-subsidized insurance for fee-for-service work carried out by private practitioners was the only way to preserve the integrity of the doctor-patient relationship. Private fee-for-service practice and the integrity of the doctor-patient relationship became the mantra of those opposing state intervention except on these terms.

In March 1943, the Federal Council, noting that neither salaried service plan had been endorsed by a state branch, adopted the New South Wales resolutions. At the same time, the Victorian branch sought to deal with what it saw as the main problems of the medical system—provision for people on moderate incomes, inadequate services in rural areas, and overcrowded outpatient departments. It proposed extending fee-for-service practice to all social groups. It would finance services from a special government fund that would pay part of the fee. In January 1944, the convocation of the Victorian branch laid down what it would accept as basic provisions of a national medical service: the existing consultant, general practitioner and hospital services had to continue; and means would have to be devised for bridging the financial gap between a complete service and universal availability. Victoria continued to be less wholeheartedly committed to fee-for-service than was New South Wales, seeing it as only one alternative to any unacceptable scheme put forward by the government.

In September 1944, the Federal Council strongly protested against introduction of any radical scheme for a national medical service during the war or for one year afterward. It resolved that in any acceptable scheme the individual would have to bear some financial responsibility, unless his financial situation was such as to preclude this possibility. It was ready to discuss a fee-for-service plan in which the individual paid a percentage of the scheduled fee, if an acceptable form of administration was in place. However, it saw a free medical service under government control as neither acceptable to it nor in the public interest. As we have seen, in November 1944 the Federal Council had entered into negotiations with Cumpston and Goode. Its representatives had indicated support for the fee-for-service principle. Yet the lack of agreement at branch level on support for the principle is revealed by the fact that the Victorian branch repudiated the stance of the BMA representatives, saying that they were pushing a scheme unlikely to be accepted by many doctors. The problem was that strong disagreement existed over the means of payment. The disagreement arose from changes in medical practice, as the advance of specialization threatened general practitioner incomes and professional independence. Support for the nonnegotiability of the fee-for-service principle had become very strong, but its dominance at this stage was not absolute.[16]

As the war drew to a close, the Chifley Labor government moved slowly on the matter of a national medical service while moving more quickly on other health-related matters, such as pharmaceutical benefits. The slow pace was determined by fiscal and constitutional considerations. Concerned with inflation, the Treasury was not keen to endorse more large expenditures. The electorate's rejection of the 1944 referendum indicated voter restiveness about centralized planning and controls. Ex-servicemen—who might have been a significant radical political force in support of the national welfare program, as was the case in some other countries, like Britain—were rewarded, because of lobbying by the Returned Servicemen's League, with special health services and pensions. Their needs were amply met by these special arrangements.

The Roman Catholic Church, which had already indicated opposition to centralized state control of hospitals, grew more critical of nationalization as the Cold War developed in the immediate postwar years. Since Labor was heavily dependent electorally on the votes of Catholics and the party leadership itself was strongly Catholic, the shift in the attitude of that church was an influential factor.

On the one hand, the government battle over health was of minor importance compared with the primary struggle to nationalize private banks and airlines. Further, the earlier, integrated scenarios of the NHMRC were now replaced by ad hoc policy shifts driven by constitutional and political considerations. On the other hand, diversity of opinion within the medical profession was replaced by united opposition to government proposals. Even some supporters of the salaried-service concept became part of this opposition, as suspicion mounted that the government was not committed to implementing the concept. Moreover, by the late 1940s the Cold War had moved the center of politics to the right. Socialized medicine was easily condemned as a Soviet-style totalitarian policy. Erstwhile advocates of a salaried service joined the opposition or ceased to voice public support.

The vociferous claims of the conservative federal opposition parties and private business interests that the Chifley Labor government's high policy—bank and airline nationalization and creation of a national shipping line—was socialism by stealth was easily extended to socialized medicine. The NHMRC plan for a salaried service that would rationally bring together preventive and curative medicine disappeared in the protracted struggle between a now-united profession and the federal Labor government over the professional autonomy and financial independence of doctors. Further, the leading public proponents of the NHMRC plan left the scene. Cumpston retired as commonwealth director general of health in May 1945, while Cilento in the same year took up a senior post with the occupation forces in Germany. Other leading public health doctors, like E.S. Morris of NSW and A.R. Southwood of South Australia, ceased to discuss publicly the key questions of method of payment and state control, although Southwood continued to advocate group clinics as the best means by which to deliver primary health care and prevention. This fundamental issue of accessible and equitable health services delivery was to surface again in the 1970s in the community health center movement (it will be discussed in the second volume of this history of public health in Australia). The weakening of leadership in public health was made worse by the premature death of Frank McCallum, Cumpston's chosen successor as director general of health, and his replacement by A.J. Metcalfe, who did not enjoy the BMA's regard as his predecessors had and who generally lacked their professional stature.

It was the conflict between the federal government and the profession over the pharmaceutical benefits legislation of 1944, not that over the national medical service, that served to unite the profession, focusing attention on broader issues of the limits of the commonwealth's constitutional powers and on the government's readiness to punish doctors refusing to cooperate. The conflict over the second Pharmaceutical Benefits Act, 1947, powerfully reinforced the profession's cohesion and its determination to resist the government's attempts to coerce it into compliance. In accord with BMA policy, 3,200 of the six thousand doctors in Australia refused to accept formularies provided by the government. The government faced unacceptable cost increases if the restricted formulary were not followed. Privately BMA leaders agreed that it covered more than 90 percent of drugs normally used, but the real issue was resistance to coercion. The government now (1948) fuelled the flames by introducing heavy fines for prescribing drugs *in* the formulary on anything other than the official prescription form. After initially supporting the BMA branches in Victoria and NSW in their condemnation of the new government penalties, South Australia and Tasmania began to urge compromise again. But the two large state branches were able to dominate the Federal Council when their representation on the council was significantly increased. A resolution was passed requiring branch approval before the council entered upon any contact with the government.

The government was keen to bring an end to the matter. It had the 1947 act amended: heavier penalties for noncompliance were introduced; an official form now had to be used for prescribing any drug in the formulary, unless the patient volunteered to forego benefits. This qualification appeared to forestall any claim that the doctor was being conscripted, although in most cases he or she would be forced to comply.

The Federal Council of the BMA asked the High Court to review the legislation. A majority of the court held that compulsory use of the form was "civil conscription" and so constitutionally invalid. With a federal election looming, the government deferred further action. Some of the BMA state branches now openly aligned themselves with the political opponents of the Labor government. In South Australia, the branch publicly supported the campaign against bank nationalization. In Victoria, individual members campaigned against the government (though the branch itself did not). In NSW, the branch funded antigovernment propaganda; five hundred general practitioners took part in a radio campaign. The free-pharmaceuticals scheme ultimately foundered on the rock of the federal constitution and the opposition of the organized profession. But the Labor government's ineptitude in handling the conflict, whether by its failure to answer BMA charges or its resort to threats of coercion, contributed to its collapse, as did the decline in political support for centralized state control in an international Cold War context.

When the federal health minister, Senator N.E. McKenna, took the initiative again in late 1948 on the question of medical services, the government's plan had moved a long way from the salaried-service concept, which was retained only as a long-term goal. He proposed a government-subsidized fee-for-service scheme, with half the scheduled fee to be paid by the patient. In response to BMA demands, patients were to be able to opt out. Essentially, the scheme covered only general practice, because specialists's fees would come under regulation only if the physicians agreed. Concerned with cost containment, the government gave the Federal Health Department means to exercise tight control of doctors who contracted into the scheme. The National Health Service Act, 1948–49, divided the country into health areas under district medical officers, who would take advice from representatives of local doctors. Regional clinics staffed on a sessional basis were to do preventive work. Remote areas would have a salaried service, but the great bulk of the population would continue to be served by private practitioners. The Liberal-Country Party Opposition and the organized profession both rejected the legislation. The BMA was unhappy about long-term competition for private practice from attractive, state-financed clinics. But the primary issue was state control. The BMA would cooperate only if the direct link between the state and private practitioners were abolished. Copayment was to be discarded. The patient would pay the fee, obtaining from the government any refund that was due. Administration would be taken from the Federal Health Department and given to a commission having a majority of doctors as members. Even so, just before the federal election, fee schedules for 192 items were gazetted by the Chifley Labor government. But in the event, this had no decisive effect on the election result; the Menzies Liberal-Country Party government came to power in December 1949. Soon after, the BMA Federal Council stated that it now had hope for the future.[17]

Constitutional obstacles, the capacity of a powerful professional group (having closed ranks) to pursue its own interests, inept behavior on the part of the Labor government at various points in the long, drawn-out negotiation process, the strength of government concern about inflation and the dominance of economic over social and health policy were all factors working against achievement of a national health service that would integrate preventive and curative work in publicly funded primary-care clinics staffed by a salaried medical workforce. Timing was also critical. There was a time of fluidity of opinion during the war when radical proposals based on the salaried-service concept and centralized planning were seriously entertained by the profession and negotiated change was possible. Constitutional difficulties delayed negotiations until the profession had united around resistance to state control in a new postwar context of waning popular enthusiasm for centralized planning and polarization, brought on by the emergent Cold War, of electoral opinion about state intervention.

A NATIONAL HEALTH SERVICE IN BRITAIN

By the 1930s, there was broad consensus in lay and professional circles in Britain that the state should facilitate access to medical services for all citizens and that the established health care system failed to provide universal access. Virtually no agreement existed in the interwar period on means by which to improve access. Some opted for the voluntary hospitals, others for national health insurance, yet others for local authority services as the platform on which to build greater provision of care. Appreciating the deficiencies of the national insurance system set up in 1911 (nonhospital medical care for workers, with no provision for dependants), the first minister of health, Dr. Christopher Addison, and his principal advisers the permanent secretary (Sir Robert Morant) and the chief medical officer (Sir George Newman), well understood the need for a unified health service. They saw it as under the control of local authorities, while a nationalized hospital system would be staffed by salaried doctors.

The Ministry of Health continued to look at the establishment of a national health service in terms of the gradual growth of local authority services. The Labor Party was also in favor of this path. As observed earlier, Addison had requested B.E. Dawson (later Lord Dawson of Penn), head of the Consultative Council, to recommend a scheme for "the systematized provision of such forms of medical and allied services as should . . . be available for the inhabitants of a given area."[18] Dawson's 1920 report did not favor unification under existing local authorities but rather ad hoc area health authorities composed of elected members and co-opted professionals. Preventive and curative services would be integrated in local primary health centers manned by general practitioners, with a second tier of health centers to be manned by consultants and specialists. The health centers would be linked to the hospital system, to which general practitioners as well as consultants would have access. The Dawson report did not address the issue of whether services should be free. The 1929 Local Government Act placed Poor Law hospital and other services under local authority control, with the result that municipal authorities now administered public health and medical services. But this attempt at unification of medical services failed in the face of proliferation and duplication of local authority services. The economic depression of the 1930s put great stress on the existing chaotic system. The dependents of most employees under the national insurance arrangements had to obtain care in municipal hospitals, while voluntary hospitals, suffering from a long-term decline in middle-class philanthropy, were in dire financial straits. They often had to concede a degree of independence in return for municipal subsidies.

In the interwar period the BMA had proposed contributory insurance as the means by which to increase provision of services, although nothing was done to implement the proposal. By the time the country went to war, there was much uncertainty as to what might be the future role of rates, taxes and contributory insurance. Two camps had emerged, with the Ministry of Health, the London County Council and the Labor Party in one, and the BMA, voluntary hospitals and the Conservatives in the other.[19]

The coming of the war and the need to provide for an anticipated large number of bombing casualties transformed the health care system. The civil defense regional administration coordinated all hospitals, as well as blood transfusion, laboratory and specialist medical services. The Emergency Hospital Scheme was so successful that soon there were calls for it to be made a

National Hospital Service. In 1941 the health minister, Ernest Brown, looked forward to involving the public and voluntary hospitals in a national service, available to all, in the postwar period. But the Beveridge plan for social security quickly broadened the objective to a comprehensive state health service. In December 1942, Sir William Beveridge, chair of the Interdepartmental Committee on Social Insurance and Allied Services, released his report on social security for the postwar era. For Beveridge, integral to social security were maintenance of employment, child allowances (to relieve poverty in large families), and a universal medical service for the prevention and cure of disease. Vested interests like the insurance industry and the medical profession were critical of the plan; the coalition government was divided; Prime Minister Winston Churchill was not keen. However, popular support was great. A national poll carried out a fortnight after the release of the report revealed that 88 percent supported the concept of universal access to medical and hospital services.

The Health Ministry and local authorities saw the projected service as an extension of existing facilities but with general practitioners becoming salaried staff members of local authorities. They would be employed in primary-care health centers. The coalition government's 1943 plan for forty authorities (existing local authorities, or amalgamations) to be responsible for all services funded by the public purse was the first proposal to realize the vision of unification of all state services under local government that the minority report of the Poor Law Commission in the 1900s and, before that, nineteenth-century reformers like Simon had held. In early 1944, H.U. Willink, the new health minister, published a white paper, *A National Health Service,* which incorporated the plan, modified in the light of discussions. Doctors and voluntary hospitals remained critical—the general practitioners not wishing to lose their professional and financial independence, and the hospitals wishing to prevent local authority control of their funds. In Parliament, Willink identified the basic principles of the plan as a comprehensive service available irrespective of means; freedom for doctors and patients to opt out; parliamentary and local authority control; and provision for professionals to influence the development of the service. Popular support remained high.

But by 1945 modification of the 1943 proposals had gone even farther. Local government control of the service was gone, as local authorities were placed under area and regional planning bodies, which would include unelected professionals. General practitioners would not become salaried staff but continue in the role of independent contractors (as established by the national insurance scheme). Voluntary hospitals would be insulated from local government financial control. The concessions to the medical profession and the hospitals widened the gulf between them on one side and the Labor party and the local authorities on the other. The bureaucrats planning the service were attacked by the BMA for supporting local government.

Although Labor was in power from mid-1945, it was unclear if the new government would implement the 1944 white paper proposals (about which it had not been happy), the less compromised proposals of the 1943 plan, or those embodied in its own *National Service for Health* of April 1943. Brushing aside his senior advisers' concern to protect the independence of the voluntary hospitals, Aneurin Bevan, the Labor minister of health, urged nationalization and regionalization of hospitals. These proposals represented the most innovative aspects of Bevan's plan. The National Health Service Act was passed in November 1946, and legislation for Scotland was passed in 1947.

The service did not come into being for another two years, during which time Bevan carried on sometimes bitter negotiations with the medical profession. Bevan decided on different administrations for hospital, public health, and general practitioner and other independent contractor services. This was done partly to mollify local authorities, who would continue to administer public health services, and the independent contractor general practitioners, who would also enjoy continuity of administration. Nationalization of hospitals probably reflected widespread concern about local government capacity to cope with a reconstruction task that included control of hospitals. Moreover, the voluntary hospitals were more likely to accept nationalization than municipal control. Regional hospital boards, each related to a natural hospital region, would implement government policy. Everyday administration of hospital groups in natural hospital districts fell to district committees (later hospital management committees). Although it lost municipal hospitals to the regional system, local government, constituted as local health authorities, retained control of a wide range of services. They were also promised control of the projected health centers, which were to accommodate independent contractors (general practitioners) as well as salaried staff, but the national system of centers failed to develop. The medical officers of health continued to be responsible for the range of established public health services like maternity and child health, domiciliary midwifery, immunization and health visiting. The general practitioner and other independent contractor services were administered by committees (later executive councils), which were basically those of the old national insurance system. The new National Health Service embodied Beveridge's requirements that it be free and available to all and offer both preventive and curative services. It would seem that one of the scheme's most valued features—to both citizens and health professionals—was relief from direct charges.

Most of the interest groups were ready to cooperate. Although the local authorities were not happy with their loss of functions, the large ones were in most cases under Labor control. The voluntary hospitals could expect to play a considerable part in hospital management and were pleased not to be under municipal control. Hospital doctors stood to gain in various ways. The consultants had long supported regionalization; private practice remained possible, and they would enjoy a substantial voice in hospital management. It was the general medical practitioners (and dental practitioners) who would not be reconciled. The BMA, which was dominated by general practitioners, was intransigent over its basic claims: that the market in medical practices continue; that payment of general practitioners be through capitation and the small salary component therefore be abolished; that controls concerning the distribution of general practitioners be abandoned; and that the highest "court of appeal" for general practitioners facing loss of contracts not be the minister.

Until quite late in the run-up to the inauguration of the National Health Service, the medical profession was overwhelmingly against participation. A compromise was reached, however, after mediation by consultants. While the ban on the sale of practices continued, greater compensation would be forthcoming from the government. For most general practitioners, the small salary component was abolished. Minor concessions to general practitioner demands were made in connection with the appeal procedure. On 5 July 1948, the National Health Service came into being, with about half a million employees and contractors—360,000 in hospitals; twenty-six thousand in the Local Health Authority sector; and fifty-five thousand in the Executive Council sector.[20] The *Times* captured the widespread sense of pride in the achievement: "This day makes history—insurance and assistance to help in all the changes and chances of life, a free national health service for all—these are the great landmarks in British social progress which we have reached this month."[21]

The coming of the National Health Service saw the public health sector lose general, poor law, tuberculosis, infectious diseases and mental and mental deficiency hospitals, as well as clinical work, the last because general practitioner services were now available to all. Where the local authorities had run comprehensive services in areas like maternity and child health, tuberculosis and mental health, they now became subsidiary to the other branches of the National Health Service. Moreover, cooperation with these branches was made more difficult by the long-standing poor relations between the medical officers of health and clinicians. Local health departments lost their sense of direction in these circumstances and never regained it before their demise in 1974.

In 1955, the Health Ministry observed that "there is still a great deal of preventive work . . . for the [domiciliary] teams to do. . . . The difficulty is of course to attract the interest of general practitioners, who are at present reluctant to make use of the Health Visitors and other domiciliary services provided by Local Health Authorities."[22] Local government had pioneered health education and promotion, and in 1927 it had created the Central Council for Health Education to assist with coordination of the work of the local authorities. The Scottish Council for Health Education had been set up in 1943. The local authorities carried out successful mass campaigns against diphtheria and tuberculosis in the postwar period. But class, occupational and regional differences in health were not addressed, in part to avoid controversy. In 1955, soon after Richard Doll and Austin Bradford Hill first pointed to the epidemiological links between smoking and lung cancer, the chief medical officer could claim that "there is no likelihood that research in the field of preventive medicine would offer any promise of early marked alteration in the country's morbidity."[23] It was hoped at the outset the National Health Service would give much weight to prevention and to positive health. But leadership was lacking. C.R. Brockington, medical officer health for the West Riding of Yorkshire and later professor of social and preventive medicine at the University of Manchester, in 1949 pointed to the preventive responsibilities incumbent on the local authorities under the National Health Service Act. He envisaged health centers becoming "centres of preventive medicine where adequate records and routine health checks become routine procedures." He believed that "at some time in the future they will become the focus of medicine." He saw "Part III of the Act . . . as a minor charter in public health. Had it been passed into law without the rest of the Act, the world of public health might have acclaimed it without reservation."[24]

The development of medicine became centered in the regional hospital boards. About one-third of a board's membership was medical but came overwhelmingly from curative medicine. The pursuit of preventive work became harder now that public health doctors, in contrast to the situation prior to the National Health Service, had to depend on another authority for clinics or consultant domiciliary visits. The balance of health services tipped decisively toward hospitals and curative medicine. Some experts favored the taking of public health from local authorities, in order to revivify prevention. Brockington stood against this, in part because it would render public health practitioners unaccountable to local communities: "The outlook of the clinician, who occupies more than a third of seats on the boards, is centred upon the individual. . . . The outlook of the medical officer of health centres upon society. If then local government in health . . . is now to be deposed, let not the throne be occupied by those who know not."[25] Traditionally, maternity and child health had been the prime focus of the health education work of local authorities, and as of the inauguration of the National Health Service, 4,700 centers were functioning. Moreover, until the advent of the service, the centers were part of a growing maternity service. But the local authorities now became junior partners to the other branches of the service.

The future of local health authority services seemed clouded. Basic to the problem was the significant increase in hospital confinements. Just under 40 percent of births in 1937, they had grown to over 64 percent twenty years later. The Royal College of Obstetricians and Gynaecologists pushed for maternity services to be placed under hospital control. It wanted to restrict the work of general practitioners and local authority medical officers. Obstetric work would be limited to qualified obstetrician-general practitioners. They would run antenatal clinics—local authority clinics were perceived as obsolescent—as well as take charge of deliveries in obstetric units. Domiciliary midwives employed by local authorities—five thousand by the mid-1950s—would join the hospitals. Both the local health authorities and the BMA rejected the college proposals. The Ministry of Health was forced to resolve the conflict. In 1956 a Maternity Services Committee was set up; it ultimately recommended a target of 70 percent hospital confinements. It also recommended that obstetrician-general practitioners gradually take over antenatal clinics from local authority medical officers. At this price, the local authority maternity and child welfare clinics continued to function.[26]

Underlying the failure to build health centers and increase community care services was the fact that spending on health lagged behind that on other social services, like housing and education, in the first ten years of the life of the National Health Service. From 29.5 percent of total social services expenditure in 1949–50, spending on the National Health Service and local welfare services fell to 25.8 percent in 1957–58. In addition, within the tripartite structure of the service, the regional hospital administration enjoyed greater status and priority in resources than the primary-care sector, run by the executive councils, or the community services, run by the local authorities.

In the first decade the hospitals received almost all of the capital investment available. By the late 1950s, they were responsible for about 60 percent of current spending, compared with the primary-care sector's 27 percent and community services' 9 percent. Another indicator is the comparative growth in professional staff. In 1949–58, medical and dental practitioners employed by local authorities grew in number by 10 percent, those in the primary-care sector by 12 percent, but those in hospitals by 32 percent. The result was that better career opportunities and higher professional status lay with hospital medicine. General practice, particularly public health medicine, seemed unexciting and lacking in prestige. Recruitment to public health medicine declined in qualitative and quantitative terms. The effect on the nonhospital services (which represented much less costly solutions to national health problems) was to confirm already low levels of initiative and morale.[27]

NATIONAL HEALTH INSURANCE IN THE UNITED STATES

When social insurance finally arrived in the United States in 1935, as a result of the New Deal's response to the economic depression, national health insurance was omitted. Except for old-age pensions, social security provision (including health care in the postwar era) remained confined to the poorer classes. The Franklin D. Roosevelt administration had not included health insurance in its social security measures because it had calculated that if it did, the Social Security Act of 1935 would not pass. Also, some of President Roosevelt's advisers saw it as a form of subsidization of doctors, who would stand to gain more than citizens. The failure of health insurance during and just after World War I had been very much due to the opposition of the medical profession. In the 1920s the income and prestige of the profession had increased notably. Early in 1935, a special meeting of the American Medical Association (AMA) House of Delegates rejected compulsory health insurance. The AMA was prepared to endorse voluntary insurance, however, if it conformed to association guidelines.

In 1937, the Technical Committee on Medical Care of the Interdepartmental Committee to Co-ordinate Health and Welfare Activities (established in 1935 to oversee proliferating federal programs) was asked to draw up plans for a national health program. The committee preferred health program grants for the states to national insurance. It emphasized the need for more public health, maternal and child health services, and for an increase in hospital capacity. Other proposals included introduction of a medical care scheme underwritten by taxes, insurance, or a combination of the two. The committee's proposals were warmly received by a 1938 national conference of labor, farmer and health professional representatives. The AMA quickly offered to support all proposals if the committee abandoned compulsory health insurance. When the committee refused, the AMA sought to sink the insurance proposal in another way—it expressed official support for the committee's proposals for an increase in public health services, provision of compensation for wages lost due to illness and federal assistance for care of people without personal resources. The American Public Health Association, split between members who saw some medical care to be legitimately part of public health and those who did not, endorsed the AMA's stand.

President Roosevelt initially was inclined to make the national health program part of his 1938 election campaign, but then decided against it. From 1938 the Roosevelt administration enjoyed less support in Congress. Early in 1939, New York senator R.F. Wagner brought in a bill that would have introduced the national health program measures recommended by the Technical Committee on Medical Care and supported by the AMA. The bill also provided for health insurance as something for the states to introduce. The AMA now opposed the bill. President Roosevelt made clear that he would be satisfied with funding of hospital construction in areas of need. This limited proposal fared no better than the larger health program, failing to pass in the House of Representatives. Opinion polls in the late 1930s and early '40s showed that although a majority endorsed national health insurance, those who had a strong preference were in the minority. There is some evidence that Roosevelt was also reluctant to support insurance in 1938–39 because of AMA opposition, even if the strength of opposition now was less than earlier in the century.[28]

Until the early 1940s, the constitutional viability of national insurance was uncertain with respect to states' rights. Even so, the Wagner-Murray-Dingell Bill of 1943 provided for national insurance that was both comprehensive and universal. Roosevelt himself the next year sought the approval of Congress for a right to medical treatment as part of a more general economic bill of rights. In late 1945, President Harry Truman proposed a scheme that, like the prewar national health program, included hospital development and expansion of public health, maternal and child health services. It also included support for medical education and research, and for universal health insurance, with public funding of membership for the poor. Although Truman stressed that the measure did not seek to change the private nature of service organization—that it was not socialization of medicine—the medical profession's reaction was hostile. The AMA proposed instead expansion of public services for the poor and of voluntary insurance for those able to afford it. Polls revealed majority support for compulsory national insurance as such—58 percent in a national poll in late 1945. But when it was compared with specific alternatives like voluntary insurance, national insurance enjoyed only minority endorsement. Congressional reaction was not encouraging. The conservative chairman of the House Committee would not allow hearings, while in the Senate the Republicans indicated that they would not be involved in hearings. Many significant players in health care, like the American Hospital Association, supported voluntary insurance. In August 1946 Truman saw his proposal for hospital construction realized, but prospects for national insurance worsened as the Republican Party took over Congress. They branded it socialized medicine, linking it to the larger issue of the threat of communism.

After Truman's victory in the 1948 presidential election (in which he had strongly supported national insurance), the AMA mounted a massive public relations campaign. This persuaded many citizens that insurance was indeed socialized medicine and the forerunner of further acts of socialization. By 1949, polls showed a decline in support from 58 to 36 percent. Attempts at compromise failed. Thus—the president having broken with southern Democrats over civil rights issues—Bernard Baruch's plan for those on low incomes to have Social Security–funded compulsory insurance while those on higher incomes would take out voluntary insurance could not proceed, despite support from the American Federation of Labor.

However, other social security measures were passed in this period; in 1950, for example, ten million more people were included in old-age and survivors' insurance. It was clear that while expansion of welfare services for the poor (along with private insurance for the better off) was acceptable, national health insurance would not get off the blocks. Supporters now pursued the lesser goal of hospital insurance for the aged. They had lost what was fundamentally an ideological battle, even when they had tried to present their case as a question of the efficient provision of resources to advance the health of the country. While supporting the principle of health insurance, the community was not clear about what form it should take and so were open to persuasion by interests opposed to national insurance. Such interests disposed of considerable campaign funds. Where the Committee for the Nation's Health had at its disposal about fifty thousand dollars a year, the AMA paid $2.25 million for its extensive public relations campaign. Business generally supported the AMA, for financial as well as ideological reasons—to avoid paying employees' insurance. Industries like pharmaceuticals also had a larger interest in preserving private medicine. Public support for capitalism was growing in the United States in the 1940s and '50s as the social trauma of the 1930s depression receded (although Cold War sentiment did not prevent Western European countries from developing national systems of insurance). Moreover, while federal intervention in support of health care continued to expand, such intervention was fragmented. Not only was funding earmarked for hospital building or medical research, but support tended to focus on particular diseases, like heart disease or cancer.[29]

The U.S. Public Health Service (USPHS) developed essentially as a manager of epidemic crises, like bubonic plague in San Francisco in the 1900s, and a manager of health care services for those too poor to buy them from private medicine. It also became a major supporter of biomedical research. In the 1920s and early 1930s, the USPHS acquired responsibility for drug rehabilitation centers, venereal disease clinics and psychiatric hospitals. When the Social Security Act, 1935, made available federal funds for maternal and child welfare services, the USPHS used such grants to the states to create local health departments. After Thomas Parran became surgeon general in 1936, the service cooperated with the Farm Security Administration in providing medical care for the rural poor. Parran's successor from 1947, Leonard Scheele, focused his efforts on developing the National Institute of Health (about which more below). Under Scheele, the National Institute of Health joined with the National Heart Institute, the National Biological Institute and National Institute of Dental Research to become the National Institutes of Health (NIH). By the mid-1950s, not only had four additional institutes been included but the NIH budget for research had expanded from thirty-seven to a hundred million dollars. From 1849, the Bureau of Indian Affairs had run a health care service of indifferent quality for Native Americans. When Native American recruits during World War II were found to have a high prevalence of tuberculosis, the National Tuberculosis Association, the AMA, the American Public Health Association and the Association of State and Territory Health Officials all pressed the USPHS to take over responsibility for their health care. This took place in 1955.[30]

The failure of the liberal push for national health insurance meant the inadequate distribution of medical services would not be corrected. From 1950 to the mid-1960s, medical policy stressed growth of resources—especially expansion of medical research and hospital infrastructure—without redistribution of medical services. Public support for primary-care expansion was negligible compared with support for high-technology medicine. Concern about those who had not shared in postwar economic prosperity led to a focus in federal policy from the mid-1960s on redistributive measures. From the 1970s, however, as economic growth faltered but inflation persisted, cost containment increasingly became a major objective of public policy.

Medical research as a federal function had begun very modestly in the Marine Hospital Service's bacteriological laboratory on Staten Island, New York, in 1887. In 1902, under federal power to regulate vaccines and sera marketed interstate, the laboratory had initiated work on biological products; at the same time, divisions of chemistry, pharmacology and zoology had been established. In 1930 the laboratory was reorganized as the National Institute of Health. In the late 1930s, cancer research and control became national concerns. In 1937 the National Cancer Institute was established as part of the National Institute of Health. At the same time the USPHS was empowered to provide funds for extramural research. Yet funds spent on research remained small. Where the Department of Agriculture spent $26.3 million in 1938, the USPHS spent a mere $2.8 million.

Wartime exigencies boosted medical research. The need for a synthetic substitute for quinine for malaria therapy in the Pacific War, isolation of blood derivatives like gamma globulin and mass production of penicillin were the more notable achievements. In mid-1941, the Office of Scientific Research and Development was created. Its Committee on Medical Research developed an extensive program of research and development, with 450 contracts let to universities and 150 to research institutes, hospitals and comparable bodies. Three years later, the USPHS was authorized to fund extramural research in areas besides cancer. At the end of the war, the National Institute of Health assumed responsibility for Committee on Medical Research projects still in progress. The National Institute of Health had research funds of $180,000 in 1945 but two years later disposed of four million dollars.

As surgeon general, Leonard Scheele worked closely with influential lobby groups pressing for greater federal funds for medical research. Mary Lasker and Florence Mahoney used their wealth and political influence in the cause. Public opinion and Congress were amenable. Mary Lasker and the American Cancer Society successfully promoted funding of research on cancer. The single-disease, or categorical, approach to funding became the way in which the national research program, following the earlier pattern of fund-raising by voluntary bodies, developed. As we have seen, the National Institute of Health became the National Institutes of Health in 1948. Five new categorical institutes were subsequently set up. By 1950, the NIH received just over forty-six million dollars, a substantial proportion of which was spent on grants to outside researchers. Federal spending on medical research had grown dramatically from three million dollars in 1941 to seventy-six million ten years later. When random, controlled trials demonstrated the efficacy of the Salk polio vaccine in 1955, community and political faith in research seemed more than vindicated. Its potential to advance the health status of the nation seemed endless. The budget of the NIH increased impressively, from eighty-one million dollars to four hundred million in 1955–60.[31] By 1967, it had grown to $1.4 billion.

The USPHS in the 1960s was not central to federal government attempts to provide medical care for the aged and the poor. Medicare and Medicaid were administered by the Department of Health, Education and Welfare. But the USPHS remained in charge of health services for Native Americans and developed its role as adviser to local health authorities in crisis situations, especially through its Centers for Disease Control (CDC) in Atlanta. (Thomas Parran had in 1946 overseen the transformation of the Office for Malaria Control in War Areas into the Communicable Disease Center, which later became the CDC.) The USPHS programs on tuberculosis and venereal disease was relocated in the CDC, monitoring of vaccines production initiated, and the epidemiological division developed. The Epidemiological Intelligence Service had from 1951 carried out surveillance of disease in the United States and internationally. The USPHS thus continued its basic role of medical management, both in health crises and in directly running services for the socially disadvantaged. At a time when public funds were going to fundamental biomedical research (and hospital expansion), not prevention, the USPHS also oversaw the management of a quickly expanding biomedical research establishment at the NIH.

In Britain, too, public health doctors were, within the National Health Service, increasingly acting as managers in the postwar period, as they grappled with the problems of coordinating a growing community service sector. Indeed, by the 1960s public health was being seen as planning of community services. Public health doctors were soon to be renamed "practitioners of community medicine." In 1974, "community physicians" replaced medical officers of health. The epidemiological transition from the long-standing dominance of infectious diseases in the disease pattern of Western countries to the dominance of chronic degenerative diseases and of accidents saw the further decline of environmental public health and an emerging focus on clinical prevention at the individual level. Where in Western countries in 1900 the primary killers had been tuberculosis, pneumonia, diarrhoeal diseases and enteritis, by the 1940s they were coronary heart disease, cancer, and accidents.

In the United States, as in Australia, the integration of preventive and curative medicine in a more efficiently organized health system was made impossible by conservative political forces within medicine and outside it. Not even national health insurance could be established. Biomedical research and high-technology medicine were the recipients of public goodwill and federal funds, in part because of the impressive wartime advances of medical science. Biomedicine trounced public health in the public relations sphere, taking the credit not only for such recent achievements but for the secular decline of infectious disease—when, as we have seen, McKeown's work had showed infectious disease mortality falling decisively long before the antibiotic era. Public health professionals failed to communicate their historical achievements in improving the health of the community, and they failed to persuade politicians to provide adequate funding. In the United States and the United Kingdom, public health became preoccupied with management of health care services. More critically, in both countries, as in Australia, public health failed to adapt conceptually to the modern epidemiological transition in a speedy fashion, or to articulate a major new preventive role in relation to the emerging chronic-disease hazards to the health of the people. The field was left wide open for clinical medicine to articulate an individually oriented, preventive approach.[32] In volume 2 of this history of public health, *The People's Health: Public Health in Australia, 1950 to the Present* the individually oriented approach is discussed at some length in the context of the evolution of preventive strategies in the 1950s and 1960s.

NOTES

1. *The World Health Report, 2000. Health Systems: Improving Performance* (Geneva: World Health Organization, 2000), 12–13.

2. Quoted in C. Thame, "Health and the State: The Development of Collective Responsibility for Health Care in Australia in the First Half of the Twentieth Century" (Ph.D. dissertation, Australian National University, Canberra, 1974), 301.

3. See M.J. Lewis, "Editor's Introduction," in J.H.L. Cumpston, *Health and Disease in Australia: A History*, ed. M.J. Lewis (Canberra: Australian Government Publishing Service [hereafter AGPS], 1989), 16.

4. D.G. Green and L.G. Cromwell, *Mutual Aid or Welfare State: Australia's Friendly Societies* (Sydney: Allen and Unwin, 1984), 24.

5. Quoted in T.H. Kewley, *Social Security in Australia, 1900–72* (Sydney: Sydney University Press, 1973), 100.

6. Ibid., 99–102, 140–49.

7. *Commonwealth Parliamentary Debates* 119 (14 September 1928), 6746.

8. S. Sax, *A Strife of Interests: Politics and Policies in Australian Health Services* (Sydney: Allen and Unwin, 1984), 35–41; F.A. Pockley, "Correspondence: The Future of Medicine as a Profession," *Medical Journal of Australia* 1 (1933), 205; L.A. Dey, "National Health Insurance," *Medical Journal of Australia* 1 (1937), 527–31.

9. Sir Walter Kinnear, *Report on Health and Pensions Insurance* (Canberra: Government Printer, 1937), 10–31; Sax, *A Strife of Interests*, 39.

10. Quoted in Lewis, "Editor's Introduction," 17.

11. Kewley, *Social Security in Australia, 1900–72*, 161–65; Sax, *A Strife of Interests*, 41–42.

12. Australian Labor Party, *Sixteenth Conference Report,* 1943, n.p.
13. J.A. Gillespie, *The Price of Health: Australian Governments and Medical Politics 1910–1960* (Cambridge: Cambridge University Press, 1991), 131–41. See Lewis, "Editor's Introduction," 29.
14. Gillespie, *The Price of Health,* 142–54.
15. Ibid. See Lewis, "Editor's Introduction," 20, 30.
16. Thame, "Health and the State," 319–29; Gillespie, *The Price of Health,* 185–93.
17. Gillespie, *The Price of Health,* 224–49. See Lewis, "Editor's Introduction," 20–21.
18. Quoted in W.W. Holland and S. Stewart, *Public Health: The Vision and the Challenge* (London: Nuffield Trust, 1998), 40.
19. C. Webster, *The Health Services since the War.* Vol. 1, *Problems of Health Care: The National Health Service before 1957* (London: Her Majesty's Stationery Office, 1988), 389–92; Holland and Stewart, *Public Health,* 40–42; D. Porter, *Health, Civilization and the State: A History of Public Health from Ancient to Modern Times* (London: Routledge, 1999), 212–14.
20. C. Webster, *The National Health Service: A Political History* (Oxford: Oxford University Press, 1998), 6–30; Holland and Stewart, *Public Health,* 73–89.
21. Quoted in Holland and Stewart, *Public Health,* 91.
22. Quoted in Webster, *Problems of Health Care,* 375.
23. Quoted in ibid., 377.
24. Quoted in Holland and Stewart, *Public Health,* 99–100.
25. Quoted in ibid., 100–101.
26. Webster, *Problems of Health Care,* 373–80; Holland and Stewart, *Public Health,* 97–103.
27. Webster, *The Health Services since the War.* Vol. 2, *Government and Health Care: The National Health Service 1958–1979* (London: Stationery Office, 1996), 7–9.
28. P. Starr, *The Social Transformation of American Medicine* (New York: Basic Books, 1982), 266–79.
29. Ibid., 280–89.
30. J. Duffy, *The Sanitarians: A History of American Public Health* (Urbana: University of Illinois Press, 1990), 279; Porter, *Health, Civilization and the State,* 285–88.
31. Starr, *The Social Transformation of American Medicine,* 335–43.
32. D. Porter, "Public Health," in *Companion Encyclopedia of the History of Medicine,* ed. W.F. Bynum and R. Porter (London: Routledge, 1993), vol. 2, 1257–58; Porter, *Health, Civilization and the State,* 289–90; E. Fee and B. Rosenkrantz, "Professional Education for Public Health in the United States," in *A History of Education in Public Health,* ed. E. Fee and R.M. Acheson (New York: Oxford University Press, 1991), 246–47.

Chapter 7

The Health System at Midcentury

PUBLIC HEALTH TAKEN FOR GRANTED

By 1950 or so, in Australia, as in the United Kingdom and the United States, curative medicine was highly esteemed by governments and citizens alike. It was widely credited with wartime achievements of grand proportions. It gained even greater standing as the antibiotic revolution proceeded in the immediate postwar years. In effect, it took the credit for the historical "defeat" of infectious diseases in Australia, Britain and America when in truth public health had been a significant contributor, long before it had become effective, to the secular decline in mortality from infection, and therefore to the general decline in mortality. Male life expectancy in England and Wales increased from twenty-seven to thirty years in 1700 to seventy-five years in 1971, with over half of the gain taking place before 1900. Decline in infectious disease mortality accounted for 86 percent of the increased life expectancy, and the bulk of this decline occurred before the coming of antibiotics.[1]

Compared with clinical medicine, public health was virtually invisible to citizens, and perhaps, invisible to citizens because it was invisible to the media. Even in the United Kingdom, where state provision of health services had gone much farther than in Australia or the United States, the National Health Service was primarily concerned with curative and rehabilitative services for the individual, not population health. The robust public health function of the prewar era went into decline as public health doctors failed to establish a significant role in the new order. In Australia, where the Menzies Liberal-Country Party government's national health care funding scheme underwrote the fee-for-service structure of private general practice, which dominated primary health care, preventive work was neglected. The constitutional division of power and the retreat from state intervention as the wartime electoral support for collective measures disappeared ended any serious chance of a nationalized medical service integrating preventive and curative work. The antibiotic therapeutic revolution seemed to promise unlimited biomedical progress and to vindicate medicine's focus on the individual patient and on hospital care.

It was, however, not just a question of the great promise of medical science and the fact that public health practitioners lost their sense of direction. There was the effect of what Simon Szreter has called "an iron law of public health history," which involves a lesson that each generation, including our own, has to relearn. The very historical successes of public health meant that public and preventive health practices in the 1950s and '60s became routine, the safety they provided taken for granted by citizens. Public health became, politically, an invisible and undervalued activity. Thus, when neoliberal governments in the 1980s in the United Kingdom and the United States sought drastically to cut state spending, public health, like other public goods such as social welfare, could be dismissively described as parasitic on the private sector. At the same time private enterprise was lauded as the engine of economic growth and so as the real source of advancement of general well-being. Strong economic growth as the provider of material wherewithal may be a necessary condition of better health. Nonetheless, the state's ameliorating influence through public health services (and state-subsidized, universal health care) on the health-destructive effects of market-driven economic growth is required if better health is to be sustained and, moreover, is to be equitably distributed among social classes.[2] But this extremely important lesson was lost in the face of a routinized and nearly invisible public health and of a dramatic and highly visible curative medicine.

Further, as observed previously, changing demography (an aging population) and changing disease patterns were altering the fundamental problems with which public health had to deal. In the longer term, the prevalence of chronic degenerative conditions, for which no biomedical cures existed, resurrected professional and government interest in prevention. The steeply rising costs of technologically driven health care reinforced official concern, from the 1970s, with prevention and public health. An era of prosperity that began in the 1950s in Australia was also an era of slowdown in health improvement. Life expectancy at birth had been growing steadily since the 1900s; now it did not improve for two decades. By the start of the 1970s, Australia was in the midst of a series of modern "epidemics"—coronary heart disease, lung cancer, traffic accidents, and alcoholism.[3] The first professional and government response was to stress individual responsibility; only much later did the economic and social-structural constraints on individual behavior change begin to be recognized. How public health in Australia (and in the United Kingdom and United States) in detail dealt with the new epidemics of affluence, as well as more traditional epidemics of tuberculosis and polio, will be discussed at length in volume 2 of this history.

A RECAPITULATION

One hundred fifty years ago, a significant step toward a state-mandated, universal health system was taken in Australia with the introduction in the colony of Victoria of the first important public health legislation. A state-subsidized health care funding system was slower to develop. It did not become truly universal until the advent of Medibank in the mid-1970s offered equal access to medical care. Rapid, poorly regulated urbanization and the growth of an industrial base for the economy in the second half of the nineteenth century produced marked degradation of the physical environment. Concentration of people in large colonial cities and towns facilitated communication of infectious diseases. Communicable diseases contributed strongly to the decimation of the Aboriginal tribes as European settlement spread across the continent.

The sanitary idea, which triumphed in the mid-nineteenth century as the collective answer to the deadly synergy of disease and poverty in urban Britain, was transported to the Australian colonies almost as soon as it appeared in the "mother country." Classic public health administrations were in place in all colonies by the turn of the century. As in Britain and America, epidemic disease (which threatened rich and poor alike) spurred the growth of state intervention to protect the health of the population.

In the 1900s, public health entered a new phase and saw limited growth of personal advisory services for subpopulations like babies and mothers. This development Australia shared with the United Kingdom and the United States. The organized medical profession supported these innovations as long as services did not threaten the incomes of private practitioners by providing treatment in addition to educational advice. The state, in an era when belief in individual responsibility for health and welfare was still dominant, did not provide extensive funding for these purposes; indeed, it relied heavily on voluntary organizations.

Humanitarian concern, especially in the case of infants, was an important motivation. But concern with what was called "national efficiency"—national economic and military capacity in a world of growing tension between European nations and empires, and the emergence of Japan as a modern power—was a strong motivator of political action as well as a source of much rhetoric across the Western world. A fit and growing—and in contemporary Australia, white—population was viewed as basic to the economic development, long-term occupation, and military defense of the island continent. The pursuit of national efficiency in this area became a significant reason for state support for infant, maternal and school health services. For public health leaders, particularly the more farsighted ones like J.H.L. Cumpston, national efficiency remained a significant superordinate goal in the 1920s, '30s and '40s. In that sense, among the public health professional elite and some of the political one, larger political goals of almost a "mercantilist" nature drove public health forward up to World War II. By the 1940s, with Labor in government, notions of social and distributive justice were also driving health policy, though as observed above, health, like social welfare, was subordinated to the objectives of macroeconomic policy.

The interwar period began with apparently good prospects for public health. The Australian army's outstanding preventive work on infectious diseases during the 1914–18 war showed the potential for prevention in peace given political will and proper organization. The national hygienists—Cumpston, J.S.C. Elkington, and R.W. Cilento—wanted to implement a national strategy to exploit this potential. Believing that the real gains in health would come from prevention, they were ready to see clinical practice remain in private hands. The leaders of the medical profession supported their plans. Thus, the Federal Committee of the British Medical Association in Australia called in 1920 for a federal health department to coordinate the activities of the states and advance research. In 1915, Cumpston had publicly called for coordination of national public health policy. Constitutionally, of course, the commonwealth possessed only the quarantine power; the states were mainly responsible for health matters. Nationalization of medicine as urged by British Fabian socialists, Cumpston told a university audience in 1919, was neither practicable nor useful. But a national public health policy under commonwealth direction would engage the basic causes of disease; it would reduce demand for clinical services. Indeed, he proposed to the federal government that the commonwealth persuade the states to transfer their powers over health, or emulate the United States and establish a federal health authority that would focus on research and education, leaving executive action to the states. Cumpston proposed at the 1920 Australasian Medical Congress creation of a national system of public health administration, with central and district staffs supported by testing laboratories across the country. Congress itself issued a call for a Federal Ministry of Health to be established immediately.

With the assistance of inducements offered by the Rockefeller Foundation, Cumpston got his Federal Health Department in 1921, and he became the founding director general of health. The national hygienists got their Royal Commission on Health in 1925. The commission recognized that the states had repeatedly failed to cooperate with the commonwealth in health matters. However, the constitutional division of powers prevented the Federal Health Department from dealing directly, as did the Health Ministry in the United Kingdom, with local government authorities. Among the commission's more significant recommendations was one to create a federal health council to facilitate commonwealth-state cooperation and another to introduce a national public health scheme promoting preventive work. The public health scheme never materialized, because the cost was considerable and the degree of commonwealth control required was not acceptable to the states. A Federal Health Council was established in 1927; however, state sensitivities meant that it saw much discussion but produced little action.

In 1930, just before Depression-induced restrictions on expenditure were locked into place, Cumpston managed to have a national school of public health established at the University of Sydney to train public health professionals and carry out research. As restrictions eased in the later 1930s, he embarked upon another project, securing establishment of the National Health and Medical Research Council (NHMRC). The 1925 royal commission had called for a health research council, and a few years later both medical researchers and the BMA had urged establishment of a medical research council. Cumpston was critical of the British Medical Research Council for alleged aloofness from the everyday applications of research. He ensured that a central concern of the NHMRC was machinery to promote cooperation in public health. Even on the research subcommittee, researchers were kept in a minority. By the time of the 1939–45 war, despite the constitutional division of power favoring the states in health, the national hygienists had created a considerable federal presence in public health. However, the grand plan for a national hygiene system directed by the commonwealth had not been realized. It was to emerge again, however, in an enhanced form in the national hygienists' 1941 proposal for a national, salaried health service integrating preventive and curative work.

As medical care in the early twentieth century became more effective and more costly, the issue of better access for the less well off emerged. The political Left and Right differed as to how this might be achieved, and in particular they disagreed about the respective roles of the state and the individual citizen in funding better access. Labor moved haltingly toward support for state-funded, state-provided services for all citizens, whereas non-Labor cleaved to a state-mandated contributory approach covering those unable to afford private fees and preserving individual responsibility for health care. As early as 1910, a New South Wales Labor government had been committed to providing a number of public medical services as a right of citizenship, like access to free primary education. Lack of resources, the disruption of peacetime priorities caused by the 1914–18 war, and the strong opposition of the organized medical profession to state-provided services allowed very little to be materially achieved. In the late 1930s, in the context of the conservative United Australia Party (UAP) government's proposed contributory national health insurance scheme, the federal Labor Party took a similar position. The Labor leader, John Curtin, told Parliament in 1938 that national health services should be approached in the same way as education and should be free to all citizens.

The UAP government had invited British expert Sir Walter Kinnear to draw up a national insurance scheme. In his 1937 plan, compulsory contributions would be made by employee, employer and the state. The self-employed, unemployed and dependants of wage earners were excluded. Medical benefits covered only general practitioner services. Labor, which wanted a tax-funded scheme, opposed the UAP scheme, as for different reasons did critics within government ranks. Although legislation was passed in 1938, negotiations with doctors over capitation fees and political leadership struggles within the government delayed introduction of the scheme. The Second World War shelved it indefinitely.

The liberal democracies early in the war pledged themselves to the defeat of the totalitarian powers and to establish a just and secure social order. In the first phase of postwar social reconstruction planning in Australia, in 1941–43, the national hygienists' proposal for a national health service—integrating preventive and curative work and using salaried doctors but not excluding private practice—dominated health services policy making. By 1944, this radical proposal was moribund. Federal Labor, in government since 1941, was now seeing health as one part of a cash benefits–based social-security system. It was thus expressing its preference for state-provided income support as the primary means of delivering welfare. It was also keen to reconcile expansion of health and welfare spending with the macroeconomic policy objective of the containment of postwar inflation. Moreover, its aim was a social justice one of equitable access to medical care, whereas the national hygienists, as public health professionals, were focused on advancing the health status of the population through efficiently organized and integrated preventive and curative services.

In 1941 the NHMRC had adopted, for discussion with the BMA, a report composed by Cumpston, Cilento and others calling for a national salaried service responsible for preventive and curative work in a nationwide network of regional centers and hospitals. An expanded version of Cumpston's prewar national public health scheme, it was driven by the idea of national efficiency rather than that of social justice. The ultimate goal was a fit and vigorous people able to develop and defend Australia.

Opposed to a salaried service, the BMA proposed instead, in 1941, private practice funded by compulsory insurance, and in 1943, by voluntary insurance. With the war now going better for the Allied cause, the Curtin Labor government began to introduce its social welfare program. When open conflict erupted with the medical profession, it did so over a lesser part of the health program. Challenged in the High Court, the Pharmaceutical Benefits Act, 1944, was found to be unconstitutional. Under the 1946 referendum, the commonwealth gained power inter alia over medical services but not to the extent of "civil conscription" of medical practitioners. This was to prove a permanent obstacle to nationalization of medicine.

The Chifley Labor government enacted the National Health Service Act of 1948–49. This envisaged the bulk of medical practice would continue on a fee-for-service basis, with the patient to be reimbursed for half the fee out of public funds. Remote areas, which found it difficult then (as now) to attract private practitioners, would have salaried doctors. The BMA remained suspicious of any involvement of the commonwealth in payment of fees, and it would not cooperate. After electoral defeat in late 1949, Labor left federal office.

If the states resisted the interwar efforts of the national hygienists to implement a rational public health scheme for Australia as a whole, they failed within their individual jurisdictions to build coherent public health policies. New problems tended in the 1920s to be dealt with on an ad hoc basis by state, municipal or voluntary action. Medical officers of health were commonly only part-time, and their distribution across states was uneven. A debilitating division existed between the local government level, which focused on environmental sanitation, and the state level, where personal health services were administered. Public health remained underresourced and understaffed in the 1940s.

In the United Kingdom and to some extent the United States, public health in the interwar period had become caught up in administration of public medical services for socially disadvantaged groups to the detriment of its main responsibility for disease prevention, at a time when, as can be seen in retrospect, a fundamental shift in disease patterns was beginning to occur. In the American case, the U.S. Public Health Service checked immigrants for physical and mental diseases. During and after World War I, and then again in the late 1930s, it was involved in national campaigns to control venereal disease. Indeed, in the 1930s and '40s, federal public health funding focused in a piecemeal way on particular diseases like venereal disease or tuberculosis, or on population subgroups like mothers and children. Under the New Deal, millions of dollars went to expand public health facilities at the state and county levels, and to train personnel to staff the growing local services. But in the immediate postwar period, hospitals and their high-technology medicine were the growing points of the American health system. Under the Hill-Burton Act of 1946 the federal government provided four billion dollars over three decades for the construction of hospital facilities. At the same time, private insurance, which was spreading, offered partial coverage for hospitalization. Hospital medicine by the start of the 1960s enjoyed high status; areas of medicine to do with primary care and prevention—like family practice, infectious diseases or pediatrics—carried much less prestige and provided lower incomes.[4]

In Britain, during the interwar period, public health doctors acquired responsibility for municipal hospitals, a significant component of national health care facilities, along with their continued responsibility for a range of personal health services. General practitioners feared that the salaried medical officers of health would encroach on the preserves of private practice. The public health doctors confidently believed that when medicine was nationalized, they would be the managers of a national service based on the local level of government and integrating curative and preventive work. But when the National Health Service arrived in the 1940s, it not only failed to make local authorities the lynchpin of the service but guaranteed a central role for general practitioners as independent contractors. Moreover, in their inter-war preoccupation with management of personal health services and institutional treatment facilities for the less well to do, the public health doctors failed to investigate the relationship between poverty and disease, an issue the importance of which was heightened by the poor performance of the economy in the 1920s and '30s. Indeed, it was academic social medicine, divorced from the workaday administrative world of public health, that dealt with the impact of social conditions on health and moved beyond public health's concern with infectious diseases to look at all significant diseases.

PUBLIC HEALTH AT MIDCENTURY

By 1950, the energy of public health to pursue its historical goal of advancing the people's health, in Australia as in the United Kingdom and the United States, was at a low ebb. The public image of curative medicine was becoming increasingly bright, while public health had faded to near invisibility. Curative medicine, backed by the growing power of biomedical research, especially in the United States, promised a world free of disease and disability and seemed confident that it would discover the "magic bullets" to destroy heart disease and even cancer, as it had discovered antibiotics to destroy bacterial infections. Public health practitioners were just beginning to adjust to the epidemiological transition to chronic "degenerative" diseases. These demanded interventions much more complex than environmental sanitation or mass immunization campaigns—interventions that had to change deeply rooted personal behaviors, and beyond that the larger social, economic and cultural factors that created the context for individual lifestyles. But epidemiology, public health's intellectual instrument of investigation, was hampered by the individualistic bias of its approach to explanation, and so to intervention. The risk-factor approach did not allow enough room for the causative role of social factors and so did not encourage interventions aimed at social, economic and environmental change. As Beaglehole and Bonita point out, this privileged medicalization over socialization of prevention.[5]

Governments were busy creating collective means, whether by direct provision of public medical services or subsidization of private insurance and private medical practice, to facilitate access to health care services. But it was curative and rehabilitative, not preventive and health-promotive, services on which, at this stage, they pinned their hopes for improvement of the health of the people.

NOTES

1. L. Garrett, *Betrayal of Trust: The Collapse of Global Public Health* (New York: Hyperion, 2000), 10.

2. S. Szreter, "Economic Growth, Disruption, Deprivation, Disease and Death: On the Importance of the Politics of Public Health for Development," *Population and Development Review* 23(4) (1997), 716–18.

3. B.S. Hetzel and S.R. Leeder, "Half a Century of Healthcare in Australia," *Medical Journal of Australia* 174 (2001), 34.

4. Garrett, *Betrayal of Trust*, 325–26; D. Porter, *Health, Civilization and the State: A History of Public Health from Ancient to Modern Times* (London: Routledge, 1999), 285–90.

5. R. Beaglehole and R. Bonita, *Public Health at the Crossroads: Achievements and Prospects* (Cambridge: Cambridge University Press, 1997), 119.

Selected Bibliography

Coward, D. *Out of Sight: Sydney's Environmental History 1851–1981.* Canberra: Department of Economic History, Research School of Social Sciences, Australian National University, 1988.

Cumpston, J.H.L. *Health and Disease in Australia: A History.* Ed. M.J. Lewis. Canberra: Australian Government Publishing Service (hereafter AGPS), 1989.

Duffy, J. *The Sanitarians: A History of American Public Health.* Urbana: University of Illinois Press, 1990.

Fildes, V., L. Marks, and H. Marland, eds. *Women and Children First: International Maternal and Infant Welfare, 1870–1945.* London: Routledge, 1992.

Gillespie, J.A. *The Price of Health: Australian Governments and Medical Politics 1910–1960.* Cambridge: Cambridge University Press, 1991.

Holland, W.W., and S. Stewart. *Public Health: The Vision and the Challenge.* London: Nuffield Trust, 1998.

Kunitz, S.J. *Disease and Social Diversity: The European Impact on the Health of Non-Europeans.* New York: Oxford University Press, 1994.

Lancaster, H.O. *Expectations of Life: A Study in the Demography, Statistics, and History of World Mortality.* New York: Springer-Verlag, 1990.

Lewis, M. *Managing Madness: Psychiatry and Society in Australia, 1788–1980.* Canberra: AGPS, 1988.

———. *A Rum State: Alcohol and State Policy in Australia.* Canberra: AGPS, 1992.

———. *Thorns on the Rose: The History of Sexually Transmitted Diseases in Australia in International Perspective.* Canberra: AGPS, 1998.

Lewis, M., S. Bamber, and M. Waugh, eds. *Sex, Disease, and Society: A Comparative History of Sexually Transmitted Diseases and HIV/AIDS in Asia and the Pacific.* Westport, Conn.: Greenwood Press, 1997.

Lewis, M.J., and S.R. Leeder. *Where to from Here? The Need to Construct a Comprehensive National Health Policy.* Sydney: Australian Health Policy Institute, University of Sydney, 2001.

MacLeod, R., and M. Lewis, eds. *Disease, Medicine and Empire: Perspectives on Western Medicine and the Experience of European Expansion.* London: Routledge, 1988.

Palmer, G.R., and S.D. Short. *Health Care and Public Policy: An Australian Analysis.* South Yarra: Macmillan Publishers Australia, 2000.

Porter, D., ed. *The History of Public Health and the Modern State.* Amsterdam, Atlanta: Editions Rodopi B.V., 1994.

Porter, R. *The Greatest Benefit to Mankind: A Medical History of Humanity from Antiquity to the Present.* London: HarperCollins, 1997.

Powles, J. "Professional Hygienists and the Health of the Nation." In *The Commonwealth of Science: ANZAAS and the Scientific Enterprise in Australia 1888–1988,* ed. R. MacLeod. Melbourne: Oxford University Press, 1988, 292–307.

Reid, J., and P. Trompf, eds. *The Health of Aboriginal Australia.* Sydney: Harcourt Brace Jovanovich, 1991.

Rosen, G. *A History of Public Health.* Baltimore: Johns Hopkins University Press, 1993.

Schofield, R., D. Reher, and A. Bideau, eds. *The Decline of Mortality in Europe.* Oxford: Clarendon Press, 1991.

Starr, P. *The Social Transformation of American Medicine.* New York: Basic Books, 1982.

Webster, C. *The Health Services since the War.* Vol. 1, *Problems of Health Care: The National Health Service before 1957.* London: Her Majesty's Stationery Office, 1988.

———. *The Health Services since the War.* Vol. 2, *Government and Health Care: The National Health Service 1958–1979.* London: Stationery Office, 1996.

Index

About the Author

MILTON J. LEWIS is Senior Research Fellow in the Department of Public Health and Community Medicine at the University of Sydney. With degrees from the University of New South Wales and the Australian National University, Lewis has worked in higher education institutions in Australia, the United Kingdom, and New Guinea. He has published widely on the history of medicine and public health. He is a member of several Australian and overseas associations concerned with the history of medicine and health, and he was chairperson of the organizing committee of the First National Conference of the Australian Society of the History of Medicine held in Sydney in 1989.